FOUNDATIONS OF PERIODONTICS

FOR THE DENTAL HYGIENIST Second Edition

FOUNDATIONS OF PERIODONTICS FOR THE DENTAL HYGIENIST

Second Edition

Jill S. Nield-Gehrig, RDH, MA

Dean Emeritus, Division of Allied Health & Public Service Education
Asheville-Buncombe Technical Community College
Asheville, North Carolina

Donald E. Willmann, DDS, MS

Professor, Department of Periodontics
University of Texas Health Science Center at San Antonio
San Antonio, Texas

Wolters Kluwer | Lippincott Williams & Wilkins
Health

Philadelphia · Baltimore · New York · London
Buenos Aires · Hong Kong · Sydney · Tokyo

Acquisitions Editor: John Goucher
Managing Editor: Kevin C. Dietz
Marketing Manager: Hilary Henderson
Production Editor: Julie Montalbano
Designer: Terry Mallon
Compositor: Maryland Composition, Inc.
Printer: R.R. Donnelley-Willard

351 West Camden Street
Baltimore, MD 21201

530 Walnut Street
Philadelphia, PA 19106

Printed in the United States of America

First Edition, 2003

Library of Congress Cataloging-in-Publication Data

Nield-Gehrig, Jill S. (Jill Shiffer)
    Foundations of periodontics for the dental hygienist / Jill S. Nield-Gehrig, Donald E. Willmann. —2nd ed.
    p. ; cm.
    Rev. ed. of: Foundations of periodontics for the dental hygienist / Jill S. Nield-Gehrig, Donald E. Willmann [editors]. c2003.
    Includes bibliographical references and index.
    ISBN-13: 978-0-7817-8487-0
    ISBN-10: 0-7817-8487-5
    1. Periodontics. 2. Dental hygienists. I. Willmann, Donald E. II. Foundations of periodontics for the dental hygienist. III. Title.
    [DNLM: 1. Periodontics. 2. Dental Hygienists. WU 240 N667f 2007]
    RK361.F675 2007
    617.6'32—dc22

                                                                                                2006024138

To purchase additional copies of this book, call our customer service department at **(800) 638-3030** or fax orders to **(301) 223-2320**. International customers should call **(301) 223-2300**.

Visit Lippincott Williams & Wilkins on the Internet: http://www.LWW.com. Lippincott Williams & Wilkins customer service representatives are available from 8:30 AM to 6:00 PM, EST.

07 08 09 10 11
1 2 3 4 5 6 7 8 9 10

Preface for Course Instructors

Foundations of Periodontics for the Dental Hygienist, 2nd edition, is written with two primary goals in mind: to create a textbook that focuses on the dental hygienist's role in periodontics and to develop a book with an instructional design that facilitates the teaching and learning of the complex subject of periodontics—as it relates to dental hygiene practice—without omitting salient concepts or "watering down" the material. Written primarily for dental hygiene students, *Foundations of Periodontics for the Dental Hygienist* also would be a valuable resource on current concepts in periodontics for the practicing dental hygienist or general dentist.

NEW INSTRUCTOR'S RESOURCE CD-ROM

The Instructor's Resource CD-ROM has a collection of instructional aids for course instructors.

1. PowerPoint Slides. The PowerPoint slides are designed to be user-friendly for a wide variety of software versions and equipment.
   - Slides may be customized by saving the slides to a computer hard drive and using the formatting features of your slide presentation software application, such as the slide design, slide color scheme, or slide background feature, to customize the slides as desired.
   - Special effects, such as progressive disclosure, may be added to the slides by using the custom animation feature of your slide presentation software application.

2. Discussion Points. This feature provides suggested discussion points for the Focus on Patients items, Patient Cases in Chapter 29, and Fictitious Patient Cases in Chapter 30.

3. Test Bank. The test bank questions can be used for quizzes or combined to make up unit tests or to create midterm and final examinations.

4. Instructor's Guide. These documents contain suggestions for student assignments and use of the Fictitious Patient Cases in Chapter 30.

STUDENT RESOURCE CD-ROM PACKAGED WITH THE BOOK

The student CD-ROM provides full-color versions of the clinical photographs by chapter. Since clinical signs of inflammation cannot be detected on the black-and-white photos in the book, students should refer to the full-color versions on the CD-ROM.

TEXTBOOK FEATURES

Foundations of Periodontics for the Dental Hygienist has many features designed to facilitate learning and teaching.

1. Module Overview and Outline. Each module begins with a concise overview of the module content. The module outline makes it easier to locate material within the module. The outline provides the reader with an organizational framework with which to approach new material.

2. Learning Objectives and Key Terms. Learning objectives assist students in recognizing and studying important concepts in each chapter. Key terms are listed at the beginning of each chapter. One of the most challenging tasks for any student is learning a whole new dental vocabulary and gaining the confidence to use new terms with accuracy and ease. The key terms list assists students in this task by identifying important terminology and facilitating the study and review of terminology in each chapter. Terms are highlighted in bold type and clearly defined within the chapter.

3. Instructional Design
   - Each chapter is subdivided into sections to help the reader recognize major content areas.
   - Chapters are written in an expanded outline format that makes it easy for students to identify, learn, and review key concepts.
   - Material is presented in a manner that recognizes that students have different learning styles. Hundreds of illustrations and clinical photographs visually reinforce chapter content.
   - Chapter content is supplemented in a visual format with boxes, tables, and flow charts.

4. Focus on Patients. The Focus on Patients items allow the reader to apply chapter content in the context of clinical practice. The cases provide opportunities for students to integrate knowledge into their clinical work.

5. Full Color Insert. The color insert contains full-color clinical photographs of the periodontal disease classifications most commonly encountered in a general dental practice.

6. Chapter Review Questions. Chapter Review Questions provide a quick review of chapter content.

7. Internet Resources in Periodontics. Chapter 28 provides an extensive list of Internet resources. Students should be encouraged to develop skills in online information gathering. With the rapid explosion of knowledge in the dental and medical sciences, a student can no longer expect to learn everything that he or she needs to know, now and forever, in a few years of professional training. Students must learn how to retrieve accurate information quickly from reliable Internet sites, such as MEDLINE.

8. Radiographic Analysis Patient Cases. Chapter 29 provides radiographs for six cases. These cases give students the opportunity to develop skills in radiographic analysis as it pertains to the hard tissues of the periodontium in health and disease.

9. Comprehensive Fictitious Patient Cases. Chapter 30 presents two fictitious patient cases. Patient assessment data pertinent to the periodontium challenges the student to interpret and use the information in periodontal care planning for the patient.

10. Glossary. A glossary at the back of the book provides quick access to common periodontal terminology.

CHAPTER SEQUENCING

The book is divided into seven major content areas:

Part 1: The Periodontium in Health
Part 2: Periodontal Pathology
Part 3: Diseases of the Periodontium
Part 4: Assessment for Clinical Decision Making
Part 5: Implementation of Therapy
Part 6: Other Aspects of Periodontal Therapy
Part 7: Resources and Patient Cases

PART 1: The Periodontium in Health

Chapter 1 provides students with an opportunity to review the structures of the periodontium. Chapter 2 is a detailed discussion of microscopic oral anatomy pertinent to understanding the periodontium in health and disease.

PART 2: Periodontal Pathology

Part 2 covers the ever-expanding body of knowledge on the important topics of pathogenesis and etiology of periodontal disease. An understanding of the etiology, mechanisms, and processes involved in periodontal disease is fundamental to successful dental hygiene practice.

PART 3: Diseases of the Periodontium

Part 3 covers the classification of periodontal diseases and conditions. Chapter 9 provides an overview of the 1999 international classification of periodontal diseases. Chapter 10 provides a detailed discussion of plaque-induced gingival diseases and nonplaque-induced gingival lesions. Chapter 11 presents detailed descriptions of the most commonly encountered types of periodontitis.

PART 4: Assessment for Clinical Decision Making

Part 4 covers the assessment and planning phases of periodontal therapy: clinical periodontal assessment, radiographic analysis, care modifications based on systemic conditions, evidence-based periodontal care, and decision making during treatment planning.

PART 5: Implementation of Therapy

Part 5 covers the implementation phase of periodontal therapy: nonsurgical periodontal therapy, patient's role in nonsurgical periodontal therapy, helping patients change behavior, nutrition, periodontal surgical concepts, chemical agents, periodontal maintenance, and dental implant maintenance.

PART 6: Other Aspects of Periodontal Therapy

Part 6 covers three topics: periodontal emergencies, documentation and insurance reporting of periodontal care, and future directions for periodontal care.

PART 7: Resources and Patient Cases

Part 7 focuses on application of periodontal concepts. These three chapters provide periodontal resources in dental literature and periodontal care, patient cases for radiographic analysis, and two fictitious patient cases.

Foundations of Periodontics for the Dental Hygienist, 2nd edition strives to present the complex subject of periodontics in a reader-friendly manner. The authors greatly appreciate the comments and suggestions from educators and students about the first edition of this book. It is our sincere hope that this textbook will help students and practitioners alike to acquire knowledge that will serve as a foundation for the prevention and management of periodontal diseases.

Jill S. Nield-Gehrig, RDH, MA
Donald E. Willmann, DDS, MS

Contributors

INSTRUCTOR'S RESOURCE CD-ROM
Chapter 10 Gingival Diseases
Chapter 20 Nutrition and Periodontal Disease

Rebecca Sroda, RDH, MS
Director of Dental Education
South Florida Community College
600 W College Drive
Avon Park, Florida 33825-9356

Chapter 4 Search for the Causes of Periodontal Disease

Sharon Logue, RDH, MPH
Coordinator, School Fluoride Mouthrinse Program
Virginia Department of Health
Division of Dental Health
109 Governor Street
Richmond, Virginia 23219

Chapter 13 Radiographic Analysis of the Periodontium

William S. Moore, DDS, MS
Division Head, Division of Oral & Maxillofacial Radiology
Department of Dental Diagnostic Science
University of Texas Health Science Center at San Antonio
7703 Floyd Curl Drive
San Antonio, Texas 78229-3900

Chapter 15 Evidence-Based Periodontal Care
Chapter 18 Content on powered devices

Carol A. Jahn, BSDH, MS
Manager, Professional Education & Communications
Waterpik Technologies, Inc
Personal Healthcare Products
25601 Enrico Fermi Ct., #J
Warrenville, Illinois 60555-2056

Chapter 19 Helping Patients Change Behavior

Dr. Rebecca Lang, EdD, RDH, CHES
Grand View College
Associate Professor, Health and Physical Education
1200 Grandview Avenue
Des Moines, Iowa 50316

Chapter 23 Section on Prevention of Root Caries

Teresa Butler Duncan, RDH, BS
Clinical Instructor
Department of Dental Hygiene
School of Health Related Professionals
The University of Mississippi Medical Center
Jackson, Mississippi 39216

Chapter 26 Documentation and Insurance Reporting of Periodontal Care

Dianne Glasscoe, RDH, BS
Professional Dental Management, Inc.
www.professionaldentalmgmt.com
285 Roderick Road
Frederick, Maryland 21704

Chapter 29 Patient Cases: Radiographic Analysis

Dr. John Preece, DDS, MS
Professor, Division of Oral & Maxillofacial Radiology
Dental Diagnostic Science
University of Texas Health Science Center at San Antonio
7703 Floyd Curl Drive
San Antonio, Texas 78229-3900

Acknowledgments

It is a great pleasure to acknowledge the following individuals whose assistance was indispensable to this second edition:

- **Rebecca Sroda,** RDH, MA, Director of Dental Education at South Florida Community College, who created the Instructor's Resource CD-ROM for this textbook.
- The faculty and dental hygiene students at Tallahassee Community College and South **Florida Community College** who use the *Foundations of Periodontics* text and contribute greatly to its improvement.
- **Cynthia R. Biron,** RDH, EMT, MA, of *DH-Meth-Ed* Dental Hygiene Education Consulting Services for her recommendations for the second edition.
- **Charles D. Whitehead,** the highly skilled medical illustrator who created all the wonderful illustrations for the book.

And finally, we would be remiss if we failed to express our gratitude to John Goucher and **Kevin Dietz** of Lippincott Williams & Wilkins for their vision and support.

Jill S. Nield-Gehrig, RDH, MA
Donald Willmann, DDS, MS

Contents

PART 1   THE PERIODONTIUM IN HEALTH

Chapter 1   Tissues of the Periodontium in Health 1

Chapter 2   Microscopic Anatomy of the Periodontium 17

PART 2   PERIODONTAL PATHOLOGY

Chapter 3   The History of Periodontal Disease 39

Chapter 4   Search for the Causes of Periodontal Disease 55

PART 3   DISEASES OF THE PERIODONTIUM

PART 4 ASSESSMENT FOR CLINICAL DECISION MAKING

PART 5 IMPLEMENTATION OF THERAPY

Liability Statement

Chapter

1 Tissues of the Periodontium in Health

Refer to the CD packaged with this book for full color versions of the clinical photographs in this chapter.

Learning Objectives

- List and describe the four tissues of the periodontium.
- Explain the function that each tissue serves in the periodontium.
- Identify the following anatomic areas of the gingiva in the oral cavity: free gingiva, gingival sulcus, interdental gingiva, and attached gingiva.
- Identify the tissues of the periodontium on an unlabeled drawing depicting the periodontium in cross section.
- Identify the following boundaries of the gingiva in the oral cavity: gingival margin, free gingival groove, and mucogingival junction. If the free gingival groove is not visible clinically, determine the apical boundary of the free gingiva by inserting a probe to the base of a sulcus on an anterior tooth.
- In the oral cavity, identify the free gingiva on an anterior tooth by inserting a periodontal probe to the base of the sulcus.
- In the oral cavity, contrast the coral pink tissue of the attached gingiva with the darker, shiny tissue of the alveolar mucosa.

■ In the oral cavity, use compressed air to detect the presence or absence of stippling of the attached gingiva.
■ Identify the structures that cause the stippled appearance of the attached gingiva.
■ Identify the alveolar process (alveolar bone) on a human skull.
■ Describe the position and contours of the alveolar crest of the alveolar bone in health.
■ Describe the nerve and blood supply to the periodontium.
■ Explain the role of the lymphatic system in the health of the periodontium.
■ Define the key terms in this chapter.
■ Demonstrate knowledge of the tissues of the periodontium by applying concepts from this chapter to the cases found in the Focus on Patients section of this chapter.

KEY TERMS

Periodontium	Free gingival groove	Alveolus
Gingiva	Mucogingival junction	Alveolar bone proper
Free gingiva	Periodontal ligament	Periosteum
Gingival sulcus	Cementum	Alveolar crest
Attached gingiva	Alveolar bone	Interproximal bone
Stippling	Cortical bone	Interradicular bone
Interdental gingiva	Fenestration	Innervation
Papillae	Dehiscence	Trigeminal nerve
Col	Cancellous bone	Anastomose

DIRECTIONS FOR USING THE CD PACKAGED WITH THIS BOOK

CD Contents:
- Full color versions of some of the drawings in the book
- Full color versions of all the clinical photographs in the book. Since the clinical signs of inflammation cannot be detected on the black and white photos in the book, you will find it helpful to view the color photographs on the CD as you study each chapter.

Opening the Photos and Drawings on the CD:
- The photographs and drawings are saved in a PDF format.
- Adobe Reader is a free software application that is used to open PDF documents. You can download Adobe Reader at http://www.adobe.com/support/downloads/main.html
- Once you have installed Adobe Reader on your computer's hard drive, double click on the CD icon to open it. Double click on the photograph or drawing that you wish to view. It will open in Reader.

CD Contents for This Chapter:
The CD contains full color versions of *figures 1-3, 1-4,* and *1-5* in this chapter. Each structure in a drawing is designated by a unique color. This will make it easier for you to tell one structure from the others on the drawing.

SECTION 1: STRUCTURES OF THE PERIODONTIUM

The **periodontium** (peri = around and odontos = tooth) is the functional system of tissues that surrounds the teeth and attaches them to the jawbone. These tissues include the gingiva, periodontal ligament, cementum, and alveolar bone (**Fig. 1-1**). Each of these tissues plays a vital role in maintaining the health and function of the periodontium (**Table 1-1**). Knowledge of the anatomy of the periodontium is a necessary foundation for understanding the concepts of (i) normal function of the periodontium, (ii) disease prevention, and (iii) the periodontal disease process.

Dental hygiene students usually are introduced to the tissues of the periodontium during the first semester or quarter of the dental hygiene curriculum. In the preclinical stages of the curriculum, mastering dental terminology and anatomy can sometimes be overwhelming and confusing. This chapter provides dental hygiene students with an opportunity to review this complex system of tissues known as the periodontium.

Table 1-1. The Periodontium

Structure	Brief Description of Its Function
Gingiva	■ Provides a tissue seal around the cervical portion (neck) of the tooth ■ Holds the tissue against the tooth during mastication
Periodontal ligament	■ Suspends and maintains the tooth in its socket
Cementum	■ Anchors the ends of the periodontal ligament fibers to the tooth so that the tooth stays in its socket ■ Protects the dentin of the root
Alveolar bone	■ Surrounds and supports the roots of the tooth

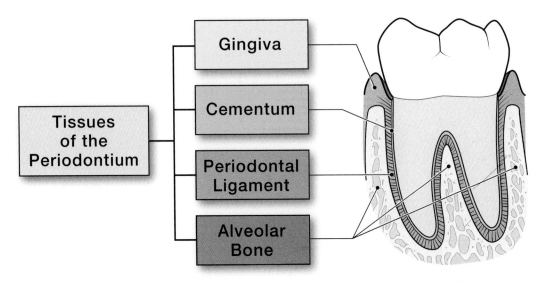

Figure 1-1. Tissues of the Periodontium. A: A graphic representation of the periodontal tissues. **B:** Tissues of the periodontium in cross section.

GINGIVA

1. **Overview of the Gingiva**
    A. Description. The **gingiva** is the tissue that covers the cervical portions of the teeth and the alveolar processes of the jaws (**Fig. 1-2**). It is composed of a thin outer layer of epithelium and an underlying core of connective tissue.
    B. Function. The gingiva provides a tissue seal around the cervical portions of the teeth and covers the alveolar processes of the jaws.
    C. Anatomic Areas. The gingiva is divided into four anatomical areas (**Fig. 1-3**).
        1. Free gingiva
        2. Gingival sulcus
        3. Interdental gingiva
        4. Attached gingiva

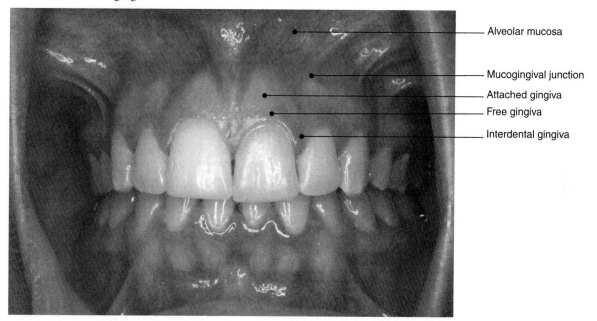

Figure 1-2. The Gingival Tissues. Photograph of healthy gingival tissues showing the free, attached, and interdental gingiva.

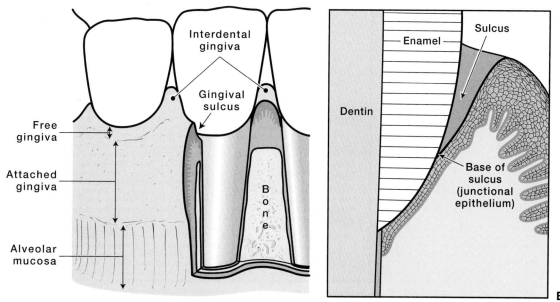

Figure 1-3. Anatomic Areas of the Gingiva. A: Diagram of the anatomic areas of the gingiva. B: Close-up view of the gingival sulcus drawn in cross section.

D. Boundaries of the Gingiva
  1. The coronal boundary, or upper edge, of the gingiva is the **gingival margin** (**Fig. 1-4**).
  2. The apical boundary, or lower edge, of the gingiva is the alveolar mucosa. The **alveolar mucosa** can be distinguished easily from the gingiva by its dark red color and smooth, shiny surface.

E. Demarcations of the Gingiva
  1. The **free gingival groove** (**Fig. 1-5**) is a shallow linear depression that separates the free and attached gingiva (this line may be visible clinically but is not obvious in many instances).
  2. The **mucogingival junction** is the clinically visible boundary where the pink attached gingiva meets the red, shiny alveolar mucosa. (Clinically visible means that this landmark can be seen in the oral cavity.)

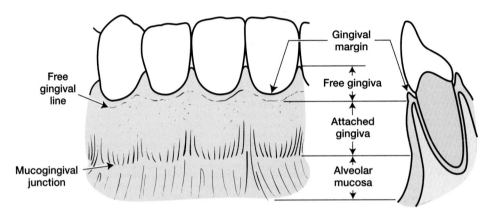

Figure 1-4. Boundaries of the Gingiva. Illustration showing the boundaries and anatomical areas of the gingiva.

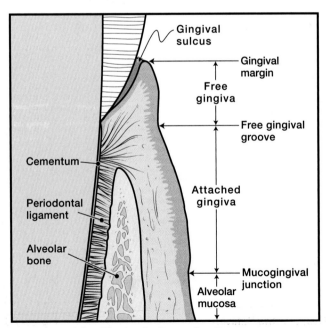

Figure 1-5. Boundaries of the Gingiva in Cross Section. The boundaries and anatomic areas of the gingiva shown in cross section.

2. **Free Gingiva.** The **free gingiva** is the unattached portion of the gingiva that surrounds the tooth in the region of the cementoenamel junction (CEJ). The free gingiva is also known as the unattached gingiva or the marginal gingiva.
   A. Location of the Free Gingiva
      1. The free gingiva is located coronal to (above) the CEJ.
      2. It surrounds the tooth in a turtleneck or cufflike manner.
   B. Characteristics of the Free Gingiva
      1. The tissue of the free gingiva fits closely around the tooth but is not directly attached to it.
      2. This tissue, because it is unattached, may be gently stretched away from the tooth surface with a periodontal probe.
      3. The free gingiva also forms the soft tissue wall of the gingival sulcus.
   C. Contour of the Free Gingival Margin
      1. The tissue of the free gingiva meets the tooth in a thin rounded edge called the **gingival margin**.
      2. The gingival margin follows the contours of the teeth, creating a scalloped (wavy) outline around them.
3. **Attached Gingiva.** The **attached gingiva** is the part of the gingiva that is tightly connected to the cementum on the cervical third of the root and to the periosteum (connective tissue cover) of the alveolar bone.
   A. Location of the Attached Gingiva. The attached gingiva lies between the free gingiva and alveolar mucosa.
   B. Width of Attached Gingiva
      1. The attached gingiva is widest in the incisor and molar regions (ranging from 3.3 to 3.9 mm on the mandible and 3.5 to 4.5 mm on the maxilla).
      2. The attached gingiva is narrowest in premolar regions (1.8 mm on mandible and 1.9 mm on maxilla).
      3. The width of the attached gingiva is not measured on the palate since clinically it is not possible to determine where the attached gingiva ends and the palatal mucosa begins **(Fig. 1-6)**.
   C. Color of the Attached Gingiva
      1. In health, the attached gingiva is pale or coral pink.
      2. The attached gingiva may be pigmented **(Fig. 1-7)**.
         a. Pigmentation occurs more frequently in dark-skinned individuals.
         b. The pigmented areas of the attached gingiva may range from light brown to black.

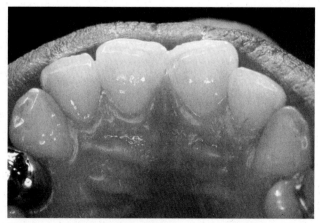

Figure 1-6. Tissue of the Palate. On the palate, the lingual gingiva is directly continuous with the keratinized masticatory mucosa of the hard palate.

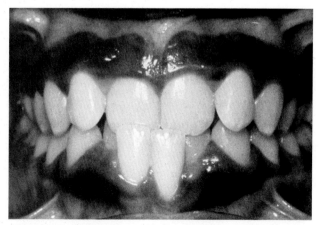

Figure 1-7. Pigmentation of the Gingiva. Pigmentation of the gingiva is seen in dark-skinned individuals. (Courtesy of Dr. Robert P. Langlais, UTHSCSA, San Antonio, TX.)

D. Texture of the Attached Gingiva
   1. In health, the surface of the attached gingiva may have a dimpled appearance similar to the skin of an orange peel. This dimpled appearance is known as **stippling** (**Fig. 1-8**). Healthy tissue may or may not exhibit a stippled appearance as the presence of stippling varies greatly from individual to individual.
   2. Stippling is caused by the presence of the connective fibers that attach the gingival tissue to the cementum and bone.

E. Function of the Attached Gingiva
   1. The attached gingiva allows the gingival tissue to withstand the mechanical forces created during activities such as mastication, speaking, and toothbrushing.
   2. The attached gingiva prevents the free gingiva from being pulled away from the tooth when tension is applied to the alveolar mucosa.

4. **Interdental Gingiva.** The **interdental gingiva** is the portion of the gingiva that fills the area between two adjacent teeth apical to the contact area (**Fig. 1-9**).
   A. Parts of Interdental Gingiva
      1. The interdental gingiva consists of two interdental **papillae**, one facial papilla, and one lingual papilla (papilla = singular noun; papillae = plural noun).
         a. The lateral borders and tip of an interdental papilla are formed by the free gingiva from the adjacent teeth.
         b. The center portion of the interdental papilla is formed by the attached gingiva.
      2. The **col** is a valleylike depression in the portion of the interdental gingiva that lies directly apical to the contact area. The col is not present if the adjacent teeth are not in contact or if the gingiva has receded.
   B. Function of Interdental Gingiva. The interdental gingiva prevents food from becoming packed between the teeth during mastication.

5. **Gingival Sulcus.** The **gingival sulcus** is the *space* between the free gingiva and the tooth surface (**Fig. 1-10**).
   A. Description. The sulcus is a V-shaped, shallow space around the tooth.
   B. Depth. The depth of a clinically normal gingival sulcus is from 1 to 3 mm, as measured using a periodontal probe.
   C. Base of Sulcus. The base of the sulcus is formed by the **junctional epithelium** (a specialized type of epithelium that attaches to the tooth surface).

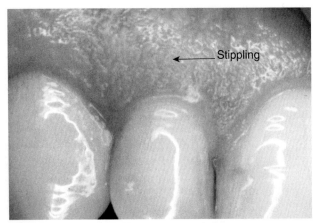

Figure 1-8. Gingival Stippling. In health, the surface of the attached gingiva may have a dimpled appearance known as gingival stippling.

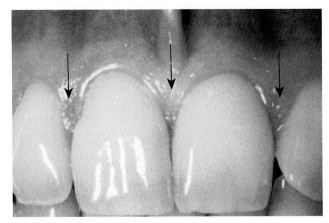

Figure 1-9. The Interdental Gingiva. The interdental tissue fills the area between two adjacent teeth.

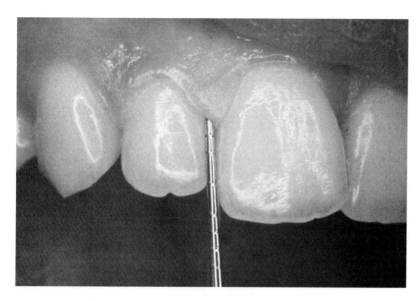

Figure 1-10. Gingival Sulcus. This photograph shows a periodontal probe inserted into the gingival sulcus, the space between the free gingiva and the tooth.

PERIODONTAL LIGAMENT

1. **Description.** The **periodontal ligament** (**PDL**) is a layer of soft connective tissue that covers the root of the tooth and attaches it to the bone of the tooth socket (**Fig. 1-11**).
   A. The PDL is composed mainly of fiber bundles.
   B. The fibers of the PDL attach on one side to the root cementum and on the other side to the alveolar bone of the tooth socket.
2. **Functions.** The periodontal ligament has five functions in the periodontium:
   A. Supportive function—suspends and maintains the tooth in its socket.
   B. Sensory function—provides sensory feeling to the tooth, such as pressure and pain sensations.
   C. Nutritive function—provides nutrients to the cementum and bone.
   D. Formative function—builds and maintains cementum and the alveolar bone of the tooth socket.
   E. Resorptive function—can remodel the alveolar bone in response to pressure, such as that applied during orthodontic treatment (braces).

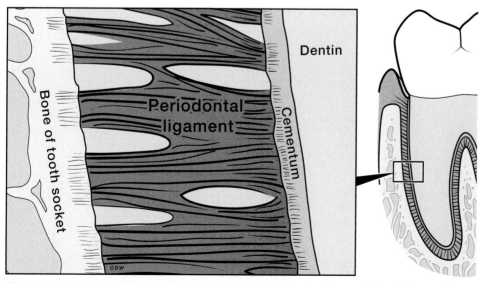

Figure 1-11. Periodontal Ligament. On **tooth side**, the ends of the periodontal ligament fibers are anchored in the cementum of the root. **On the bone side**, the ends of the periodontal ligament fibers are anchored in the alveolar bone of the tooth socket.

ROOT CEMENTUM

1. **Description.** Cementum is a thin layer of hard, mineralized tissue that covers the surface of the tooth root.
2. **Characteristics of Cementum**
   A. Cementum is light yellow.
   B. It overlies and is attached to the dentin of the root.
   C. Cementum is a bonelike tissue that is more resistant to resorption than bone. Resistance to resorption (loss of substance) is an important characteristic of cementum that makes it possible for the teeth to be moved during orthodontic treatment. The high resistance of cementum to resorption allows the pressure applied during orthodontics to cause resorption of alveolar bone, for tooth movement, without resulting in root resorption.
   D. Cementum does not have its own blood or nutrient supply; it receives its nutrients from the periodontal ligament.
3. **Functions of Cementum in the Periodontium.** Cementum performs several important roles in the periodontium and, therefore, conservation of cementum should be a goal of periodontal instrumentation.
   A. Cementum anchors the ends of the periodontal ligament fibers to the tooth; without cementum, the tooth would fall out of its socket.
   B. The outer layer of cementum protects the underlying dentin and seals the ends of the open dentinal tubules.
   C. Cementum formation compensates for tooth wear at the occlusal or incisal surface due to attrition; cementum is formed at the apical area of the root to compensate for occlusal attrition.

ALVEOLAR BONE

1. **Description**
   A. The alveolar bone or alveolar process is the bone of the upper or lower jaw that surrounds and supports the roots of the teeth (Fig. 1-12).
   B. The existence of alveolar bone is dependent on the presence of teeth; when teeth are extracted, in time, the alveolar bone resorbs. If teeth do not erupt, the alveolar bone does not develop.
2. **Function of Alveolar Bone in the Periodontium.** The alveolar bone forms the bony sockets that provide support and protection for the roots of the teeth.

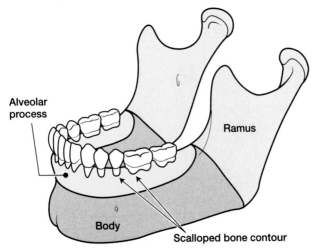

Figure 1-12. The Mandible. The three anatomic areas of the mandible are the ramus, body, and the alveolar process.

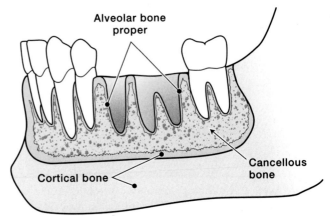

Figure 1-13. Layers of the Alveolar Process. A lateral section of the mandible reveals the three bony layers: the alveolar bone proper, cancellous bone, and cortical bone.

3. **Layers that Compose the Alveolar Process.** When viewed in cross section, the alveolar process is composed of three layers of hard tissue and covered by a thin layer of connective tissue (**Fig. 1-13**).
    A. The **alveolar bone proper** (or **cribriform plate**) is the thin layer of bone that lines the socket to surround the root of the tooth.
        1. The **alveolus** is the bony socket; a cavity in the alveolar bone that houses the root of a tooth (alveolus, singular; alveoli, plural) (**Fig. 1-14**).
        2. The alveolar bone proper has numerous holes that allow blood vessels from the cancellous bone to connect with the vessels of the periodontal ligament space.
        3. The ends of the periodontal ligament fibers are embedded in the alveolar bone proper.
    B. The **cortical bone** is a layer of compact bone that forms the hard, outside wall of the mandible and maxilla on the facial and lingual aspects. This cortical bone surrounds the alveolar bone proper and gives support to the socket.
        1. The buccal cortical bone is thin in the incisor, canine, and premolar regions; cortical bone is thicker in molar regions.
        2. Since the cortical plate is only on the facial and lingual sides of the jaw, it will not show up in a radiograph; only the cancellous bone and the alveolar bone proper can be seen on a radiograph.
        3. The **alveolar crest** is the most coronal portion of the alveolar process.
            a. In health, the alveolar crest is located 1 to 2 mm apical to (below) the CEJ of the teeth (**Fig. 1-15**).
            b. When viewed from the facial or lingual aspect, the alveolar crest meets the teeth in a scalloped (wavy) line that follows the contours of the CEJs.
    C. The **cancellous bone** (or **spongy bone**) is the latticelike bone that fills the interior portion of the alveolar process (between the cortical bone and the alveolar bone proper). The cancellous bone is oriented around the tooth to form support for the alveolar bone proper.
    D. The **periosteum** is a layer of connective soft tissue covering the outer surface of bone; it consists of an outer layer of collagenous tissue and an inner layer of fine elastic fibers.

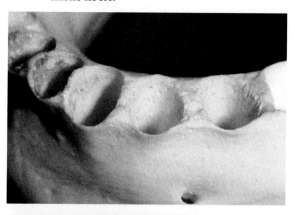

Figure 1-14. Alveoli of the Mandible. The alveoli are the sockets in the alveolar bone that house the roots of the teeth. (Courtesy of Dr. Don Rolfs, Periodontal Foundations, Wenatchee, WA)

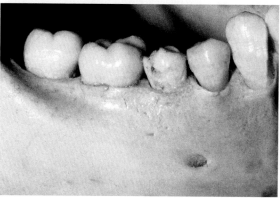

Figure 1-15. Bony Contours. The alveolar crest meets the teeth in a scalloped line that follows the contours of the cementoenamel junctions. (Courtesy of Dr. Don Rolfs, Periodontal Foundations, Wenatchee, WA)

SECTION 2: NERVE SUPPLY, BLOOD SUPPLY, AND LYMPHATIC SYSTEM

NERVE SUPPLY TO THE PERIODONTIUM

1. **Description.** The **innervation** of the periodontium—nerve supply to the periodontium—is derived from the branches of the **trigeminal nerve (Fig. 1-16)**.
   A. The trigeminal nerves have sensory, motor, and intermediate roots that attach directly to the brain.
   B. The trigeminal nerve is responsible for the sensory sensibility of most of the skin of the front part of the face and head, the teeth, oral cavity, maxillary sinus, and nasal cavity.
   C. The motor function of the trigeminal nerve is essential for the act of chewing.
2. **Functions of the Nerve Supply to the Periodontium**
   A. Nerve receptors in the gingiva, alveolar bone, and periodontal ligament register pain, touch, and pressure.
   B. Nerves in the periodontal ligament provide information about movement and tooth position. These nerves provide the sensations of light touch or pressure against the teeth and play an important role in the regulation of chewing forces and movements. When biting down on something hard, it is the nerves of the periodontal ligament that are stimulated, allowing the individual to experience a sense of pressure with the teeth against the hard object.
3. **Innervation of the Gingiva**
   A. Innervation of the gingiva of the maxillary arch is from the superior alveolar nerves (anterior, middle, and posterior branches), infraorbital nerve, and the greater palatine and nasopalatine nerves.
   B. Innervation of the gingiva of the mandibular arch is from the mental nerve, buccal nerve, and the sublingual branch of the lingual nerve.
4. **Innervation of the Teeth and Periodontal Ligament**
   A. Innervation of the teeth and periodontal ligament of the maxillary arch is from the superior alveolar nerves (anterior, middle, and posterior branches).
   B. Innervation of the teeth and periodontal ligament of the mandibular arch is from the inferior alveolar nerve.

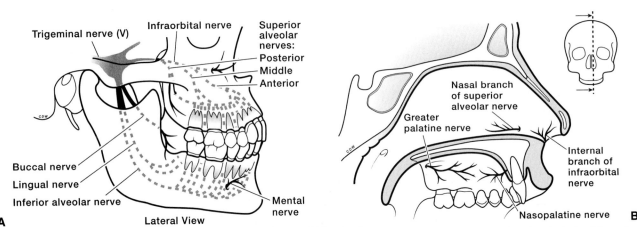

Figure 1-16. Nerve Supply to the Periodontium (Lateral View). A: The nerve supply to the periodontium is derived from the branches of the trigeminal nerve. **B:** Nerve innervation to the palate.

BLOOD SUPPLY TO THE PERIODONTIUM

1. **Description.** The vessels of the periodontium **anastomose** (join together) to create a complex *system of blood vessels* that supply blood to the periodontal tissues. This network of blood vessels acts as a unit, supplying blood to the soft and hard tissues of the maxilla and mandible. It is the proliferation of this rich blood supply to the gingiva that accounts for the dramatic color changes that are seen in gingivitis.

2. **Function.** The major function of the complex network of blood vessels of the periodontium is to transport oxygen and nutrients to the tissue cells of the periodontium and to remove carbon dioxide and other waste products from the cells for detoxification and elimination.

3. **Vascular Supply to the Periodontium (Fig. 1-17)**
   A. Maxillary gingiva, periodontal ligament, and alveolar bone
      1. Anterior and posterior superior alveolar arteries
      2. Infraorbital artery
      3. Greater palatine artery
   B. Mandibular gingiva, periodontal ligament, and alveolar bone
      1. Inferior alveolar artery
      2. Branches of the inferior alveolar artery: the buccal, facial, mental, and sublingual arteries

4. **Vascular Supply to the Teeth and Periodontal Tissues**
   A. The major arteries
      1. Superior alveolar arteries—maxillary periodontal tissues
      2. Inferior alveolar artery—mandibular periodontal tissues
   B. Branch arteries (**Figs. 1-18 and 1-19**)
      1. The dental artery: a branch of the superior or inferior alveolar artery
      2. Intraseptal artery: enters the tooth socket
      3. Rami perforantes: terminal branches of the intraseptal artery; they penetrate the tooth socket and enter the periodontal ligament space where they anastomose (join) with the blood vessels from the alveolar bone and periodontal ligament
      4. Supraperiosteal blood vessels: located in the free gingiva and are the main supply of the blood to the free gingiva; these vessels anastomose with blood vessels from the alveolar bone and periodontal ligament
      5. Subepithelial plexus: branches of the supraperiosteal blood vessels located in the connective tissue beneath the free and attached gingiva
      6. Periodontal ligament vessels: supply the periodontal ligament and form a complex network of vessels that surrounds the root
      7. Dentogingival plexus: a fine-meshed network of blood vessels located in the connective tissue beneath the gingival sulcus

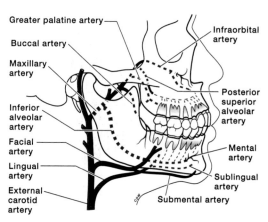

Greater palatine artery
Buccal artery
Maxillary artery
Inferior alveolar artery
Facial artery
Lingual artery
External carotid artery
Infraorbital artery
Posterior superior alveolar artery
Mental artery
Sublingual artery
Submental artery

Figure 1-17. Vascular Supply to the Periodontium. A complex network of blood vessels supplies blood to the periodontium.

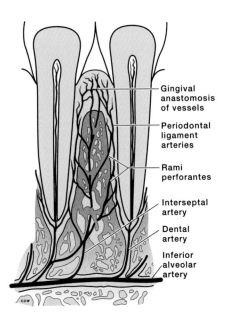

Figure 1-18. Branch Arteries. The branch arteries supply blood to the teeth and periodontium.

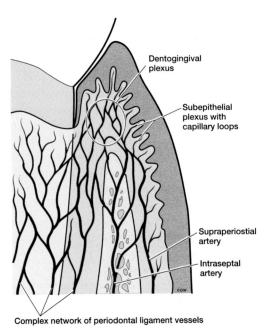

Figure 1-19. Network of Vessels. A fine network of vessels supplies blood to gingiva, gingival connective tissue, and periodontal ligament.

LYMPHATIC SYSTEM AND THE PERIODONTIUM

1. **Description.** The **lymphatic system** is a network of lymph nodes connected by lymphatic vessels that plays an important role in the body's defense against infection.
2. **Function. Lymph nodes** (pronounced: limf nodes) are small bean shaped structures located on either side of the head, neck, armpits, and groin. These nodes filter out and trap bacteria, fungi, viruses, and other unwanted substances to safely eliminate them from the body.
3. **Lymph Drainage of the Periodontium.** The lymph from the periodontal tissues is drained to the lymph nodes of the head and neck (**Fig. 1-20**).
   A. Submandibular lymph nodes—drain most of the periodontal tissues
   B. Deep cervical lymph nodes—drain the palatal gingiva of the maxilla
   C. Submental lymph nodes—drain the gingiva in the region of the mandibular incisors
   D. Jugulodigastric lymph nodes—drain the gingiva in the third molar region

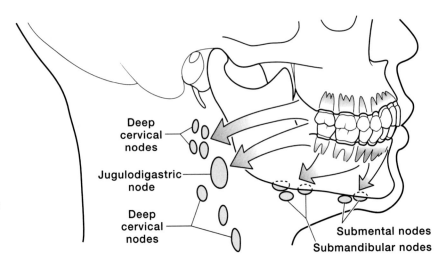

Figure 1-20. Lymphatic System of the Periodontium. The lymph from the periodontium is drained to the lymph nodes of the head and neck.

CHAPTER SUMMARY STATEMENT

The gingiva, periodontal ligament, cementum, and alveolar bone make up a system of tissues that surround the teeth and attach them to the alveolar bone. Each tissue of the periodontium plays a vital role in the functioning and retention of the teeth.

- The gingiva provides a tissue seal aroung the cervical portion of the teeth and covers the alveolar process.
- The periodontal ligament supports the tooth in its socket, provides nutrients and sensory feeling to the tooth, and maintains cementum and the alveolar bone of the tooth socket.
- The cementum anchors the periodontal ligament to the tooth and seals the ends of the open dentinal tubules. Cementum formation compensates for tooth wear due to occlusal attrition.
- The alveolar bone forms the bony sockets that provide support and protection for the roots of the teeth.

SECTION 3: FOCUS ON PATIENTS

CASE 1
A patient involved in an automobile accident receives a penetrating wound involving the oral cavity. The wound enters the alveolar mucosa near the apex of a lower premolar tooth and extends from the surface mucosa all the way through the tissues to the premolar tooth root. List periodontal tissues most likely injured by this penetrating wound.

CASE 2
A patient who has lost a maxillary lateral incisor tooth is scheduled to have a dental implant placed. The dental implant placement will require the clinician to prepare a hole with a drill in the bone formerly occupied by the lateral incisor tooth. Name the types of bone that will most probably be penetrated by the drill.

CASE 3
A dentist injects local anesthetic before working on a maxillary molar tooth. The injection results in complete loss of sensation in the molar tooth and in most of the gingiva surrounding the molar tooth. Name the nerves that most likely have been affected by the injection of the local anesthetic.

SECTION 4: CHAPTER REVIEW QUESTIONS

1. Which of the following is NOT one of the tissues of the periodontium?
   A. Periodontal ligament
   B. Body of the mandible
   C. Gingiva
   D. Cementum

2. Cementum is NOT necessary to the health of the periodontium because the underlying dentin will protect the root if the cementum is removed by toothbrush abrasion or from dental procedures.
   A. True
   B. False

3. Which tissue of the periodontium may be pigmented in dark skinned individuals?
   A. Free gingiva
   B. Attached gingiva
   C. Periodontal ligament
   D. Alveolar mucosa

4. Healthy gingival tissue ALWAYS has a dimpled appearance known as stippling.
   A. True
   B. False

5. One function of the attached gingiva is to prevent the free gingiva from being pulled away from the tooth when tension is applied to the alveolar mucosa.
   A. True
   B. False

6. Which of the following forms the base of a gingival sulcus?
   A. Interdental gingiva
   B. Attached gingiva
   C. Junctional epithelium
   D. Periodontal ligament

7. On the tooth side, the periodontal ligament fibers are embedded in which of the following structures?
   A. Alveolar bone
   B. Attached gingiva
   C. Interdental gingiva
   D. Cementum

8. Cementum does not have its own blood supply; it receives its nutrients from the periodontal ligament.
   A. True
   B. False

9. Which of the following is the thin layer of bone that lines the tooth socket?
   A. Alveolus
   B. Alveolar bone proper
   C. Cortical bone
   D. Cancellous bone

Chapter

2 Microscopic Anatomy of the Periodontium

Refer to the CD packaged with this book for full color versions of some of the illustrations in this chapter.

Learning Objectives

■ Define the term epithelial tissue and describe its function in the body.
■ List and define the layers that comprise the stratified squamous epithelium of the skin.
■ Define keratin and describe its function in the epithelium.
■ Define the term cell junction and describe its function in the epithelial tissues.
■ Compare and contrast the terms desmosome and hemidesmosome.
■ Describe the epithelium–connective tissue interface found in most tissues of the body, such as the interface between the epithelium and connective tissues of the skin.
■ Describe the function of connective tissue in the body.

- List and define the layers that comprise the stratified squamous epithelium of the gingiva.
- Identify the three anatomic areas of the gingival epithelium on an unlabeled drawing of the anatomic areas of the gingival epithelium.
- Define the term oral epithelium and describe its location and function in the gingival epithelium.
- Define the term sulcular epithelium and describe its location and function in the gingival epithelium.
- Define the term junctional epithelium and describe its location and function in the gingival epithelium.
- State which of the anatomic areas of the junctional epithelium have an uneven, wavy epithelium–connective tissue interface **in health** and which have a smooth junction in **health**.
- State the level of keratinization present in each of the three anatomical areas of the junctional epithelium (keratinized, nonkeratinized, or parakeratinized).
- Identify the enamel, gingival connective tissue, junctional epithelium, internal basal lamina, external basal lamina, epithelial cells, desmosomes, and hemidesmosomes on an unlabeled drawing depicting the microscopic anatomy of the junctional epithelium and surrounding tissues.
- Describe the function of the gingival connective tissue.
- Define the term supragingival fiber bundles and describe their function in the periodontium.
- Given an unlabeled drawing showing the supragingival fiber groups, label each of the fiber groups by name.
- Define and describe the significance of the biologic width.
- Define the term periodontal ligament and describe its function in the periodontium.
- Identify the principal fiber groups of the periodontal ligament on an unlabeled drawing.
- Define the term Sharpey's fibers.
- Define the term cementum and describe its function in the periodontium.
- State the three relationships that the cementum may have in relation to the enamel at the cementoenamel junction.
- Define the term alveolar bone and describe its function in the periodontium.

KEY TERMS

Histology
Cells
Extracellular matrix
Epithelial tissue
Stratified squamous epithelium
Keratinized layer
Keratinization
Nonkeratinized layers
Basal cell layer
Basal lamina
Cell junctions
Desmosome
Hemidesmosome
Connective tissue
Extracellular ground substance
Epithelium–connective tissue interface
Epithelial ridges
Connective tissue papillae
Gingival epithelium
Oral epithelium

Parakeratinized
Sulcular epithelium
Junctional epithelium
Laminae
Internal basal lamina
External basal lamina
Dental pellicle
Collagen fibers
Supragingival fiber bundles
Dentogingival unit
Biologic width
Periodontal ligament
Fiber bundles of the periodontal ligament
Sharpey's fibers
Cementum
OMG (overlap, meet, gap)
Alveolar bone (alveolar process)
Osteoblasts
Osteoclasts

SECTION 1: HISTOLOGY OF BODY TISSUES

Histology is a branch of anatomy concerned with the study of the microscopic structures of tissues. Knowledge of the microscopic characteristics of tissues is a prerequisite for understanding the microscopic anatomy of the periodontium. Section 1 reviews the microscopic anatomy of the epithelial and connective tissues of the body.

MICROSCOPIC ANATOMY OF TISSUES

Tissues comprise cells and an extracellular matrix.
1. **Cells** are the smallest structural unit of living matter capable of functioning independently. There are 100 trillion cells in the human body.
2. **Extracellular matrix** is a meshlike material that surrounds the cells. This material helps to hold cells and tissues together and provides a medium within which cells can migrate and interact with one another. The extracellular matrix consists of ground substance and fibers.
    A. The ground substance is a gellike material that fills the space between the cells.
    B. The fibers consist of collagen, elastin, and reticular fibers.

MICROSCOPIC ANATOMY OF EPITHELIAL TISSUE

1. **Description.** The **epithelial tissue** is the tissue that makes up the outer surface of the body (skin) and lines the body cavities such as the mouth, stomach, and intestines (mucosa). The skin and mucosa of the oral cavity are made up of **stratified squamous epithelium**—a type of epithelium that comprises flat cells arranged in several layers.
2. **Composition of Epithelial Tissue** (Fig. 2-1)
    A. Plentiful Cells. Most of the volume of epithelial tissue consists of many closely packed epithelial cells. Epithelial cells are bound together into sheets.
    B. Sparse Extracellular Matrix
        1. The extracellular matrix component of epithelial tissue is small.
        2. The extracellular matrix consists mainly of a thin mat called the basal lamina, which underlies the cellular sheets. The **basal lamina** is a thin mat of extracellular matrix that separates the epithelial sheets from the underlying connective tissue.
    C. Epithelial sheets almost always rest on a supporting bed of connective tissue.

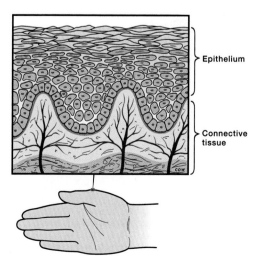

Figure 2-1. Stratified Squamous Epithelium and Connective Tissue of the Skin. The epithelium of the skin consists of many closely packed epithelial cells and a thin basal lamina. The epithelium of the skin rests on a supporting bed of connective tissue. The epithelium does not contain blood vessels; nourishment is received from blood vessels in the underlying connective tissue.

3. **Keratinization. Keratinization**—the process by which epithelial cells on the surface of the skin become stronger and waterproof.
   A. Keratinized Layer
      1. **Keratinized epithelial cells** have no nuclei and form a tough, resistant layer on the surface of the skin. The most heavily keratinized epithelium of the body is found on the palms of the hands and soles of the feet.
      2. **Nonkeratinized epithelial cells** have nuclei and act as a cushion against mechanical stress and wear. Nonkeratinized epithelial cells are softer and more flexible. Nonkeratinized epithelium is found in areas such as the mucosal lining of the cheeks—permitting the mobility needed to speak, chew, and make facial expressions.
4. **Blood Supply.** Epithelial tissues do not contain blood vessels; nourishment is received from blood vessels contained in the underlying connective tissue (**Fig. 2-1**).

EPITHELIAL CELL JUNCTIONS

Neighboring epithelial cells attach to one another by specialized cell junctions that give the tissue strength to withstand mechanical forces and to form a protective barrier.
1. **Definition. Cell junctions** are cellular structures that mechanically attach a cell and its cytoskeleton to its neighboring cells or to the basal lamina.
2. **Purpose.** Cell junctions bind cells together so that they can function as a strong structural unit. Tissues, such as the epithelium of the skin that must withstand severe mechanical stresses have the most abundant number of cell junctions.
3. **Forms of Epithelial Cell Junctions**
   A. **Desmosome**—a specialized cell junction that connects two neighboring epithelial cells and their cytoskeletons together. You might think of desmosomes as being like the snaps used to close a denim jacket. Instead of fastening the front of a jacket together, desmosomes fasten cells together (**Fig. 2-2**).
      1. A cell-to-cell connection
      2. An important form of cell junction found in the gingival epithelium
   B. **Hemidesmosome**—a specialized cell junction that connects the epithelial cells to the basal lamina (**Fig. 2-2**).
      1. A cell-to-basal lamina connection
      2. An important form of cell junction found in the gingival epithelium

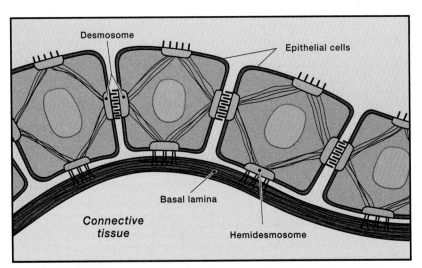

Figure 2-2. Epithelial Cells and Basal Lamina. Epithelial cells attach to each other with specialized cell junctions called desmosomes. Hemidesmosomes attach the epithelial cells to the basal lamina.

MICROSCOPIC ANATOMY OF CONNECTIVE TISSUE

The epithelium rests on a supporting bed of connective tissue (**Fig. 2-3**). The **basal lamina** is a thin, tough sheet that separates the epithelial tissue from the underlying connective tissue.

1. **Description. Connective tissue** fills the spaces between the tissues and organs in the body. It is made up of a large amount of material that surrounds the cells and relatively few cells.
2. **Composition of Connective Tissue (Fig. 2-3)**
    A. Sparse Cells. Connective tissue cells are sparsely distributed in the extracellular matrix.
        1. Fibroblasts (fiber-builders)—cells that form the extracellular matrix (fibers and ground substance) and secrete it into the intercellular spaces
        2. Macrophages and neutrophils—phagocytes (cell-eaters) that devour dying cells and microorganisms that invade the body
        3. Lymphocytes—cells that play a major role in the immune response
    B. Plentiful Extracellular Matrix. The extracellular matrix—a rich gellike substance containing a network of strong fibers—is the major component of connective tissue. The network of fiber matrices, rather than the cells, gives connective tissue the strength to withstand mechanical forces.
3. **Types of Connective Tissue**
    A. Loose connective tissue
    B. Cartilage
    C. Bone (including the alveolar bone of the periodontium)
    D. Bone marrow
    E. Tonsils and lymph nodes
    F. Fat
    G. Dental tissues (cementum, dentin, and pulp)—all dental tissues of the tooth are specialized forms of connective tissue *except enamel*. Enamel is an epithelial tissue.

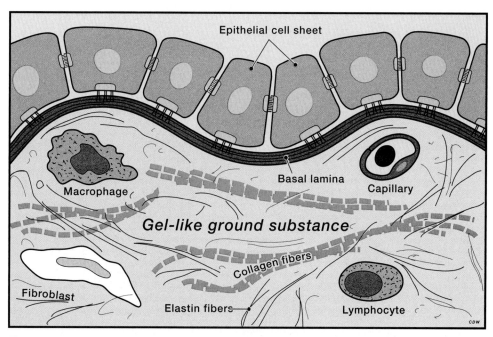

Figure 2-3. Microscopic Anatomy of Connective Tissue. Connective tissue comprises a gel-like substance, protein fibers, and connective tissue cells.

EPITHELIAL–CONNECTIVE TISSUE BOUNDARY

1. **Description.** The **epithelial–connective tissue interface** is the boundary where the epithelial and connective tissues meet.
2. **Characteristics of the Epithelial–Connective Tissue Boundary.**
   A. **Wavy Boundary.** In most places in the body, the epithelium meets the connective in a wavy, uneven manner (**Fig. 2-4**).
      1. **Epithelial ridges**—deep extensions of epithelium that reach down into the connective tissue. The epithelial ridges are also known as rete pegs.
      2. **Connective tissue papillae**—fingerlike extensions of connective tissue that extend up into the epithelium.
   B. Smooth Boundary
      1. Some specialized epithelial tissues in the body meet the connective tissue in a smooth interface that has no epithelial ridges or connective tissue papillae.
      2. Some anatomical areas of the gingiva have an epithelial–connective tissue interface that is smooth. The anatomy of the gingival epithelial and connective tissues is described in detail in Section 2.
3. **Function of the Wavy Tissue Boundary**
   A. The wavy tissue interface enhances the adhesion of the epithelium to the connective tissue by increasing the surface area of the junction between the two tissues. This strong adhesion of the epithelium allows the skin to resist mechanical forces.
   B. The wavy junction between the epithelium and connective tissue also increases the area from which the epithelium can receive nourishment from the underlying connective tissue. The epithelium does not have its own blood supply; blood vessels are carried close to the epithelium in the connective tissue papillae.

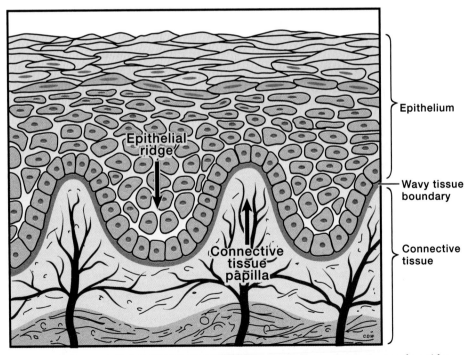

Figure 2-4. Uneven Epithelial–Connective Tissue Interface. In most cases, the epithelium meets the connective tissue at an uneven, wavy border. Epithelial ridges extend down into the connective tissue. Connective tissue papillae extend upward into the epithelium.

SECTION 2: HISTOLOGY OF THE GINGIVA

Knowledge of the microscopic anatomy of the gingiva is a requirement for understanding the periodontium in health and in disease. At first glance, the microscopic anatomy of the periodontium may seem to be impossibly complicated. The anatomy of the periodontium, however, is much like that of tissues elsewhere in the body. This section reviews the microscopic anatomy of the gingival epithelium, junctional epithelium, and gingival connective tissues.

MICROSCOPIC ANATOMY OF GINGIVAL EPITHELIUM

The **gingival epithelium** is a specialized stratified squamous epithelium that functions well in the wet environment of the oral cavity. The microscopic anatomy of the gingival epithelium is similar to the epithelium of the skin. The gingival epithelium has three anatomical areas (**Fig. 2-5**):

1. Oral epithelium
2. Sulcular epithelium
3. Junctional epithelium

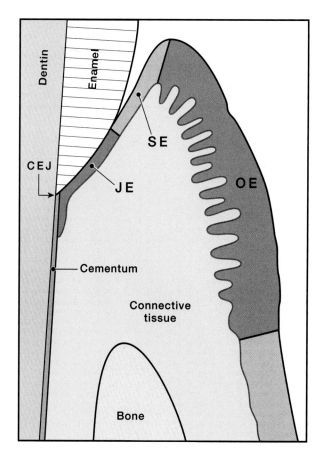

Figure 2-5. Three Areas of the Gingival Epithelium.
The gingival epithelium has three distinct areas:
- JE—junctional epithelium at the base of the sulcus
- SE—sulcular epithelium that lines the sulcus
- OE—oral epithelium covering the free and attached gingiva

1. **Oral epithelium (OE)**—epithelium that covers the outer surface of the free gingiva and attached gingiva; it extends from the crest of the gingival margin to the mucogingival junction (Fig. 2-5).
    A. Keratinization. The OE may be *keratinized or parakeratinized* (partially keratinized).

      B. Interface with Gingival Connective Tissue. The junction of the OE with the connective tissue has *a wavy interface* that has epithelial ridges.

  2. Sulcular epithelium (SE)—epithelial lining of the gingival sulcus; it extends from the crest of the gingival margin to the coronal edge of the JE (**Fig. 2-6**).

      A. Keratinization. The SE is a thin, *nonkeratinized epithelium.*

         1. The SE is permeable allowing fluid to flow from the gingival connective tissue into the sulcus. This fluid is known as the **gingival crevicular fluid**. The flow of gingival crevicular fluid is slight in health and increases in disease.

      B. Interface with Gingival Connective Tissue. In health, the junction of the SE with the connective tissue has a *smooth interface* with no epithelial ridges (no wavy junction).

  3. Junctional epithelium (JE)—epithelium that forms the base of the sulcus and joins the gingiva to the tooth surface (**Fig. 2-6**).

      A. Length and Width of JE

         1. The JE ranges from 0.71 to 1.35 mm in length.[1]

         2. The JE is about 15 to 30 cells thick at the coronal zone—the zone that attaches highest on the crown of the tooth.

         3. The JE tapers to 4 to 5 cells thick at the apical zone.

      B. Keratinization of JE

         1. The JE is a thin, nonkeratinized epithelium.

         2. Nonkeratinized epithelial cells of both the sulcular and junctional areas of the gingival epithelium make them a less effective protective covering. Thus, the sulcular and junctional areas provide the easiest point of entry for bacteria or bacterial products to invade the connective tissue of the gingiva.

      C. Juntional Epithelium Interface with Gingival Connective Tissue. In health, the JE has a *smooth tissue interface* with the connective tissue (no wavy junctions).

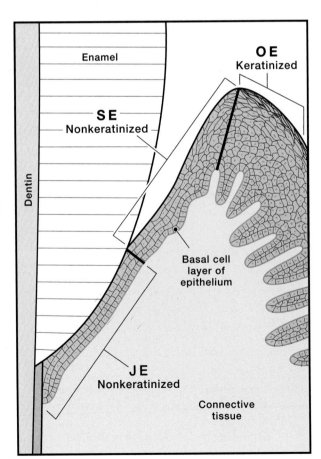

Figure 2-6. Microscopic Anatomy of the Three Areas of the Gingival Epithelium. Interface with Connective Tissue.

■ JE (junctional epithelium)—these epithelial cells join the gingiva to the tooth surface at the base of the sulcus.

■ SE (sulcular epithelium)—these epithelial cells extend from the edge of the junctional epithelium coronally to the crest of the gingival margin.

■ OE (oral epithelium)—these epithelial cells form the outer layer of the free and attached gingiva.

MICROSCOPIC ANATOMY OF JUNCTIONAL EPITHELIUM

1. **Why a Tooth Needs a Junctional Epithelium**
   A. A Break in the Epithelial Protective Covering
      1. The body is protected by a continuous sheet of epithelium that covers its outer surfaces and lines the body cavities, including the oral cavity.
      2. The teeth penetrate this protective covering by erupting through the epithelium, thus creating an opening through which microorganisms can enter the body.
   B. An Epithelial Seal
      1. The body attempts to seal the opening created when a tooth penetrates the epithelium by attaching the epithelium to the tooth.
      2. The word junction means connection; thus, the epithelium that is connected to the tooth is termed the JE.
2. **Components of Junctional Epithelium**
   A. Plentiful Cells. The JE consists of layers of closely packed epithelial cells. The epithelial cells of the JE are nonkeratinized—have nuclei—and are connected to their neighboring epithelial cells by desmosomes.
      1. **Internal basal lamina**—a thin mat of extracellular matrix between the epithelial cells of the JE and the tooth surface.
      2. **External basal lamina**—a thin mat of extracellular matrix between the epithelial cells of the JE and the gingival connective tissue.
         a. A membrane, called the **dental pellicle**, lies between the tooth and the internal basal lamina (**Fig. 2-8**). The dental pellicle is also called the dental cuticle or acquired pellicle.
         b. The dental pellicle forms during the late stages of tooth eruption and thickens with age. The components of dental pellicle are not known.
   B. Sparse Extracellular Matrix. The extracellular matrix consists mainly of two basal laminae (**Fig. 2-7**). **Laminae**—the plural form of the word lamina.

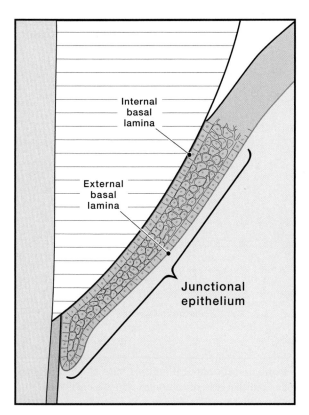

Figure 2-7. Basal Laminae of the Junctional Epithelium. The junctional epithelium has two basal laminae. The internal basal lamina attaches to the tooth surface. The external basal lamina attaches to the underlying gingival connective tissue.

JUNCTIONAL EPITHELIUM—CONNECTIVE TISSUE INTERFACE

1. **Attachment of Junctional Epithelium to the Tooth Surface**
   A. The epithelial cells of the JE attach to the *tooth surface* using *hemidesmosomes* and the *internal basal lamina* (Fig. 2-8).
      1. The internal basal lamina is a thin sheet of extracellular matrix adjacent to the tooth surface.
      2. The epithelial cells attach to the tooth surface by four to eight hemidesmosomes per micron at the coronal zone and two hemidesmosomes per micron in the apical zone of the JE.[2] The apical zone is the area of the JE with the least adhesiveness.
   B. The attachment of the hemidesmosomes and internal basal lamina to the tooth surface is not static; rather, the cells of the JE appear to be capable of moving along the tooth surface.
2. **Attachment of the Junctional Epithelium to the Underlying Gingival Connective Tissue**
   A. The epithelial cells of the JE attach to the underlying *gingival connective tissue* using *hemidesmosomes* and the *external basal lamina* (Fig. 2-8).
   B. In health, the JE has a *smooth tissue interface* with the connective tissue (no wavy junctions).
3. **Functions of Junctional Epithelium**
   A. The JE attaches the gingiva to the enamel and/or the cementum of the tooth, thus providing a seal at the base of the gingival sulcus or periodontal pocket.
   B. The JE provides a protective barrier between the plaque biofilm and the connective tissue of the periodontium.

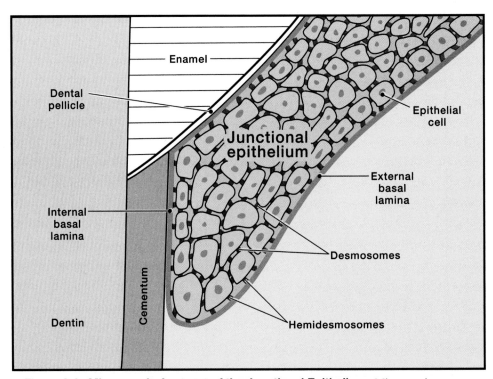

Figure 2-8. Microscopic Anatomy of the Junctional Epithelium. Microscopic structures of the junctional epithelium (JE) include the epithelial cells, desmosomes, external and internal basal laminae, hemidesmosomes, and dental pellicle.

MICROSCOPIC ANATOMY OF GINGIVAL CONNECTIVE TISSUE

1. **Function.** The gingival connective tissue of the free and attached gingiva provides solidity to the gingiva and attaches the gingiva to the cementum of the root and the alveolar bone. The gingival connective tissue is also known as the lamina propria.
2. **Components of the Gingival Connective Tissue.** In contrast to the gingival epithelium (which has an abundance of cells and sparse extracellular matrix), the gingival connective tissue has an abundance of extracellular matrix and few cells.
   A. Cells. Cells comprise about 5% of the gingival connective tissue, including fibroblasts (fiber building cells) and immune cells such as neutrophils, macrophages, and lymphocytes.
   B. Extracellular Matrix
      1. Protein fibers account for about 55% to 65% of the gingival connective tissue. Most of these are **collagen fibers** that form a dense network of strong, ropelike cables that secure and hold the gingival connective tissues together.
      2. Gellike material between the cells makes up about 30% to 35% of the gingival connective tissue. This gellike material helps to hold the tissue together.
3. **Supragingival Fiber Bundles (Gingival Fibers)**—the network of ropelike collagen fiber bundles located coronal to (above) the crest of the alveolar bone.
   A. Characteristics of the Fiber Bundles
      1. The fiber bundles are embedded in the gellike ground substance of the extracellular matrix.
      2. The attachment of the JE to the tooth is strengthened by the supragingival fiber bundles that brace the gingival margin against the tooth surface.
      3. Together the JE and the gingival fibers are referred to as the **dentogingival unit**. The dentogingival unit acts to provide structural support to the gingival tissue.
   A. Functions of the Fiber Bundles
      1. Brace the free gingiva firmly against the tooth and reinforce the attachment of the JE to the tooth.
      2. Provide the free gingiva with the rigidity needed to withstand the frictional forces that result during mastication.
      3. Unite the free gingiva with the cementum of the root and alveolar bone.
      4. Connect adjacent teeth to one another to control tooth positioning within the dental arch.
   B. Classification of Fiber Groups. The supragingival fiber bundles are classified based on their orientation, sites of insertion, and the structures that they connect **(Figs. 2-9 and 2-10)**.
      1. Alveologingival—extend from the periosteum of the alveolar crest into the gingival connective tissue. These fiber bundles attach the gingiva to the bone.
      2. Circular—encircle the tooth in a ringlike manner coronal to the alveolar crest and are not attached to the cementum of the tooth. These fiber bundles connect adjacent teeth to one another.
      3. Dentogingival—embedded in the cementum near the cementoenamel junction (CEJ) and fan out into the gingival connective tissue. These fibers act to attach the gingiva to the teeth.
      4. Periostogingival—extend laterally from the periosteum of the alveolar bone. These fibers attach the gingiva to the bone.
      5. Intergingival—extend in a mesiodistal direction along the entire dental arch and around the last molars in the arch. These fiber bundles link adjacent teeth into a dental arch unit.
      6. Intercircular—encircle several teeth. These fiber groups link adjacent teeth into a dental arch unit.
      7. Interpapillary—are located in the papillae coronal to (above) the transseptal fiber bundles. These fiber groups connect the oral and vestibular interdental papillae of posterior teeth.

8. Transgingival—extend from the cementum near the CEJ and run horizontally between adjacent teeth. These fiber bundles link adjacent teeth into a dental arch unit.

9. Transseptal—pass from the cementum of one tooth, over the crest of alveolar bone, to the cementum of the adjacent tooth. These fiber bundles connect adjacent teeth to one another and secure alignment of teeth in the arch.

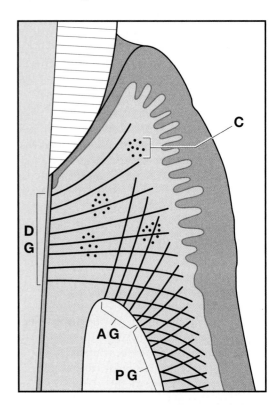

Figure 2-9. Supragingival Fiber Groups.

■ C—circular
■ AG—alveologingival
■ DG—dentogingival
■ PG—periostogingival

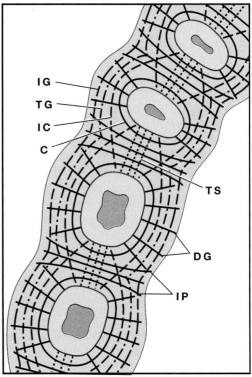

Figure 2-10. Supragingival Fiber Groups of the Mandibular Arch (Occlusal View, Looking Down on the Mandibular Arch).

■ C—circular
■ IG—intergingival
■ IC—intercircular
■ IP—interpapillary
■ DG—dentogingival
■ TG—transgingival
■ TS—transseptal

BIOLOGIC WIDTH

1. **Description.** The **biologic width** includes that portion of the tooth surface that is covered by the JE and the connective tissue including the supragingival fiber bundles (**Fig. 2-11**).

2. **Length of the Biologic Width.** Approximately 2 mm of vertical space is needed to contain the JE and the supragingival fiber bundles.
   A. The length of JE is approximately 1 mm.[3]
   B. The approximate vertical space taken up by the supragingival fiber groups is approximately 1 mm in length.

3. **Significance.** The biologic width is an important consideration in the design of dental restorations and crowns. The margin of a restoration or crown must never be placed so close to the alveolar bone that it encroaches on the biologic width (**Fig. 2-12**).

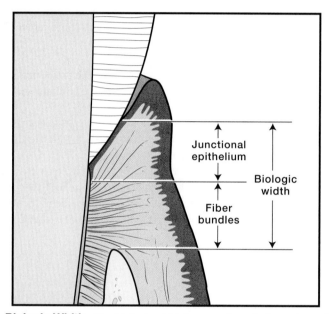

Figure 2-11. Biologic Width. The biologic width is approximately 2 mm in vertical length and contains the junctional epithelium and the gingival fiber bundles.

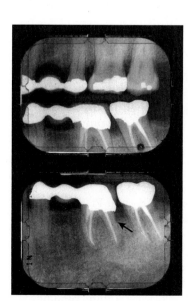

Figure 2-12. Encroachment on Biologic Width.
These radiographs show a fixed bridge on the mandibular left posterior sextant.
- On the premolar, the margins of the crown do not encroach on the biologic width.
- On the molar crown, the distal margin extends into the biologic width resulting in an area of localized bone loss (indicated on the lower radiograph with an arrow).
(Courtesy of Dr. John Preece, UTHSCSA, San Antonio, TX.)

Section 3 reviews the microscopic anatomy of the periodontal ligament, cementum, and alveolar bone. Knowledge of the microscopic anatomy of these structures is a prerequisite to understanding the characteristics of the periodontium in health and in disease.

MICROSCOPIC ANATOMY OF PERIODONTAL LIGAMENT

1. **Definition.** The **periodontal ligament (PDL)** is a thin sheet of fibrous connective tissue located between the tooth and its bony socket. The PDL connects to the tooth and the bony wall of the tooth socket.
2. **Components of the Periodontal Ligament**
   A. Cells. The cells of the PDL are mainly fibroblasts with some cementoblasts and osteoblasts.
   B. Extracellular Matrix.
      1. The extracellular matrix of the PDL is similar to the extracellular matrix of other connective tissue. This rich gellike substance contains specialized connective fibers.
      2. Fiber Bundles. The fiber bundles of the PDL are a specialized connective tissue that surrounds the root of the tooth and connects it with the alveolar bone. These fibers are the largest component of the PDL.
         a. The ropelike collagen fiber bundles of the PDL stretch across the space between the cementum and the alveolar bone of the tooth socket (**Fig. 2-13**).
         b. The collagen fiber bundles are anchored on one side in the cementum covering the tooth root; on the other side, they are embedded in the bone of the tooth socket.
   C. Blood Vessels and Nerve Supply. The PDL has a rich supply of nerves and blood vessels.
3. **Description of the Periodontal Ligament**
   A. In health, the PDL surrounds the entire root of the tooth and fills the space between the root and the bony tooth socket.
   B. The thickness of the PDL ranges from 0.05 to 0.25 mm depending on the age of the patient and the function of the tooth.
4. **Functions of the Periodontal Ligament**
   A. Supportive function—major function
      1. Attaches the tooth to its bony socket.
      2. Suspends the tooth in its socket, separating it from the socket wall, so that the root does not collide with the bone during mastication.
   B. Sensory function—the PDL is supplied with nerve fibers that transmit tactile pressure (such as a tap with dental instrument against tooth) and pain sensations.
   C. Nutritive function—the PDL is supplied with blood vessels that provide nutrients to the cementum and bone.
   D. Formative function—the PDL contains cementoblasts (cementum builders) that produce cementum throughout the life of the tooth, while the osteoblasts (bone builders) maintain the bone of the tooth socket.
   E. Resorptive function—in response to severe pressure, cells of the PDL (osteoclasts) can produce rapid bone resorption and, sometimes, resorption of cementum.
5. **Fiber Bundles of the Periodontal Ligament**—the specialized connective tissue that surrounds the root of the tooth and connects it with the alveolar bone.
   A. Principal Fiber Groups of the PDL. These fiber bundles are classified into five groups based on their location and orientation (**Fig. 2-13**).
      1. **Alveolar crest fiber group**—extend from the cervical cementum, running downward in a diagonal direction, to the alveolar crest. This fiber group resists horizontal movements of the tooth.

2. **Horizontal fiber group**—located apical to the alveolar crest fibers. They extend from the cementum to the bone at right angles to the long axis to the root. This fiber group resists horizontal pressure against the crown of the tooth.

3. **Oblique fiber group**—located apical to the horizontal group. They extend from the cementum to the bone, running in a diagonal direction. This fiber group resists vertical pressures that threaten to drive the root into its socket.

4. **Apical fiber group**—extend from the apex of the tooth to the bone. This fiber group secures the tooth in its socket and resists forces that might lift the tooth out of the socket.

5. **Interradicular fiber group** (seen only in multirooted teeth)—extend from the cementum in the furcation area of the tooth to the interradicular septum of the alveolar bone. These fiber groups help to stabilize the tooth in its socket.

B. Sharpey's Fibers

1. The ends of the PDL fibers that are embedded in the cementum and alveolar bone are known as **Sharpey's fibers (Fig. 2-14)**.

2. The attachment of the fiber bundles occurs when the cementum and bone are forming. As cementum forms, the tissue hardens around the ends of the periodontal fibers (Sharpey's fibers) surrounding them with cementum. The same process occurs during bone formation. As the bony wall of the tooth socket hardens, it surrounds the ends of the periodontal fibers with bone. The ends of the fiber bundles become trapped in the bone that forms around them.

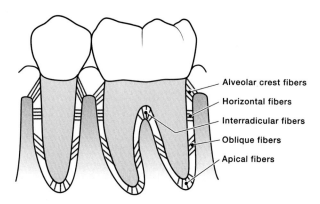

Alveolar crest fibers

Horizontal fibers

Interradicular fibers

Oblique fibers

Apical fibers

Figure 2-13. Principal Fiber Groups of the Periodontal Ligament. These fibers are classified as the alveolar crest, horizontal, interradicular, oblique, and apical.

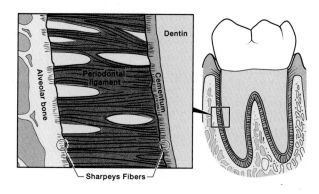

Dentin

Alveolar bone

Periodontal ligament

Cementum

Sharpeys Fibers

Figure 2-14. Sharpey's Fibers. The ends of the periodontal ligament fibers that are embedded in the alveolar bone and the cementum are known as Sharpey's fibers.

MICROSCOPIC ANATOMY OF CEMENTUM

1. **Definition. Cementum** is a calcified layer of connective tissue that covers the root of the tooth.
2. **Functions of Cementum**
   A. Seals and covers the open dentinal tubules and acts to protect the underlying dentin (**Fig. 2-15**).
   B. Attaches the periodontal fibers to the tooth.
   C. Compensates for attrition of teeth at their occlusal or incisal surfaces. Over time, teeth experience wear at their occlusal or incisal surfaces. Cementum is formed at the apical areas of the roots to compensate for loss of tooth tissues due to attrition.

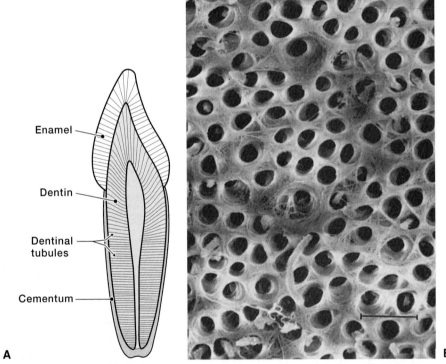

A

B

Figure 2-15. Dentinal Tubules. A: Diagram showing the numerous dentinal tubules that penetrate the dentin. B: A scanning electron micrograph of the cross section of dentinal tubules adjacent to the pulp chamber of a human tooth. The black line engraved in the lower right is 10 mm long. (From Melfi RC., *Permar's Oral Embryology and Microscopic Anatomy.* 10th ed. Philadelphia: Lippincott Williams & Wilkins: 2000:120, Figure 5-8 with permission.)

3. **Components of Mature Cementum**
   A. Organic matrix—composed of a framework of densely packed collagen fibers held together by the gellike extracellular ground substance
   B. Mineralized portion—made up of hydroxyapatite crystals (calcium and phosphate)
   C. Contains no blood vessels or nerves (Hypersensitivity of the root surface occurs when the cementum is removed exposing the dentin. It is the dentin that is sensitive to brushing or the touch of a dental instrument.)
4. **Types of Cementum**
   A. Acellular cementum
      1. Contains no cementocytes within its mineralized tissue
      2. First to be formed and covers approximately the cervical third or half of the root
      3. No new acellular cementum is produced during the life of the tooth
      4. Thickness ranges from 30 to 60 μm[4]
         Until recently, intentional aggressive removal of cementum was the standard of care for treatment of cementum exposed by the apical migration of the JE.

Intentional removal of cementum on the coronal half of the root should be avoided; over the course of many years, over zealous instrumentation can result in removal of all cementum and exposure of the underlying dentin. Conservation of cementum is ideal since loss of cementum is accompanied by exposure of the dentinal tubules and by a loss of attachment of PDL fibers to the root surface.

    5. Sharpey's fibers make up most of the structure of acellular cementum

  B. Cellular cementum

    1. Contains cementocytes within its mineralized tissue

    2. Formed after the tooth has erupted and is less calcified than acellular cementum

    3. Deposited in intervals throughout the life of the tooth (thickness increases with age)

    4. Thickness ranges from 150 to 200 μm[4]

    5. Sharpey's fibers make up a smaller portion of cellular cementum

5. Cementoenamel Junction. The cementum covering the root may have any one of three relationships with the enamel of the tooth crown. In order of frequency, the cementum may overlap the enamel, meet the enamel, or there is a gap between the cementum and enamel. This order of frequency is known as the **OMG** (overlap, meet, gap) **(Fig. 2-16)**.

  A. Overlap—in 60% of all cases, the cementum overlaps the enamel for a short distance.

  B. Meet—in 30% of all cases, the cementum meets the enamel.

  C. Gap—in 10% of all cases, there is a small gap between the cementum and enamel (exposing the dentin in this area). The patient may experience discomfort (dentinal sensitivity) during instrumentation. The use of local anesthesia may be helpful during instrumentation, and desensitization of sensitive areas should be performed following instrumentation.

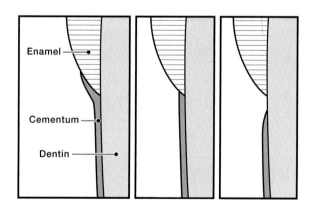

Figure 2-16. Relationship of Cementum to Enamel at the Cementoenamel Junction. In order of frequency, the cementum may: (1) overlap the enamel, (2) meet the enamel, or (3) not meet, leaving a gap between the cementum and enamel.

MICROSCOPIC ANATOMY OF ALVEOLAR BONE

1. Definiton. The **alveolar bone** or **alveolar process** is the bone of the upper or lower jaw that surrounds and supports the roots of the teeth **(Fig. 2-17)**.

2. Function of Alveolar Bone in the Periodontium. The alveolar bone forms the bony sockets that provide support and protection for the roots of the teeth.

3. Characteristics of Alveolar Bone

  A. Alveolar bone is mineralized connective tissue made by cells called osteoblasts (bone builders).

  B. Bone is rigid because calcium salts are deposited in its extracellular matrix.

  C. The alveolar bone has blood vessels and nerve innervation.

  D. Bone constantly undergoes periods of bone formation and resorption (loss).

4. **Components of Alveolar Bone**
   A. Major cell types
      1. Osteoblasts (bone builders)—cells that manufacture the organic matrix and initiate the mineralization of bone
      2. Osteoclasts (bone consumers)—cells that remove the mineral materials and organic matrix of bone
   B. Extracellular matrix
      1. Collagen fibers and gellike substance forms the major component of the alveolar bone
      2. Mineralized portion—calcified by deposition of the mineral salt hydroxyapatite
   C. Blood, lymph vessels, and nerves

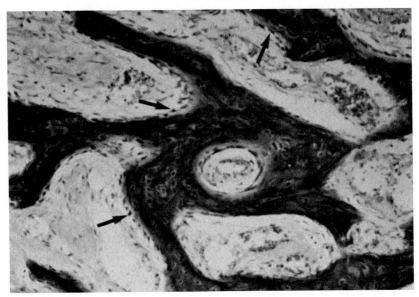

Figure 2-17. Anatomy of Alveolar Bone. A histologic section through a mandibular first molar and its alveolar process. (From Melfi RC. *Permar's Oral Embryology and Microscopic Anatomy.* 10th ed. Philadelphia: Lippincott Williams & Wilkins: 2000:215, figure 9-10 with permission.)

CHAPTER SUMMARY STATEMENT

Knowledge of the microscopic anatomy of the periodontium is fundamental in understanding the (1) function of the periodontium in health and (2) changes that occur during the periodontal disease process. The JE plays an important role in the health of the periodontium by attaching the gingival epithelium to the tooth via hemidesmosomes and an internal basal lamina. In health, the PDL, cementum, and alveolar bone act as a functional unit to support and maintain the teeth in the oral cavity.

SECTION 4: FOCUS ON PATIENTS

CASE 1

A clinician penetrates the oral mucosa with a needle before injecting a local anesthetic. The needle tip stops in the loose connective tissue underlying the surface structures. Name the layers of epithelium that have been penetrated by the needle.

CASE 2

A clinician finds it necessary to use a unique type of injection to achieve total anesthesia of a tooth being treated. The injection involves sliding a small-diameter needle into the PDL space to a point halfway down the tooth root. Name the PDL fibers most likely encountered by the needle tip during insertion.

CASE 3

Gum recession exposes a portion of tooth root on a maxillary canine tooth. Microscopic examination of the cementum in the area of the crown margin on the canine will reveal what possible relationships between the level of cementum and the level of the tooth crown?

References

1. Listgarten M. Electron microscopic study of the gingivo-dental junction of man. *Am J Anat.* 1966; 119:147–177.
2. Sabag N, Saglie R, Mery C. Ultrastructure of the normal human epithelial attachment to the cementum root surface. *J Periodontol.* 1981;52:94–95.
3. Gargiuo AW, Wentz FM, Orban B. Dimensions and relationships of the dentogingival junction in humans. *J Periodontol.* 1961;3:87.
4. Avery JK. *Essentials of Oral Histology and Embryology: A Clinical Approach.* 2nd ed. St. Louis: C.V. Mosby; 2000.

Suggested Readings

Hassell TM. Tissues and cells of the periodontium. *Periodontol 2000.* 1993;3:9–38.

Karring T, Loe H. The three-dimensional concept of the epithelium-connective tissue boundary of gingiva. *Acta Odontol Scand.* 1970;28:917–933.

Mariotti A. The extracellular matrix of the periodontium: dynamic and interactive tissues. *Periodontol 2000.* 1993;3:39–63.

Schroeder HE. *Oral Structural Biology. Embryology, Structure and Function of Normal Hard and Soft Tissues of the Oral Cavity and Temporomandibular Joints.* Stuttgart: Thieme-Flexibook; 1991.

Schroeder HE, Listgarten MA. Fine structure of the developing epithelial attachment of human teeth. *Monogr Dev Bio.,* 1971;2:1–134.

Schroeder HE, Listgarten MA., The gingival tissues: The architecture of periodontal protection. *Periodontol 2000.,* 1997;13:91–120.

Schroeder HE, Munzel-Pedrazzoli S. Morphometric analysis comparing junctional and oral epithelium of normal human gingiva. *Helv Odontol Acta.* 1970;14:53–66.

Schroeder HE, Munzel-Pedrazzoli S, Page R. Correlated morphometric and biochemical analysis of gingival tissue in early chronic gingivitis in man. *Arch Oral Biol,* 1973;18:899–923.

Schroeder HE, Theilade J. Electron microscopy of normal human gingival epithelium. *J Periodontal Res.* 1966;1:95–119.

SECTION 5: CHAPTER REVIEW QUESTIONS

1. Which of the following tissues serves as a covering tissue for the outer surfaces of the body and a lining tissue for body cavities such as the mouth, stomach, and intestines?
   A. Basal lamina
   B. Connective tissue
   C. Epithelial tissue
   D. Keratinized tissue

2. Which of the following tissues fills the spaces between the tissues and organs of the body?
   A. Basal lamina
   B. Connective tissue
   C. Epithelial tissue
   D. Keratinized tissue

3. Which of these epithelial layers comprises cells with nuclei that act as a cushion against mechanical stress and wear?
   A. Nonkeratinized layer
   B. Keratinized layer
   C. Extracellular ground layer
   D. Collagen layer

4. Epithelial cell junctions are cellular structures that can attach:
   A. An epithelial cell to a neighboring epithelial cell
   B. An epithelial cell to a basal lamina
   C. An epithelial cell to elastin fibers
   D. Both (a) and (b).

5. The function of cell junctions is to:
   A. Make it easy for cells to detach from each other to facilitate migration of cells
   B. Allow cells to bind together to function as a strong structural unit
   C. Fill the spaces between neighboring epithelial cells
   D. Both (a) and (b).

6. A cell junction that connects an epithelial basal cell to the basal lamina is termed:
   A. Hemidesmosome
   B. Desmosome
   C. Epithelial ridge
   D. Connective tissue papilla

7. In MOST places in the body, the epithelium meets the connective tissue in a wavy, uneven junction.
   A. True
   B. False

8. The deep extensions of epithelium that reach down into the connective tissue are termed:
   A. Hemidesmosomes
   B. Desmosomes
   C. Epithelial ridges
   D. Connective tissue papillae

9. Connective tissue comprises a gellike substance, fibers, and few cells.
   A. True
   B. False

10. The sulcular and junctional epithelium are keratinized epithelial tissues.
    A. True
    B. False

11. The epithelium that forms the base of the sulcus and joins the gingiva to the tooth is called the:
    A. Oral epithelium
    B. Sulcular epithelium
    C. Junctional epithelium
    D. Squamous epithelium

12. In the junctional epithelium, epithelial cells attach to neighboring epithelial cells via:
    A. Desmosomes
    B. Hemidesmosomes
    C. External basal lamina
    D. Internal basal lamina

13. The junctional epithelium attaches to the tooth surface via the:
    A. Desmosomes and the internal basal lamina
    B. Desmosomes and the external basal lamina
    C. Hemidesmosomes and the internal basal lamina
    D. Hemidesmosomes and the external basal lamina

14. The junctional epithelium attaches to the connective tissue via the:
    A. Desmosomes and the internal basal lamina
    B. Desmosomes and the external basal lamina
    C. Hemidesmosomes and the internal basal lamina
    D. Hemidesmosomes and the external basal lamina

15. Which of the following is NOT a function of the supragingival fiber bundles?
    A. Brace the free gingiva against the tooth
    B. Suspends the tooth in its bony socket
    C. Allow the free gingiva to withstand the frictional forces
    D. Connect adjacent teeth to one another

16. The biologic width is the distance from the _____ to the _____ . (Fill in the blanks).

17. The periodontal ligament is a thin sheet of fibrous tissue located between the _____ and the _____ . (Fill in the blanks).

18. An important function of the cementum of the tooth is to attach the periodontal ligament fibers to the tooth.
    A. True
    B. False

19. Alveolar bone is mineralized connective tissue.
    A. True
    B. False

Chapter

3 The History of Periodontal Disease

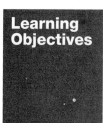
Learning Objectives

- Define the term pathogenesis.
- Define the term periodontal disease and contrast it with the term periodontitis.
- Name and define the two types of periodontal disease.
- Compare and contrast the clinical and histologic characteristics of the periodontium in health, gingivitis, and periodontitis.
- Looking in a patient's mouth, point out visible clinical signs of health, gingivitis, and/or periodontal disease.
- Looking in a patient's mouth with periodontal disease, point out any visible clinical signs of periodontal disease. Using a periodontal probe, measure the depth of the sulcus or pockets on the facial aspect of one sextant of the mouth. Using the information gathered visually and with the periodontal probe, explain whether this patient's disease is gingivitis or periodontitis.
- Describe the position of the crest of the alveolar bone in gingivitis.
- Describe the position of the junctional epithelium in health, gingivitis, and periodontitis.
- Describe the epithelial-connective tissue junction in health, gingivitis, and periodontitis.

- Explain why there is a band of intact transseptal fibers even in the presence of severe bone loss.
- Describe the progressive destruction of alveolar bone loss that occurs in periodontitis.
- Compare and contrast horizontal and vertical bone loss.
- Describe the pathway of inflammation that occurs in horizontal bone loss.
- Describe the pathway of inflammation that occurs in vertical bone loss.
- Define the terms active disease site and inactive disease site.
- Define the term attachment loss.
- Define the term gingival pocket. Explain why a gingival pocket sometimes is referred to as a false pocket.
- Define the term periodontal pocket.
- Name the two types of periodontal pockets.
- Given a drawing of a periodontal pocket, determine whether the pocket illustrated is a suprabony or infrabony pocket.

KEY TERMS

Pathogenesis
Periodontal disease
Gingivitis
Subclinical gingivitis
Periodontitis
Apical migration of the
    junctional epithelium

Inflammation
Horizontal bone loss
Vertical bone loss
Attachment loss
Disease site
Inactive disease site
Active disease site

Gingival pocket
Periodontal pocket
Suprabony pocket
Infrabony pocket

SECTION 1: PATHOGENESIS OF PERIODONTAL DISEASE

THREE BASIC STATES OF THE PERIODONTIUM

It is important to recognize the differences among health, gingivitis, and periodontitis (**Fig. 3-1**). This section provides an overview of these three basic states at the clinical and microscopic levels.

1. **Pathogenesis** is the sequence of events that occur during the development of a disease or abnormal condition.
2. **Periodontal disease** is a bacterial infection of the periodontium.
   A. Marked changes occur in the periodontium as the result of the body's response to bacterial invasion of the junctional epithelium and gingival connective tissue.
   B. The microscopic changes seen in periodontal disease can be divided into three distinct stages: (i) subclinical gingivitis, (ii) gingivitis, and (iii) periodontitis.
   C. The term *periodontal disease* should not be confused with the term *periodontitis*. Gingivitis and periodontitis are types of periodontal diseases.
3. Gingivitis is a bacterial infection that is confined to the gingiva. The damage that occurs in gingivitis results in reversible destruction to the tissues of the periodontium.
   A. Subclinical gingivitis is a stage of periodontal disease that only can be detected microscopically. There are no **clinically visible signs** at this stage of the disease— that is, there are no signs of gingivitis that are visible to the clinician's naked eye.
   B. Clinical gingivitis is periodontal disease that is characterized by changes that have clinically visible signs.
4. Periodontitis is a bacterial infection of all parts of the periodontium including the gingiva, periodontal ligament, bone, and cementum. The damage that occurs in periodontitis results in irreversible destruction to the tissues of the periodontium.

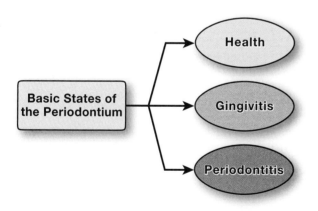

Figure 3-1. Three Basic States of the Periodontium. In the absence of disease, the periodontium is healthy. The two basic categories of periodontal disease are gingivitis and periodontitis.

PERIODONTIUM IN HEALTH

1. **Clinical Picture of Healthy Gingiva (Fig. 3-2)**
   A. Color: Pink, may be pigmented, and is resilient in consistency.
   B. Gingival Margin
      1. Scalloped outline
      2. Located coronal to (above) the cementoenamel junction (CEJ).
   C. Interdental Papillae: Firm and occupy the embrasure spaces apical to the contact areas.
   D. Absence of Bleeding: No bleeding upon probing.
   E. Sulcus: Probing depths range from 1 to 3 mm.

2. **The Microscopic Picture of Healthy Gingiva**
   A. Junctional Epithelium: The junctional epithelium (JE) is firmly attached by hemidesmosomes to the enamel slightly coronal to (above) the CEJ.
   B. Epithelial–Connective Tissue Junction: The JE has no epithelial ridges.
   C. Gingival Fibers: Intact supragingival fiber bundles support the JE.
   D. Alveolar Bone: The crest of the alveolar bone is intact and located 2 to 3 mm apical to (below) the base of the JE.
   E. Periodontal Ligament Fibers: Intact periodontal ligament fiber bundles stretch between the bony walls of the tooth socket to the cementum of the root.
   F. Cementum: Cementum is normal.

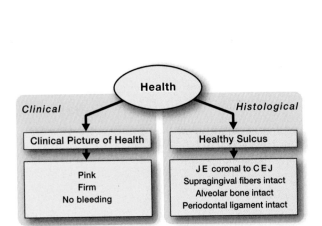
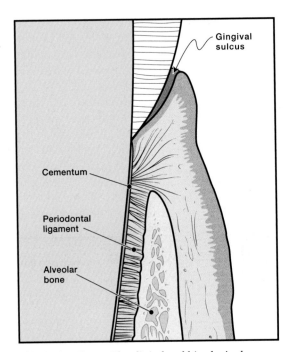

Figure 3-2. Characteristics of Healthy Periodontium. The clinical and histologic characteristics of the tissues of the periodontium in health.

GINGIVITIS—REVERSIBLE TISSUE DAMAGE

1. **Characteristics of Gingivitis. Gingivitis** is *a type of periodontal disease* characterized by changes in the color, contour, and consistency of the gingival tissues (**Fig. 3-3**).
   A. Gingivitis is observed clinically from 4 to 14 days after plaque accumulates in the gingival sulcus.
   1. **Acute gingivitis** is a gingivitis that lasts for a short period of time. Acute gingivitis often is characterized by fluid in the gingival connective tissues that results in swollen gingiva.
   2. **Chronic gingivitis** is a gingivitis that lasts for months or years.
      a. When gingivitis is chronic, the body may attempt to repair the tissue damage by forming new collagen fibers in the gingival connective tissue.
      b. Excess collagen fibers lead to gingival tissues that are enlarged and fibrotic (leathery) in consistency.
      c. The excess collagen fibers conceal the redness caused by the increased blood flow, making the tissue appear less red.
   B. Gingival enlargement may be caused by swelling (acute gingivitis) or fibrosis (chronic gingivitis).
      1. Tissue enlargement causes the gingival margin to cover more of the crown of the tooth and results in deeper probing depths.

   2. This enlargement of the gingival tissue is said to produce a false or gingival pocket.

   3. A **gingival pocket** has a sulcus depth over 3 mm. This increased probing depth is caused solely by enlarged gingival tissue. Microscopically, the JE remains in its normal position coronal to CEJ on the tooth in a gingival pocket.

C. The tissue damage in gingivitis is reversible—that is, the body can repair the damage.

D. In many cases, gingivitis may persist for years without ever progressing to the next stage, periodontitis. In some cases, a combination of risk factors may result in gingivitis progressing to periodontitis.

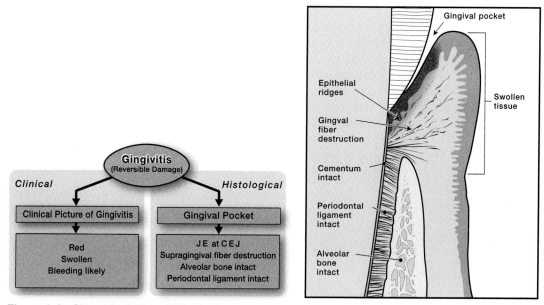

Figure 3-3. Characteristics of Gingivitis. The clinical and histologic characteristics of gingivitis. Some reversible tissue damage occurs in gingivitis.

2. Clinical Picture of Gingivitis
   A. Color: The gingival tissue is usually red or reddish blue.
      1. The blood flow increases in the gingival connective tissue and the gingival blood vessels become engorged with blood, causing the gingiva to appear red.
      2. If the gingivitis persists, the gingival blood vessels may become congested. This slow-moving blood flow causes the gingiva to have a bluish color.
   B. Gingival Margin
      1. The gingival margin is swollen and loses its knife-edge adaptation to the tooth.
      2. Gingival tissue may cover more of the crown of the tooth due to tissue swelling or fibrosis.
   C. Interdental Papillae: The interdental papillae often are bulbous and swollen.
   D. Bleeding: There is bleeding upon gentle probing.
   E. Sulcus: Probing depths may be greater than 3 mm due to swelling of the tissues. It is important to note that there is NO apical migration of the junctional epithelium in gingivitis.

3. The Microscopic Picture of Gingivitis (Table 3-1)
   A. Junctional Epithelium: The hemidesmosomes still attach to the enamel coronal to the CEJ.
   B. Epithelial–Connective Tissue Junction
      1. The JE extends epithelial ridges down into the connective tissue.
      2. *Such extension of the epithelial ridges only can occur because destruction of the gingival fibers creates space for the growing epithelium.*

C. Gingival Fibers: Damage has occurred to the supragingival fiber bundles. This damage is reversible if the bacterial infection is brought under control.

D. Alveolar Bone: The bacterial infection has not progressed into the alveolar bone. There is no destruction of alveolar bone.

E. Periodontal Ligament Fibers: The bacterial infection has not progressed into the periodontal ligament fibers.

F. Cementum: Cementum is normal.

PERIODONTITIS—PERMANENT TISSUE DESTRUCTION

1. **Characteristics of Periodontitis. Periodontitis** is *a type of periodontal disease* that is characterized by the (i) apical migration of the junctional epithelium, (ii) loss of connective tissue attachment, and (iii) loss of alveolar bone (**Fig. 3-4**).

   A. The tissue damage of periodontitis is permanent.

   B. The tissue destruction of periodontitis is not a continuous process. Rather, the disease process occurs in an intermittent manner with extended periods of disease inactivity followed by short periods of destruction.

   C. Tissue destruction progresses at different rates throughout the mouth. Destruction does not occur in all parts of the mouth at the same time, but instead, destruction usually occurs in only a few specific sites (tooth surfaces) at a time.

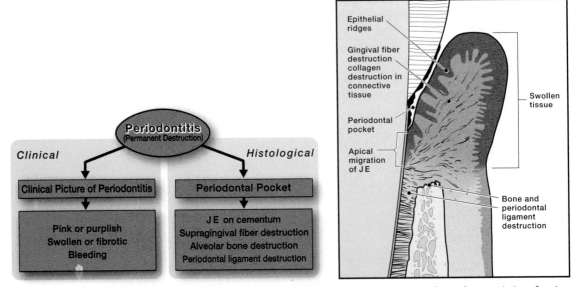

Figure 3-4. Characteristics of Periodontitis. Clinical and histologic characteristics of periodontitis. Permanent tissue damage occurs in periodontitis.

2. **Clinical Picture of Periodontitis**

   A. Color: The gingival tissue shows visible alternations in color, contour, and consistency.

      1. Edematous tissue (spongy tissue)—bluish- or purplish-red with a smooth, shiny appearance.

      2. Fibrotic tissue (firm, nodular tissue)—light pink with a leathery consistency. Beginning clinicians often mistakenly interpret this light pink color as a sign of tissue health.

   B. Gingival Margin

      1. The gingival margin may be swollen or fibrotic and does not have a close knife-edged adaptation to the tooth.

2. The position of the gingival margin varies greatly in periodontitis. The margin may be apical to the cemento-enamel junction (**recession**) resulting in a portion of the root being visible in the mouth.

C. Interdental Papillae: The interdental papillae may not fill the interdental embrasure spaces.

D. Bleeding: There often is bleeding upon probing, and suppuration (a discharge of pus) may be visible.

E. Pocket: Probing depths are 4 mm or greater in depth because the junctional epithelium is attached to the root surface.

   1. Pus may be evident upon probing.
   2. Pain is usually absent; however, probing may cause some pain due to ulceration of the pocket epithelium.

3. **The Microscopic Picture of Periodontitis** (Table 3-1)

A. Junctional Epithelium

   1. The junctional epithelium is located on the cementum, apical to—below—its normal location. Movement of the junctional epithelium apical to its normal location is termed the **apical migration of the junctional epithelium**.
   2. The coronal-most portion of the junctional epithelium detaches from the tooth surface. As the bacterial infection progresses, the apical portion of the junctional epithelium moves further in an apical direction along the root surface creating a periodontal pocket.
   3. The extracellular matrix of the gingiva and the attached collagen fibers at the apical edge of the junctional epithelium are destroyed.

B. Epithelial–Connective Tissue Junction

   1. The *junctional* epithelium proliferates and extends epithelial ridges into the connective tissue.
   2. The *sulcular* epithelium of the pocket wall thickens and extends epithelial ridges deep into the connective tissue. Small ulcerations of the pocket epithelium expose the underlying inflamed connective tissue.

Table 3-1. Histologic Changes in Disease

Disease State	Histology
Gingival Disease	Epithelial ridges extend down into connective tissue Destruction to supragingival fiber bundles
Periodontal Disease	**Changes in Epithelial Tissues:** Junctional epithelium located apical to the cementoenamel junction Junctional epithelium grows along the root surface Sulcular epithelium thickens and extends epithelial ridges down into the connective tissue **Changes in Connective Tissues and Alveolar Bone:** Collagen destruction Destruction of supragingival fiber bundles Destruction of periodontal ligament fibers; transseptal fibers regenerate and remain intact Junctional epithelium grows over the root surface in areas where periodontal ligament is destroyed Root cementum is exposed to the plaque biofilm Destruction of alveolar bone

C. Gingival Connective Tissue
   1. Changes in the gingival connective tissue are severe. Collagen destruction in the area of inflammation is almost complete.
   2. There is widespread destruction of the supragingival fiber bundles, reducing them to fiber fragments. The destruction of the periodontal ligament fiber bundles makes it easier for the junctional epithelium to migrate apically along the root surface.
   3. The transseptal fiber bundles, however, are regenerated continuously across the crest of bone. A band of intact transseptal fibers separates the site of inflammation from the remaining alveolar bone even in cases of extensive bone loss (**Fig. 3-5**).
   4. Epithelium grows over the root surface in areas where the fiber bundles have been destroyed. *The loss of fiber attachment is permanent because the epithelium growing over the root surface prevents the reinsertion of the periodontal ligament fibers in the cementum.*
D. Alveolar Bone: There is permanent destruction of the alveolar bone that supports the teeth. Tooth mobility may be present.
E. Periodontal Ligament Fibers: There is permanent destruction of some or all of the periodontal ligament fiber bundles.
F. Cementum: Cementum within the periodontal pocket is exposed to dental plaque biofilm.

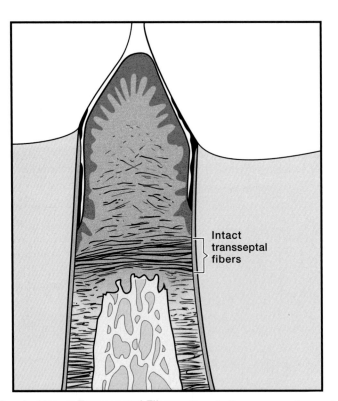

Figure 3-5. Band of Intact Transseptal Fibers. Even in the presence of severe horizontal bone loss, there is an intact band of transseptal fibers above the remaining alveolar bone.

SECTION 2: PATHOGENESIS OF BONE DESTRUCTION

Inflammation is the body's reaction to injury or invasion by disease-producing organisms. The inflammatory process that occurs in periodontitis results in permanent destruction to the tissues of the periodontium, including the destruction of gingival connective tissue, periodontal ligament, and alveolar bone. This section discusses the patterns of bone destruction that occur in periodontitis. The pattern of bone destruction that occurs depends on the pathway of inflammation as it spreads from the gingiva into the alveolar bone. It is important to understand the changes that occur in the alveolar bone because it is the reduction in bone height that eventually results in tooth loss.

CHANGES IN ALVEOLAR BONE HEIGHT IN DISEASE

1. **Reduction in Bone Height**
   A. In Health and Gingivitis—the crest of the alveolar bone is located approximately 2 mm apical to (below) the CEJs of the teeth (**Fig. 3-6**).
   B. In Periodontitis—bone destruction may be marked (**Fig. 3-7**). As periodontal disease progresses (worsens) tooth loss may occur from lack of alveolar bone support (**Fig. 3-8**).

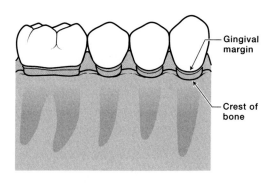

Figure 3-6. Level of Alveolar Crest in Health and Gingivitis. In health, the crest of the alveolar bone is located approximately 2 mm apical to the cementoenamel junction.

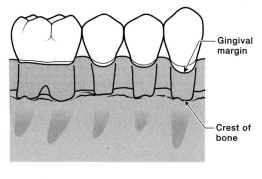

Figure 3-7. Level of Alveolar Crest in Disease. In periodontitis, the crest of the alveolar bone is located more than 2 mm apical to the cementoenamel junction.

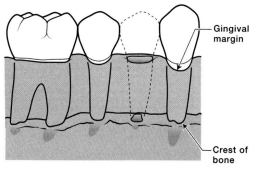

Figure 3-8. Level of Alveolar Crest as Disease Progresses. There is a progressive alveolar bone loss in periodontitis. Bone destruction may eventually lead to tooth mobility or loss due to insufficient bone support for the teeth.

PATTERNS OF BONE LOSS IN PERIODONTAL DISEASE

1. **Patterns of Bone Loss.** The two types of bone loss are (i) horizontal and (ii) vertical bone loss.
   A. **Horizontal Bone Loss**
      1. **Horizontal bone loss** is the most common pattern of bone loss (**Fig. 3-9**). This type of bone loss results in a fairly even, overall reduction in the height of the alveolar bone.
      2. This type of bone loss produces a suprabony pocket. Types of pockets are discussed in Section 3 of this chapter.
   B. **Vertical Bone Loss**
      1. **Vertical bone loss** is a less common pattern of bone loss (**Fig. 3-10**). This type of bone loss results in an uneven reduction in the height of the alveolar bone, with bone resorption progressing more rapidly in the bone next to the root surface. Vertical bone loss is also known as angular bone loss.
      2. This uneven pattern of bone loss leaves a trenchlike area of missing bone alongside the root.
      3. This type of bone loss produces an infrabony pocket.

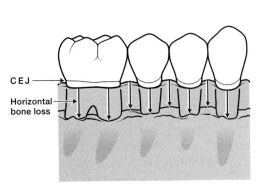
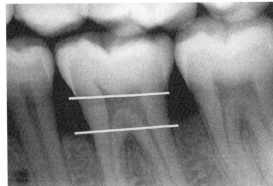

Figure 3-9. Horizontal Pattern of Bone Loss. Horizontal bone loss results in a practically even overall reduction in the height of the alveolar bone. On a radiograph, horizontal bone loss is bone destruction that is parallel to an imaginary line drawn between the cementoenamel junctions (CEJs) of adjacent teeth.

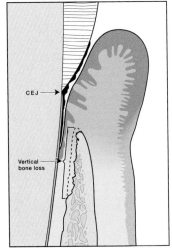
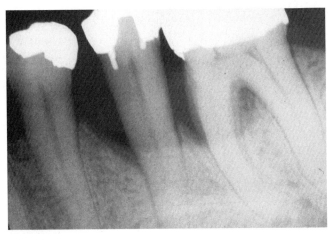

Figure 3-10. Vertical Pattern of Bone Loss. Vertical bone loss results in an uneven reduction in bone height, resulting in a trench-like area of missing bone alongside the root. On the radiograph, this type of bone loss appears as an uneven reduction in bone height.

PATHWAYS OF INFLAMMATION INTO BONE

1. **Pathway of Inflammation in Horizontal Bone Loss**
   A. In horizontal bone loss, inflammation spreads into the tissues in this order: (i) within the gingival connective tissue along the connective tissue sheaths surrounding the blood vessels, (ii) into the alveolar bone, and (iii) finally, into the periodontal ligament space (**Fig. 3-11A**).
   B. Inflammation usually spreads in this manner because it is the *path of least resistance*. The periodontal ligament fiber bundles act as an effective barrier to the spread of inflammation. Thus, the inflammation spreads into the alveolar bone and then into the periodontal ligament space.

2. **Pathway of Inflammation in Vertical Bone Loss**
   A. In vertical bone loss, inflammation spreads into the tissues in this order (i) within the gingival connective tissue, (ii) directly into the periodontal ligament space, and (iii) finally, into the alveolar bone (**Fig. 3-11B**).
   B. Inflammation spreads in this manner whenever the crestal periodontal ligament fiber bundles are weakened and no longer present an effective barrier. Prior events such as occlusal trauma can be responsible for the weakened condition of the fiber bundles.

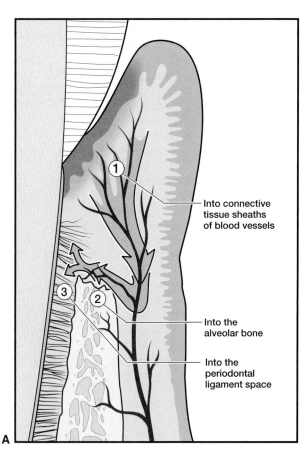
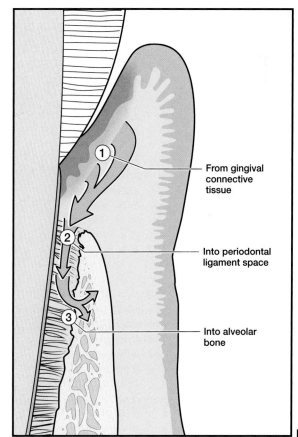

Figure 3-11. Pathway of Inflammation into Alveolar Bone.
A: In horizontal bone loss, inflammation spreads through the tissues in this order:
1—Into the gingival connective tissue
2—Into the alveolar bone
3—Finally, into the periodontal ligament
B: In vertical bone loss, inflammation spreads through the tissues in this order:
1—Into the gingival connective tissue
2—Into the periodontal ligament
3—Finally, into the alveolar bone

SECTION 3: PERIODONTAL POCKETS

CHARACTERISTICS OF PERIODONTAL POCKETS

1. Attachment Loss in Periodontal Pockets
   A. Attachment loss is the destruction of the fibers and bone that support the teeth.
   B. Tissue destruction does not spread only in an apical (vertical) direction but also in a lateral (side-to-side) direction.
   C. *A pocket on different root surfaces of the same tooth can have different depths.* The loss of attachment may vary from surface to surface of the tooth, with the base of the pocket exhibiting very irregular patterns of tissue destruction (Fig. 3-12).
2. A disease site is an area of tissue destruction. A disease site may involve only a single surface of a tooth, for example, the distal surface of a tooth. The disease site may involve several surfaces of the tooth or all four surfaces (mesial, distal, facial, and lingual).
   A. Inactive disease site—a disease site that is stable, with the attachment level of the junctional epithelium remaining the same over time.
   B. Active disease site—a disease site that shows continued apical migration of the junctional epithelium over time.
3. The disease activity of each site in the mouth should be assessed using a periodontal probe and recorded in the patient chart at regular intervals (scheduled check-up appointments).
4. A periodontal pocket is an area of tissue destruction left by the disease process. The pocket is much like a demolished home that is left after a hurricane.
   A. The presence of a periodontal pocket does not indicate necessarily that there is active disease at that site. Likewise, a demolished house does not necessarily indicate that a hurricane still is pounding the shoreline. A demolished house may indicate that the hurricane is still active or that a hurricane passed through a day, a week, or a year ago.
   B. The majority of pockets in most adult patients with periodontitis are inactive disease sites.

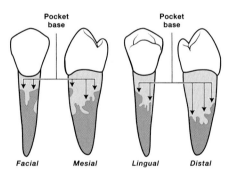

Figure 3-12. Irregular Pattern of Attachment Loss. The amount of attachment loss can vary greatly on different surfaces of the same tooth. The base of a pocket may exhibit very irregular patterns of destruction.

TYPES OF POCKETS

1. **Gingival Pockets.** A gingival pocket is a deepening of the gingival sulcus *solely as a result of gingival enlargement.*
   A. Also known as a pseudopocket, meaning false pocket, because there is no destruction of the periodontal ligament fibers or alveolar bone in a gingival pocket.
   B. There is no apical migration of the JE in a gingival pocket. The JE remains coronal to the CEJ.
   C. The increased probing depth is due to (i) swelling of the tissue or (ii) enlargement due to increased collagen fibers in the connective tissue.

2. **Periodontal Pockets**
    A. A periodontal pocket is a pathologic deepening of the gingival sulcus *as the result of the (i) apical migration of the junctional epithelium, (ii) destruction of the periodontal ligament fibers, and (iii) destruction of alveolar bone.*
    B. There are two types of periodontal pockets. The type of periodontal pocket is determined based on *the relationship of the junctional epithelium to the crest of the alveolar bone.*
        1. Suprabony Pocket
            a. Suprabony pockets occur when there is horizontal bone loss (even loss of bone).
            b. The JE, forming the base of the pocket, is located *coronal* to (above) the crest of the alveolar bone (**Fig. 3-13**).
        2. Infrabony Pocket
            a. Infrabony pockets occur when there is vertical bone loss (uneven loss of bone).
            b. The JE, forming the base of the pocket, is located *apical* to (below) the crest of the alveolar bone. The base of the pocket is located within the cratered-out area of the bone alongside of the root surface (**Fig. 3-14**).

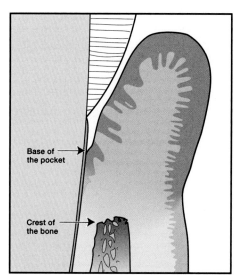

Figure 3-13. Suprabony Pocket.
Characteristics of a suprabony pocket are (i) horizontal bone loss and (ii) a pocket base located coronal to (above) the crest of the alveolar bone.

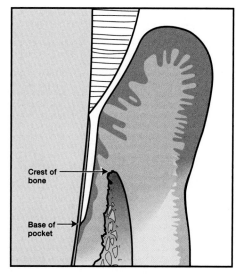

Figure 3-14. Infrabony Pocket.
Characteristics of an infrabony pocket are (i) vertical bone loss and (ii) a pocket base located below the crest of the alveolar bone within a trenchlike area of the bone.

CHAPTER SUMMARY STATEMENT

Periodontal pathogenesis is the sequence of events that occurs during the development of periodontal disease. The two types of periodontal disease are gingivitis and periodontitis. Gingivitis is a *reversible condition* that is characterized by changes in the color, contour, and consistency of the gingiva. There is no apical migration of the junctional epithelium or bone loss in gingivitis. Periodontitis results in some extent of *permanent tissue destruction* characterized by pocket formation, destruction of the periodontal ligament fibers, and resorption of alveolar bone. The pattern of alveolar bone loss and periodontal ligament destruction depends on the pathway that the inflammatory process takes as it spreads from the gingiva into the alveolar bone. It is the destruction of periodontal ligament fibers and resorption of alveolar bone that leads to tooth mobility and the possibility of tooth loss.

SECTION 4: FOCUS ON PATIENTS

CASE 1

Examination of a patient reveals swelling and redness of the gingival margin. In addition, the gingival papillae are slightly enlarged. Gentle probing elicits bleeding, and probing depths measure 4 to 5 mm in some sites. What additional information would you need about the condition of this patient to assign a diagnosis of either gingivitis or periodontitis?

CASE 2

Your patient has 6- to 7 mm attachment loss on all surfaces of the maxillary first molar. Which of the tissues of the periodontium have experienced tissue destruction surrounding this tooth?

CASE 3

Your dental team provides appropriate therapy for a periodontitis patient. When you began treatment, your initial findings were redness and edema (swelling) of the gingiva, bleeding on probing, periodontal pockets, and attachment loss. Successful control of the periodontal disease in the patient should <u>not</u> be expected to result in elimination of which of these initial clinical findings?

Suggested Readings

The pathogenesis of periodontal diseases. *J Periodonto.*, 1999;70:457–470.

Akiyoshi M, Mori K. Marginal periodontitis: A histological study of the incipient stage. *J Periodonto.*, 1967;38:45–52.

Listgarten MA. Pathogenesis of periodontitis. *J Clin Periodontol.* 1986;13:418–430.

Page RC, Offenbacher S, Schroeder HF, et al. Advances in the pathogenesis of periodontitis: summary of developments, clinical implications and future directions. *Periodontol 2000.* 1997;14:216–248.

Payne WA., Page RC, Ogilvie AL, et al. Histopathologic features of the initial and early stages of experimental gingivitis in man. *J Periodontal Res.* 1975;10:51–64.

Takata T, Donath K. The mechanism of pocket formation. A light microscopic study on undecalcified human material. *J Periodontol.* 1988;59:215–221.

Waerhaug J. Anatomy, physiology and pathology of the gingival pocket. *Rev Belge Med Dent.*, 1966; 21:9–15.

Waerhaug J., The angular bone defect and its relationship to trauma from occlusion and downgrowth of subgingival plaque. *J Clin Periodontol.* 1979;6:61–82.

SECTION 5: CHAPTER REVIEW QUESTIONS

1. The sequence of events that occur during the development of a disease is termed:
   A. Pathogenesis
   B. Periodontal disease
   C. Periodontitis
   D. Pericardium

2. Which of the following are types of periodontal disease?
   A. Gingivitis
   B. Periodontitis
   C. Both (a) and (b)

3. In gingivitis, the position of the junctional epithelium is _____ to the cementoenamel junction.
   A. Apical
   B. Coronal
   C. Distal
   D. Mesial

4. Which of the following structures is intact in gingivitis?
   A. Supragingival fiber bundles
   B. Periodontal ligament fibers
   C. Alveolar bone
   D. All of the above
   E. Only (b) and (c)
   F. None of the above

5. Increased probing depth of a gingival pocket is the result of which of the following?
   A. Enlarged tissue
   B. Apical migration of the junctional epithelium
   C. Destruction of the periodontal ligament fibers
   D. All of the above
   E. Only (a) and (b)

6. The epithelial–connective tissue junction of the junctional epithelium is wavy in which of the following states?
   A. Health
   B. Gingivitis
   C. Periodontitis
   D. All of the above
   E. Only (b) and (c)

7. Permanent destruction of the tissues of the periodontium occurs in which state?
   A. Gingivitis
   B. Periodontitis
   C. Periodontal disease
   D. Only (a) and (c)

8. Which pattern of bone loss results in a fairly even, overall reduction in the height of the alveolar bone?
   A. Horizontal bone loss
   B. Vertical bone loss
   C. Both (a) and (b)

Chapter

4 Search for the Causes of Periodontal Disease

Learning Objectives

- Describe variables associated with periodontal disease that an epidemiologist might include in a research study.
- Define prevalence and incidence as measurements of disease within a population.
- Discuss historical and current theories associated with the progression of periodontal disease.
- Describe how clinical dental hygiene practice can be affected by epidemiologic research.

KEY TERMS

Epidemiology
Prevalence
Incidence
Etiology

Periodontal pathogens
Risk factors
Intermittent disease
   progression

Periodontal pathology
Multifactorial etiology

SECTION 1: RESEARCHING PERIODONTAL DISEASE

Many generations of researchers have asked the question, "What causes periodontal disease?" while clinicians have asked, "What is the best care for my patients with periodontal disease?" This chapter discusses the study of disease in the population (epidemiology) and reviews historical and current perspectives on the causes and progression of periodontal disease.

EPIDEMIOLOGY: THE STUDY OF DISEASE

1. **Epidemiology** is the study of the health and disease within the total population (rather than an individual) and the risk factors that influence health and disease.
   A. Factors that increase host susceptibility to periodontal disease are known as **risk factors**.
   B. Through research of population groups, epidemiologists strive to identify the risk factors associated with disease such as heredity, gender, physical environment, systemic factors, socioeconomic status, and personal behavior.
   C. An understanding of the risk factors associated with a certain disease can lead to theories of the cause of that disease and then to treatment standards for patient care.
2. **Epidemiology of Periodontal Disease**
   A. A large percentage of the adult population has periodontal disease. Epidemiologists study periodontal disease to determine its occurrence in the population and to identify risk factors for periodontal disease. Some of the questions epidemiologists ask when researching periodontal disease are illustrated in **Figure 4-1**.
   B. Epidemiologic research also provides current information to the clinical dental hygienist about methods and behaviors that are successful in the treatment and prevention of periodontal disease.
   C. Studies can be designed to look at the disparities or inequities of disease patterns.[1] For instance a study may explore why more periodontal disease is found in a specific segment of the population than in another group of people. Oral diseases occur disproportionately more among individuals with low socioeconomic status and with poor general health.[2]

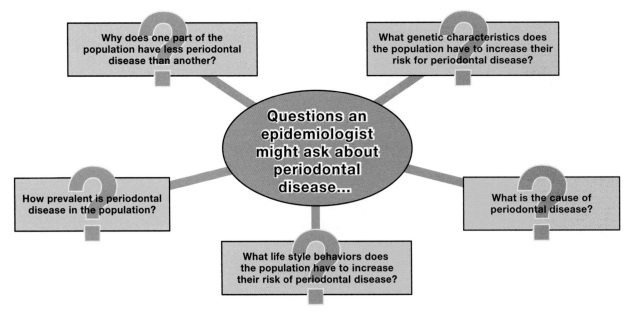

Figure 4-1. Researching Periodontal Disease. This diagram illustrates the types of questions asked by epidemiologists when studying periodontal disease.

PREVALENCE AND INCIDENCE OF DISEASE

1. **Definitions**
   A. **Prevalence** refers to the number of all cases (both old and new) of a disease that can be identified within a specified population at a given point in time.

   For example: In 2002 a study of 100 white adults, age 35 to 45, was done with a prevalence of 50% of this population being recorded as having bleeding upon probing. The Gingival Bleeding Index (GBI) was used to record bleeding. This prevalence information does not indicate how long these adults have had gingival bleeding upon probing.
   B. **Incidence** is the number of *new disease cases* in a population that occur during a given interval of time.

   For example, a follow-up study in 2003 of the same above adult population indicated an incidence of 10 additional cases recorded as bleeding upon probing. Now the new prevalence of bleeding upon probing with this population is 60%.
2. **Measuring the Prevalence of Disease**
   A. The prevalence of periodontal disease in the U.S. adult population is determined by performing clinical examinations on cross-sections of groups using indices. Refer to **Table 4-1** for a list of indices commonly used to assess periodontal disease.

Table 4-1. Commonly Used Periodontal Indices

Index	Measurement
Community and Periodontal Index of Treatment Needs (CPITN) (Federation Dentaire Internationale: Ainamo et al.)	Assesses probing depths and bleeding; developed to attain more uniform worldwide epidemiologic data; may be used for measuring group periodontal needs
Eastman Interdental Bleeding Index (EIBI) (Abrams, Caton, and Polson) (Caton and Polson)	Assesses presence of inflammation and bleeding in the interdental area upon toothpick insertion
Gingival Bleeding Index (GBI) (Carter and Barnes)	Assesses presence of gingival inflammation by bleeding from interproximal sulcus within 10 seconds of flossing
Gingival Index (GI) (Loe and Silness)	Assesses severity of gingivitis based on color, consistency, and bleeding on probing
Periodontal Screening & Recording (PSR) (American Academy of Periodontology and the American Dental Association)	Assesses periodontal health in a rapid manner including probing depths, bleeding, and presence of hard deposits

B. The items in a study to be measured are the variables. The clinical examinations may include the variables of probing depth, clinical attachment level (CAL), and interpretation of radiographic bone levels (BL). Many studies use sample groups numbering in the thousands. Several groups are then compared and statistically analyzed (**Fig. 4-2**). Epidemiologists will have different approaches to research and will include different variables in studies. The selected population can be studied over time.

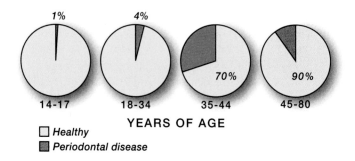

Figure 4-2. Prevalence of Periodontal Disease.
Periodontal disease in various age groups. (Data used to develop this graphic from Oliver RC, Brown LJ, Loe H. Periodontal diseases in the United States population. *J Periodontol.* 1998; 69:269–278.)

3. **Variables Associated with the Prevalence of Disease.** Research findings show that variables associated with the prevalence of periodontal disease include a person's gender, race, socioeconomic status, and age.
   A. Gender
      1. Males have a greater prevalence and severity of periodontal disease than females.
      2. There has been some speculation that females have a tendency to practice better and more frequent self-care than males. These differences in self-care behaviors may lead to the greater prevalence of disease in males.
   B. Educational Level and Socioeconomic Status
      1. Black and Hispanic males living in the United States have poorer periodontal health and a greater incidence of periodontal disease than white males.
      2. There is a greater incidence of periodontal disease in individuals with lower levels of education and income.
      3. Underdeveloped countries have a higher incidence of chronic periodontitis, possibly due to a lack of adequate information about disease prevention.
   C. Age
      1. Research studies have shown that the severity of periodontal disease increases with age; however, the exact role that age plays in periodontal disease is difficult to assess.
         a. As an individual lives longer, the chances increase that he will be exposed to additional risk factors for periodontal disease. Such risk factors include systemic illness, medications, stress, and smoking.
         b. The higher incidence of periodontal disease in the elderly, therefore, may not be due to age, but rather other risk factors to which an individual has been exposed during his or her long life.
      2. Diminished dexterity is sometimes a problem in elderly individuals and can impact the individual's ability to perform self-care. Limited dexterity may also shorten the length of time that self-care is performed on a daily basis.
   D. Access to Dental Care. Individuals who desire care or need care may not have access to dental care. Barriers to obtaining dental care include transportation—traveling long distances to a dental office—and the financial expense of dental care.

4. **Difficulties in Measurement of Periodontal Disease**
   A. It is far easier to evaluate a population for prevalence and incidence of dental caries than for periodontal disease because caries lends itself for more objective measurement. The development and process of caries is well known and involves only tooth structure.
   B. Periodontal disease, on the other hand, involves both hard and soft tissues and has multiple variables that must be considered, such as:
      a. Soft tissue color changes
      b. Tissue swelling
      c. Loss of alveolar bone and periodontal ligament fibers that support the teeth (loss of attachment)
      d. Amount of bleeding
      e. Probing depths
   C. The multiple variables used to define periodontal disease make the numbers for prevalence and incidence of periodontal disease less specific, more of a range, and more subject to change.
5. **What the Research Shows**
   A. Research on periodontal disease indicates it is one of the most widespread diseases in adult Americans, with most individuals who have periodontal disease being unaware of its presence.
   B. Currently it is estimated that 67 million Americans have some form of periodontitis.[3]
   C. Periodontal disease has been found to be the leading cause of tooth loss in adults older than age 45.
   D. The presence of periodontal disease is measured clinically in several ways. One way is by calculation of the loss of periodontal attachment. Loss of attachment is the term used to describe the destruction of periodontal ligament fibers and alveolar bone that support the teeth. **Figure 4-3** shows that attachment loss of 4 mm or more affects approximately half of adults aged 50 to 59.[4]
   E. Twenty-three percent of 65- to 74-year-olds have or have had severe periodontal disease. At all ages men are more likely than women to have severe bone loss, and at all ages people at the lowest socioeconomic levels have more severe periodontal disease.[2]
   F. By age 60 to 69 less than half of all adults in the United States have retained 21 teeth or more (**Fig. 4-4**).[4]

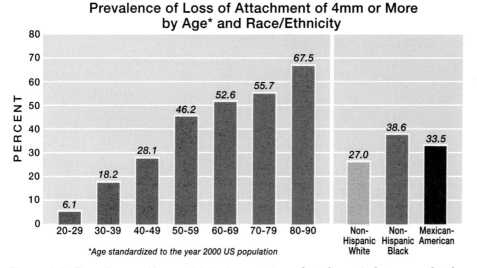

Figure 4-3. Prevalence of Loss of Attachment. Loss of attachment is the term used to describe the destruction of periodontal ligament fibers and alveolar bone that support the teeth. (Data source for graph: The Third National Health and Nutrition Examination Survey (NHANES III) 1988–1994, National Center for Health Statistics. Centers for Disease Control and Prevention.)

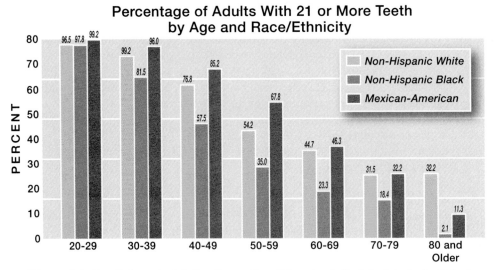

Figure 4-4. Tooth Loss in Adults. By age 60 to 69 less than half of all adults in the United States have retained 21 teeth or more. (Data source for graph: The Third National Health and Nutrition Examination Survey (NHANES III) 1988–1994, National Center for Health Statistics. Centers for Disease Control and Prevention.)

SECTION 2: MULTIPLE RISK FACTORS FOR PERIODONTAL DISEASE

Etiology is the study of all factors that may be involved in the development of a disease. Over time, researchers have changed their ideas on the causes—etiology—of periodontal disease. This chapter presents a brief historical review of how the understanding of disease risk factors has evolved over the years (**Table 4-2**). Awareness of past theories of etiology are helpful in understanding why recommendations for the prevention and treatment of periodontal disease have changed so much over the years. A 50-year-old patient who has received regular dental care over the years would have first visited a dental office in the 1950s (assuming that his of her first dental visit was by the age of 10).

Table 4-2. Theories on the Etiology of Periodontal Disease

Theory	Risk Factors	Focus of Professional Care
Calculus (Before 1960)	Calculus deposits	Removal of calculus deposits
Plaque (1965–1985)	Bacterial plaque	Removal or disruption of bacterial plaque
Host–Bacterial Interaction (Current)	Many risk factors— a complex interaction of bacterial plaque, host response, and other risk factors	Identification and control of bacterial, host, local, and systemic risk factors

HISTORICAL PERSPECTIVES ON DISEASE RISK FACTORS

1. **Calculus as Risk Factor—Before 1960**
   A. Theory. Before 1960, clinicians believed that periodontal disease was caused solely by the presence of calculus deposits that act as a mechanical irritant to the tissue (**Fig. 4-5**).
   B. Treatment Before 1960
      1. Professional Care. Professional prophylaxis was scheduled every 6 months to remove accumulated calculus deposits.
      2. Patient Self-Care. Patients were advised to brush three times per day to remove food particles.

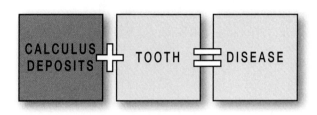

Figure 4-5. Calculus Theory. Before 1960, clinicians believed that periodontal disease was caused solely by the presence of calculus deposits.

2. **Bacterial Plaque as Risk Factor—1965 to 1985**
   A. Theory. Bacteria in dental plaque cause periodontal disease (**Fig. 4-6**).
      1. The classic research study by Löe et al.[5] demonstrated that an accumulation of bacterial plaque is important in the development of gingivitis.
      2. In the years 1975 to 1985, research focused on the composition of plaque. Researchers hoped to determine which particular bacterial species were responsible for specific types of periodontal disease. **Periodontal pathogens** are bacteria that are capable of infecting the tissues of the periodontium.
      3. During this time period, many clinicians believed that:
         a. Daily plaque control efforts *alone* could prevent or control periodontal disease.
         b. If patients did not respond to treatment, they were at fault, probably due to infrequent or inadequate self-care.
   B. Treatment 1965 to 1985
      1. Professional Care. Professional prophylaxis was scheduled two to three times per year.
      2. Patient Self-Care. The patient was instructed in self-care techniques and taught that prevention and control of periodontal disease depended on his or her daily plaque control efforts. If disease was not prevented or controlled, the patient was at fault for failing at plaque control.

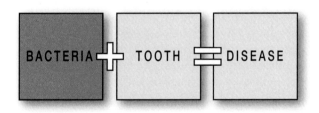

Figure 4-6. Bacterial Theory. During the years 1965 to 1985, most clinicians believed that the adequate daily plaque removal could prevent or control periodontal disease.

CURRENT VIEWS ON DISEASE RISK FACTORS

In recent years, advances in research have led to a fundamental change in our understanding of periodontal disease and have led to the development of a new theory about the risk factors involved in periodontal disease. Researchers now believe that the presence of bacterial plaque, alone, is not enough to cause periodontal disease.

1. **The Host–Bacterial Interaction as Risk Factor—Current.** It is the interaction of the host (patient) with the pathogenic bacteria that controls whether or not periodontal disease is present (**Fig. 4-7**).
   A. *A bacterial infection alone is insufficient to result in periodontal disease. The host response plays a critical role in the tissue destruction seen in periodontitis. Current research findings suggest that everyone is not equally susceptible to periodontal disease. Some individuals are more at risk than others.*
   B. Factors that increase host susceptibility to periodontal disease are known as **risk factors**.
   C. *Risk factors for periodontal disease include local oral conditions, habits, systemic disease, and genetic factors.*

Figure 4-7. Host–Bacterial Interaction Theory. Current research has shown that it is the interaction of the patient with the dental plaque that controls whether or not periodontal disease is present.

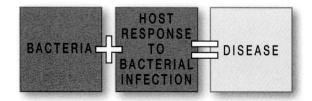

2. Current Views on Treatment
   A. Professional Care
      1. Today, the treatment of periodontal disease is directed at managing the bacterial, local, and systemic etiologic factors for periodontal disease.
      2. Periodontal maintenance appointments (recall appointments) should be scheduled as frequently as needed to assist the patient in controlling disease.
      3. Treatment may involve not only the periodontal debridement of root surfaces and the pocket environment, but when appropriate, professional care includes referral to a physician for management of systemic disease or other risk factors.
   B. Patient Self-Care
      1. The patient is educated about the role of bacterial plaque in periodontal disease and in plaque control techniques.
      2. If the disease continues to progress, the patient is not at fault for his or her failure to control the disease; instead, risk factors are identified and eliminated or controlled whenever possible. More frequent appointments for professional periodontal maintenance (recall visits) are recommended to assist the patient in controlling disease.

HISTORICAL PERSPECTIVES ON DISEASE PROGRESSION

For years, clinical researchers have been trying to find an answer to the question, "How does untreated periodontal disease progress?" In this context, **disease progression** means that the disease gets worse. Data from ongoing studies suggest that the pattern of disease progression may vary from (i) one individual to another, (ii) one site to another in a person's mouth, and (iii) one type of periodontal disease to another.

1. **Continuous Progression Theory (Historical View of Disease Progression: Prior to 1980)**
   A. The continuous disease progression theory states that periodontal disease progresses throughout the entire mouth in a slow and constant rate over the adult life of the patient (**Fig. 4-8**). This theory suggests that:
      a. All cases of untreated gingivitis lead to periodontitis.
      b. All cases of periodontitis progress at a slow and steady rate of tissue destruction.
   B. Research studies conducted in the early 1980s indicated that periodontal disease does not progress at a constant rate nor affect all areas of the mouth simultaneously. The continuous progression theory does not accurately reflect the complex nature of periodontal disease.

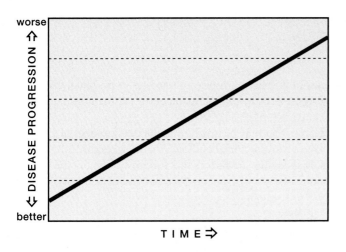

Figure 4-8. The Continuous Disease Model of Disease Progression (Prior to 1980). In the past, clinicians believed that periodontal disease progresses (worsens) throughout the entire mouth in a slow and constant rate over the life of the patient. It was believed that all cases of untreated gingivitis led to periodontitis.

2. **Intermittent Progression Theories (Current View)**
   A. **Intermittent disease progression** theories state that periodontal disease is characterized by periods of disease activity and inactivity (remission) (**Fig. 4-9**).
      1. Tissue destruction is sporadic, with short periods of tissue destruction alternating with periods of disease inactivity (no tissue destruction). The period of inactivity with no disease progression may last for months or for a much longer period of time.
      2. Tissue destruction progresses at different rates throughout the mouth. Destruction does not occur in all parts of the mouth at the same time. Instead, tissue destruction occurs in only a few specific sites (tooth surfaces) at a time.
      3. In the majority of cases, untreated gingivitis does not progress to periodontitis.
      4. Different forms of periodontitis progress at widely different rates.
      5. Susceptibility to periodontitis varies greatly from individual to individual and appears to be determined by the host response to periodontal pathogens.

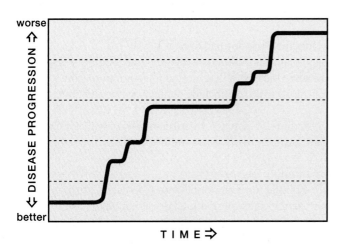

Figure 4-9. Intermittent Disease Progression Theory. Current research suggests that periodontal disease is characterized by periods of disease activity and inactivity. Furthermore, destruction does not occur in all parts of the mouth at the same time.

SECTION 3: PERIODONTAL PATHOLOGY

Periodontal pathology is the study of the characteristics and causes of periodontal diseases, as well as, the changes that occur in the structure and function of the periodontium due to disease.

1. **Etiology** is the study of all factors that may be involved in the development of a disease. Periodontal diseases have a **multifactorial etiology**; that is, it results from the interaction of many factors. **Risk factors** are factors that modify or amplify the likelihood of developing periodontal disease. Risk factors for periodontal disease are discussed in detail in Chapters 5, 6, 7, and 8.
2. **Risk Factors for Periodontal Disease**
   A. **Dental Plaque Biofilm**
      1. It has been known for years that periodontal disease is a bacterial infection. The presence of bacteria is necessary for periodontal disease to occur.
      2. A number of other factors that can (i) increase the risk of developing gingivitis or periodontitis or (ii) increase the risk of developing more severe disease when gingivitis or periodontitis are already established. These include: certain systemic diseases or conditions and the host response to the bacterial infection (**Fig. 4-10**).

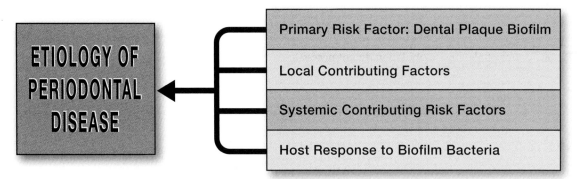

Figure 4-10. Multifactorial Etiology of Periodontal Disease. Periodontal disease results from the interaction of many factors.

   B. **Local Contributing Factors for Periodontal Disease**
      1. Local contributing factors for periodontal disease are oral conditions that increase an individual's susceptibility to periodontal infection in specific sites.
      2. Examples of local contributing factors include dental calculus and faulty restorations.
   C. **Systemic Conditions.** Systemic risk factors for periodontal disease include tobacco use, diabetes mellitus, osteoporosis, hormone alteration, stress, and prescription medications.
   D. **Host Inflammatory and Immune Response**
      1. Although bacteria are essential for periodontal disease to occur, the presence of bacteria alone is insufficient to cause periodontal disease. Rather, it is the body's response to bacteria that is responsible for the tissue destruction seen in periodontitis.
      2. The way that the body reacts to bacteria is known as the **host response**.
      3. It is the complex interaction between the bacteria and the host response to these bacteria that determines the onset and severity of periodontal disease.

CHAPTER SUMMARY STATEMENT

Advances in research have led to many changes in the understanding, prevention, and treatment of periodontal disease. In the future, ideas about causes and treatment will continue to be refined and changed as researchers delve further into the mysteries of periodontal disease. The presence of bacterial plaque combined with the existence of multiple risk factors increase a person's chance of developing periodontal disease. Chapters 5 through 8 discuss the various risk factors for periodontal disease in detail.

SECTION 4: FOCUS ON PATIENTS

CASE 1
You find a newspaper article that estimates that in your home state 73% of state residents have some form of periodontal disease. You would like to use this statistic in a homework assignment. When you include this information in your homework assignment should you describe this statistic as incidence or prevalence of periodontitis?

CASE 2
Two individuals who have exactly the same level of plaque control and exactly the same amount of plaque accumulation do not necessarily develop the same severity of periodontal disease. How do you explain this fact?

CASE 3
Your dental team has a new patient who has gingivitis. The patient has poor plaque control, generalized calculus deposits, poorly controlled diabetes mellitus, a history of smoking cigarettes, and inadequate dietary intake of calcium. In your patient counseling how would you characterize the likelihood that the patient will develop periodontitis in the future and what might you tell the patient about this?

References

1. Centers for Disease Control and Prevention. Department of Health and Human Services, Morbidity and Mortality Weekly Report. *Surveillance for Dental Caries, Dental Sealants, Tooth Retention, Edentulism, and Enamel Fluorosis—United States, 1988–1994 and 1999–2002.* Surveillance Summaries, Volume 54, 2005.
2. United States. Public Health Service. Office of the Surgeon General. and National Institute of Dental and Craniofacial Research (U.S.), *Oral health in America: A report of the Surgeon General.* NIH publication no. 00-4713. Bethesda, MD.: National Institute of Dental and Craniofacial Research: U.S. Public Health Service Dept. of Health and Human Services. 2000:xxiv, 308.
3. Golub LM, Ryan ME, Williams RC. Modulation of the host response in the treatment of periodontitis. *Dent Today.* 1998;17:102–106, 108–109.
4. Centers for Disease Control and Prevention (CDC). National Center for Health Statistics (NCHS). National Health and Nutrition Examination Survey Data (NHANES III); 1988–1994. Hyattsville, MD: U.S. Department of Health and Human Services, Centers for Disease Control and Prevention. 2002.
5. Löe H, Theilade E, Jensen SB. Experimental gingivitis in man. *J Periodontol.* 1965; 36:177–187.

SECTION 5: CHAPTER REVIEW QUESTIONS

1. Which of the following terms describes the new cases of a disease that occur within a given interval of time?
   A. Prevalence
   B. Epidemic rate
   C. Incidence
   D. Disparities

2. Which of the following statements is an accurate, current view regarding risk factors for periodontal disease?
   A. Bacterial plaque alone is the cause of periodontal disease
   B. Host response plays a critical role in the progression of periodontal disease
   C. Patient self-care has no effect on the progression of periodontal disease
   D. Daily plaque control alone can prevent periodontal disease

3. The following statements regarding epidemiological research are true EXCEPT:
   A. Variables such as socioeconomic status are included in periodontal studies
   B. Measuring for presence of periodontal disease is easier than measuring dental caries
   C. Periodontal disease is one of the most widespread diseases in adult Americans
   D. Research indicates that black and Hispanic U.S. males have more periodontal disease that white males

4. Your patient presented with early stages of periodontal disease. An example of a <u>local or environmental risk factor</u> you might investigate would be:
   A. Any systemic diseases
   B. Presence of plaque at the gingival margin
   C. Family members with periodontal disease
   D. Presence of faulty margins on dental restorations

5. Intermittent disease progression refers to:
   A. Periods of disease activity and inactivity
   B. Flossing every other day
   C. Disease progression during adolescence
   D. Disease progression in the mouth in a slow and constant rate

5 Microbiology of Periodontal Disease

Learning Objectives

- Define the terms innocuous, pathogenic, virulent, gram-positive, and gram-negative.
- Define the term biofilm and explain the advantages to a bacterium of living in a biofilm.
- Name three everyday examples of biofilms in the environment.
- Name and describe the components of the biofilm structure.
- Given a drawing of a mature biofilm, label the following: bacterial microcolonies, fluid channels, extracellular slime layer, dental pellicle, and tooth surface.
- Explain the significance of the extracellular slime layer to a bacterial microcolony.
- Explain the purpose of the fluid channels in a biofilm.
- Explain why chemicals are not effective in controlling or eliminating biofilms.
- Define the term dental bacterial plaque.
- List and describe the four phases in the development of the dental plaque biofilm.

■ Define the term bacterial bloom.
■ State the most effective ways to control dental plaque biofilms.
■ Explain why frequent periodontal instrumentation is vital in the control of dental plaque biofilms located within periodontal pockets.
■ Describe how the numbers of bacteria vary from health to disease in the periodontium.
■ Name four microorganisms that have been studied for many years in regard to their association with periodontal disease.
■ Given a drawing of the subgingival plaque biofilm, label the three zones of bacteria.
■ Name and describe the function of four bacterial virulence factors.
■ Explain to a patient the importance of self-care in the prevention and control of periodontal diseases.

KEY TERMS

Bacterium/bacteria
Innocuous
Pathogenic
Gram-positive bacteria
Gram-negative bacteria
Aerobic bacteria
Anaerobic bacteria
Facultative anaerobic bacteria
Biofilm
Mushroom-shaped microcolonies

Extracellular slime layer
Bacterial plaque
Fimbriae
Pellicle
Bacterial blooms
Mixed infection
Actinobacillus actino-mycetemcomitans
Bacteroides forsythus (Tannerella forsythensis)
Fusobacterium nucleatum

Porphyromonas gingivalis
Tooth-attached plaque
Epithelial-attached plaque
Unattached plaque
Virulence factors
Lipopolysaccharide (LPS)
Exotoxins
Bacterial enzymes

SECTION 1: BACTERIA

Bacteria are the primary etiologic agents in periodontal disease. The bacteria in dental plaque play a key role in the initiation and progression of periodontal disease. More than 500 bacterial strains may be found in dental plaque.[1] These bacteria have evolved to survive in the environment of the tooth surface, gingival epithelium, and oral cavity. Section 1 provides a brief review of basic bacterial characteristics. Knowledge of these characteristics is needed to understand the bacteria found in the oral cavity.

CHARACTERISTICS OF BACTERIA

1. **Description**
   A. **Bacterium** (plural, **bacteria**). First described in the mid-1670s by Anton van Leeuwenhoek, a Dutch scientist, bacteria are the simplest organisms and can be seen only through a microscope (**Fig. 5-1**).
   B. There are thousands of kinds of bacteria, most of which are harmless to humans.
      1. **Innocuous**—species of bacteria that are not harmful.
      2. **Pathogenic**—species of bacteria that are capable of causing disease. Another term for pathogenic bacteria is virulent bacteria. In the oral cavity, innocuous and pathogenic bacteria live together in a symbiotic relationship.
   C. Bacteria have existed on earth for longer than any other organisms and are still the most abundant type of cell.
   D. Bacteria can replicate quickly. This ability to divide quickly enables populations of bacteria to adapt rapidly to changes in their environment.

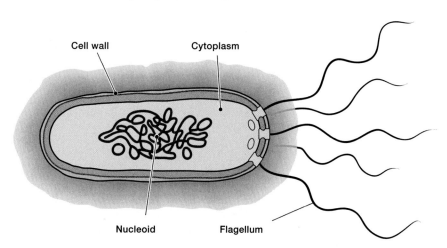

Figure 5-1. Bacterium. Structures of a typical bacterial cell.

2. **Structure of the Bacterial Cell Wall.** A tough protective layer called a **cell wall** encloses nearly all bacteria. The cell wall maintains the overall shape of the bacterial cell. The composition of the cell wall is an important characteristic used in identifying and classifying bacteria.
   A. **Gram-positive bacteria**
      a. Have a thick, single cell wall
      b. Retain a purple color when stained with a dye known as crystal violet
   B. **Gram-negative bacteria**
      a. Have double cell walls
      b. Do not stain purple with crystal violet
      c. Believed to play an important role in the tissue destruction seen in periodontitis

WHERE BACTERIA LIVE

Bacteria live almost everywhere, even in environments where other life forms cannot survive. Bacteria are always present on the skin and in the digestive and respiratory systems of humans.

1. **Response to Gaseous Oxygen.** Most bacteria may be placed into one of three groups based on their response to gaseous oxygen (O_2).
   A. Aerobic bacteria—require oxygen to live.
   B. Anaerobic bacteria—cannot live in the presence of oxygen.
   C. Facultative anaerobic bacteria—can exist either with or without oxygen.
2. **Bacterial Lifestyles**
   A. Free-Floating Bacteria
      1. Bacteria may be free-floating. These free-floating bacteria are also known as planktonic bacteria.
      2. Until recently, most research done on bacteria was conducted on free-floating bacteria.
   B. Attached Bacteria
      1. Bacteria can attach to surfaces and to one another. *Communities of bacteria that attach to each other and to a surface are described as living in a biofilm* (**Fig. 5-2**).
      2. Once a bacterium attaches to a surface, it activates a whole different set of genes that give the bacterium different characteristics from those that it had as a free-floating organism.
      3. It has been estimated that more than 99% of all bacteria on earth live as attached bacteria.[2]

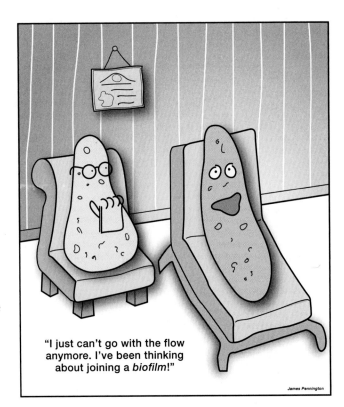

Figure 5-2. Bacterial Lifestyles. Complex communities of bacteria that are attached to a surface are described as living in a biofilm.
(Cartoon courtesy of James Pennington, MSU Center for Biofilm Engineering, Bozeman, MT.)

"I just can't go with the flow anymore. I've been thinking about joining a *biofilm*!"

James Pennington

SECTION 2: BIOFILMS

Until recently, bacteria were studied as they grew on culture plates in a laboratory. Recent advances in research technology have allowed researchers to study bacteria in their natural environment. These studies have revealed that most bacteria live in complex communities called biofilms. Furthermore, biofilm bacteria have unique characteristics that make them extremely difficult to kill.

WHAT ARE BIOFILMS AND WHERE DO THEY FORM?

1. **Description**
   A. A **biofilm** is a well-organized community of bacteria that (i) adheres to surfaces and (ii) is embedded in an extracellular slime layer.
   B. Biofilms can be formed by a single bacterial species, but usually biofilms consist of many species of bacteria as well as other organisms and debris.
   C. Biofilms form rapidly on almost any surface that is wet.
2. **Biofilm Environments**
   A. Biofilms are everywhere in nature. Biofilm may seem like a new term, but we encounter biofilms on a regular basis. The plaque that forms on teeth, the slime in fish tanks, and the slime deposit that clogs the sink drain are all examples of biofilms. The slimy rocks in a stream are biofilm coated.
   B. Biofilms can exist on any solid surface that is exposed to a bacteria-containing fluid.
      1. Biofilms can be found on medical and dental implants, indwelling intravenous and urinary catheters, contact lenses (**Fig. 5-3**), and prosthetic devices such as heart valves, biliary stents, pacemakers, and artificial joints.
      2. Legionnaire's disease, which killed 29 people in 1976, was the result of a bacterial biofilm in the hotel's air conditioning system.
   C. Biofilms thrive in dental unit water and suction lines and have been shown to be the primary source of contaminated water delivered by dental units (**Fig. 5-4**).
      1. Stagnant fluid flow allows free-floating bacteria to attach to the tubing walls in the dental unit and form intricate biofilms.
      2. Like other biofilms, these bacterial biofilms are embedded in an extracellular slime layer that protects the bacteria from physical or chemical destruction.

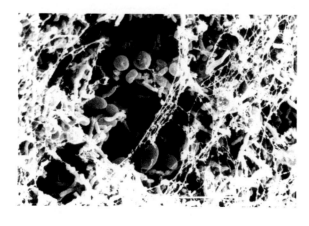

Figure 5-3. Contact Lens Biofilm. This scanning electron micrograph shows biofilm formation on the inside of a contact lens case.
(Micrograph courtesy of Drs. Louise McLaughlin-Borlace and John Dart of the Institute of Ophthalmology, University College, London, England.)

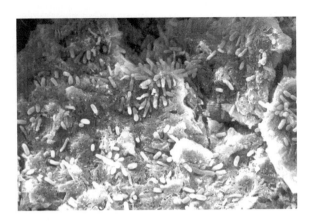

Figure 5-4. Biofilm on Dental Equipment. This scanning electron micrograph shows biofilm formation from the inside of a high volume suction line from a dental unit.
(Micrograph courtesy of Professor Jean Barbeau, Faculty of Dentistry, University of Montreal, Montreal, Canada.)

HOW BACTERIA LIVE IN BIOFILMS

1. **Biofilm Structure**
   A. Bacterial Microcolonies
      1. The bacteria in a biofilm are not distributed evenly. As the bacteria attach to a surface and to each other, they cluster together to form **mushroom-shaped microcolonies** that are attached to the tooth surface at a narrow base (**Fig. 5-5**).
      2. Each microcolony is a tiny independent community containing thousands of compatible bacteria. Different microcolonies may contain different combinations of bacterial species.

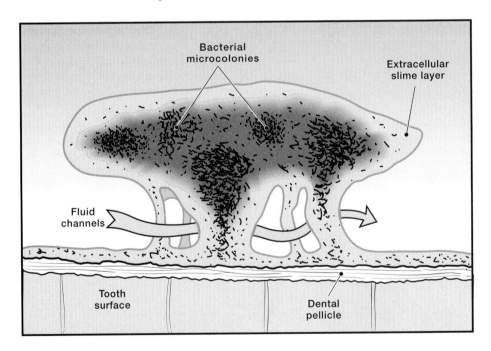

Figure 5-5. Biofilm. This illustration shows the structure of a mature biofilm: bacterial microcolonies, extracellular slime layer, and fluid channels.

   B. Extracellular Slime Layer
      1. The **extracellular slime layer** is a protective barrier that surrounds the mushroom-shaped bacterial microcolonies.
      2. The slime layer protects the bacterial microcolonies from antibiotics, antimicrobials, and the body's immune system.
   C. Fluid Channels
      1. A series of fluid channels penetrate the extracellular slime layer.
      2. These fluid channels provide nutrients and oxygen for the bacterial microcolonies and facilitate movement of bacterial metabolites, waste products, and enzymes within the biofilm structure (**Fig. 5-6**).
   D. A Primitive Communication System. The bacterial microcolonies use chemical signals to communicate with each other (**Fig. 5-7**).

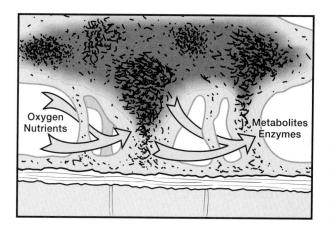

Figure 5-6. Fluid Channels.
Fluid channels in the biofilm facilitate the movement of nutrients, oxygen, bacterial byproducts, and enzymes within the biofilm structure.

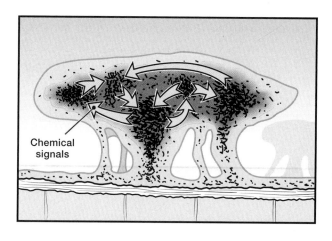

Figure 5-7. Biofilm Communication System.
The bacteria in a biofilm use chemical signals to communicate with each other.

REMOVING BIOFILMS

1. **Control and Removal of Biofilms**
   A. Bacterial microcolonies are protected from their external environment by one another and by the extracellular slime layer. Bacteria living in a biofilm are unusually resistant to antibiotics (administered systemically), antimicrobials (administered locally), and the body's defense system.
   B. *Antibiotic doses that kill free-floating bacteria, for example, need to be increased as much as 1500 times to kill biofilm bacteria* (and at these high doses, the antibiotic would kill the patient before the biofilm bacteria!).[2,3]
   C. It is likely that several mechanisms are responsible for biofilm resistance to antibiotics and antimicrobial agents.
      1. The slime layer may prevent the drugs from penetrating fully into the depth of the biofilm.
      2. Bacteria can develop resistance to antimicrobial drugs by producing a thicker protective slime layer.
      3. The slime layer may protect the bacteria against leukocytes (defensive cells of the body's immune system).
      4. Because of the protective slime layer, substances released by leukocytes in response to the invading bacteria are more damaging to the surrounding body tissue than to the biofilm bacteria.
   D. Biofilms can be destroyed, however, by simply wiping them off (disrupting their attachment to a surface). *The most successful means currently available for biofilm infection control is the physical removal of the biofilm.*

SECTION 3: THE DENTAL PLAQUE BIOFILM

Dental Plaque Biofilm. *Recent technical advances have led to the recognition that dental plaque is a biofilm.* Dental **bacterial plaque** is a biofilm that adheres tenaciously to tooth surfaces, restorations, and prosthetic appliances. The dental plaque biofilm has the same complex structure as biofilms found elsewhere: bacterial microcolonies, extracellular slime layer, and fluid channels.

DENTAL PLAQUE BIOFILM: PATTERN OF FORMATION

The pattern of plaque biofilm development can be divided into four phases: (i) attachment of bacteria to a solid surface, (ii) initial colonization, (iii) secondary colonization, and (iv) formation of the mature subgingival plaque biofilms (**Fig. 5-8**).

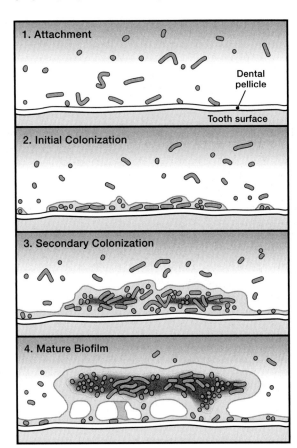

Figure 5-8. **Formation of Dental Plaque Biofilm.** The dental plaque biofilm forms in four distinct stages.

1. **Initial Attachment of Bacteria to Pellicle.**
    A. Within a few hours after pellicle formation, bacteria begin to attach to the outer surface of the pellicle. Bacteria connect to the pellicle and each other with hundreds of hairlike structures called **fimbriae.**
    B. The **pellicle** is a thin coating of salivary proteins that attach to the tooth surface within minutes after a professional cleaning.
        1. Its purpose is to protect the enamel from acidic activity.
        2. The pellicle acts like double-sided adhesive tape, adhering to the tooth surface on one side and providing a sticky surface on the other side that facilitates attachment by bacteria to the tooth surface.

2. Initial Colonization of the Tooth Surface—New Bacteria Join In

    A. Once bacteria stick to the tooth, they begin producing substances that stimulate other free-floating bacteria to join the community.

    B. Within the first 2 days in which no further cleaning is undertaken, the tooth's surface is colonized predominantly by gram-positive bacteria.

3. Secondary Colonization: Extracellular Slime Layer and Microcolony Formation

    A. Production of an Extracellular Slime Layer.

        1. It appears that the act of attaching to the tooth surface stimulates the bacteria to excrete a slimy, gluelike substance.

        2. This extracellular slime layer helps to anchor bacteria to the tooth surface and provides protection for the attached bacteria.

    B. Microcolony Formation

        1. Once the surface of the tooth has been covered with attached bacteria, the biofilm grows primarily through cell division of the adherent bacteria (rather than through the attachment of new bacteria).

        2. Next, the proliferating bacteria begin to grow away from the tooth.

        3. Bacterial blooms are periods when specific species or groups of species grow at rapidly accelerated rates.

4. Mature Biofilm: Mushroom-Shaped Microcolonies.

    A. The bacteria cluster together to form *mushroom-shaped microcolonies* that are attached to the tooth surface at a narrow base.

    B. The result is the formation of complex collections of different bacteria linked to one another (**Fig. 5-9**).

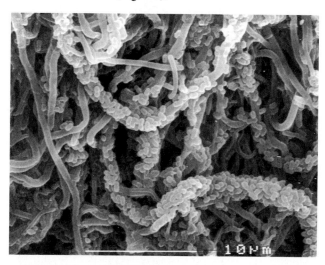

Figure 5-9. Complex Collections of Bacteria. Bacteria in a mature biofilm form complex patterns. One common array of bacteria has a corncob appearance that is created when a central rod-shaped bacterium becomes surrounded by many round cocci. (Courtesy of Ziedonis Skobe, PhD, Head, Biostructure Core Facility, The Forsyth Institute, Boston, MA.)

CONTROL AND REMOVAL OF DENTAL PLAQUE BIOFILM

1. Bacteria in mature biofilm live in a protected, safe environment.

    A. The biofilm provides the bacteria with an advantage that permits long-term survival within the sulcus or pocket environment. *The protective extracellular slime matrix makes bacteria extremely resistant to antibiotics, antimicrobial agents, and the body's immune response.*

    B. As with other biofilms, subgingival plaque is remarkably resistant to antibiotic and antimicrobial therapy.

        1. Bacteria living in mature biofilms are not easily destroyed by antimicrobial agents [4].

        2. Antimicrobial agents work best when used in conjunction with mechanical cleaning that removes or disrupts the dental plaque biofilm.

    C. *Control of bacteria in dental plaque biofilms is best achieved by the physical disruption of plaque (such as: brushing, flossing, and periodontal instrumentation).*

2. **Physical removal of dental plaque biofilms is essential.**
    A. Because of the structure of biofilms, physical removal of bacterial plaque biofilms is the most effective means of control.
        1. The mature dental plaque biofilm is a very complex structure of bacterial microcolonies, extracellular slime layer, and fluid channels.
        2. It takes some time for all four stages of biofilm formation to occur and for the mature biofilm to form.
        3. Mechanical cleaning forces the bacteria to start over with initial attachment, initial colonization, secondary colonization and finally, to become a mature biofilm.
        4. In areas that are cleaned regularly, a mature biofilm will not be able to develop. The cleaner the tooth surface, the less complex the bacterial formation.
    B. Toothbrushes and floss cannot reach the subgingival plaque biofilm located within pockets. For this reason, frequent periodontal instrumentation of subgingival root surfaces by a dental hygienist or dentist is an essential component in the treatment of periodontitis.

BACTERIA ASSOCIATED WITH HEALTH AND DISEASE

All periodontal infections are associated with—caused by—multiple bacteria. That is, periodontal disease is a **mixed infection**. For this reason, if might be helpful to think of a bacterial soup of different bacteria within the biofilm.[5]

1. **Bacteria Associated with Health**
    A. In health, the number of bacteria that can be cultured from <u>an individual healthy sulci</u> is between 100 to 1,000 bacteria.[1,5]
    B. *In health, approximately 75% to 80% of the bacteria are gram-positive.* Most of the remaining bacteria are gram-negative.
    C. Most of the bacteria in a healthy site are **nonmotile**—not capable of movement.
    D. The bacteria found in periodontal diseases are found in healthy sulci but they make up a small proportion of the total bacteria in the site.

2. **Bacteria Associated with Gingivitis**
    A. In gingivitis, the number of bacteria that can be cultured <u>from an individual site</u> ranges from 1,000 to 100,000 bacteria.[5]
    B. *The bacteria found in chronic gingivitis consist of almost equal proportions of gram-positive and gram-negative bacteria.*

3. **Bacteria Associated with Periodontitis**
    A. Periodontitis is associated with an enormous number of gram-negative bacteria.
        1. *In periodontitis, the number of bacteria that can be cultured <u>from an individual site</u> ranges from 100,000 to 100,000,000 bacteria.*
        2. Researchers have estimated the potential biofilm load in a patient with 28 teeth and generalized periodontitis. If the patient has 28 teeth and one considers the tooth roots to be circular with an average of 5 mm of biofilm on each tooth, the total mouth biofilm would cover an area about the size of the back of an adult human hand.[6]
        3. The bacteria associated with periodontitis are different from those found in periodontal health.
    B. The bacterial composition of periodontitis differs significantly from patient to patient and from site to site within the same mouth. *Chronic periodontitis is associated with high proportions of gram-negative and motile bacteria.*

PERIODONTAL PATHOGENS

Although more than 500 bacterial species have been isolated from periodontal pockets, it is likely that only a small percentage of these bacteria are periodontal pathogens.

■ Several microorganisms have been strongly associated with chronic periodontitis.[7] Refer to **Table 5-1** for a list of periodontal pathogens commonly found in periodontitis.

■ In the future, dental health care providers may have diagnostic tests and treatments specifically directed at these periodontal pathogens.

■ Four bacterial pathogens have been studied for many years in regard to their association with periodontal disease: *Actinobacillus actinomycetemcomitans, Bacteroides forsythus (Tannerella forsythensis), Fusobacterium nucleatum,* and *Porphyromonas gingivalis.*

Table 5-1. Bacteria Strongly Associated with Chronic Periodontitis

Bacteria	Gram Stain/Motility
Actinobacillus actinomycetemcomitans (serotype a)	Gram-negative, nonmotile
Streptococcus intermedius	Gram-positive, nonmotile
Campylobacter rectus	Gram-negative, motile
Eubacterium nodatum	Gram-positive, nonmotile
Fusobacterium nucleatum, subspecies *nucleatum*	Gram-negative, nonmotile
Fusobacterium nucleatum, subspecies *polymorphum*	Gram-negative, nonmotile
Prevotella intermedia	Gram-negative, nonmotile
Peptostreptococcus micros	Gram-positive, nonmotile
Prevotella nigrescens	Gram-negative, nonmotile
Porphyromonas gingivalis (previously known as *Bacteroides gingivalis*)	Gram-negative, nonmotile
Bacteroides forsythus (Tannerella forsythensis)	Gram-negative, nonmotile
Treponema denticola	Not applicable, motile

Data in Table 5-1 from Socransky SS, Haffajee AD. Dental biofilms: difficult therapeutic targets. *Periodontol 2002.* 2002;28:12–55.

1. *Actinobacillus actinomycetemcomitans (frequently abbreviated as Aa)*
   A. This microorganism has been strongly associated with aggressive periodontitis and is found in approximately 25% of chronic periodontitis cases.
   B. *A. actinomycetemcomitans* is capable of evading normal host immune response and of destroying gingival connective tissue and bone.
   C. Recent studies indicate that in family units—in which one of the parents has periodontitis and *A. actinomycetemcomitans*—that *it is highly likely that the A. actinomycetemcomitans will be transmitted from that patient to the children in the family.*[8]
      1. Several studies have demonstrated that the same clonal types of bacteria are present in family members, but different clonal types are found in unrelated individuals. Kissing is the primary means by which saliva and its bacterial contents are transmitted.[9–12] This means that the common contact of saliva in families puts children and couples at risk for contracting periodontal disease from another family member.
      2. Familial transmission should not be confused with contagion. There is little or no evidence that periodontal infections are contagious. The term contagious refers to a disease that may be transmitted by direct or indirect contact. Periodontal pathogens appear to be transmissible but only after long-term exposure and directly via the saliva.
2. *Bacteroides forsythus (Tannerella forsythensis)*
   A. *B. forsythus* commonly is found in subgingival plaque samples from deep periodontal pockets.
   B. This microorganism is associated with aggressive periodontitis.

   3. *Fusobacterium nucleatum*
      A. *F. nucleatum* is found in the early stages of gingivitis and is a prominent component of the subgingival plaque in periodontitis with severe attachment loss.
      B. This organism is capable of initiating early inflammatory changes in the tissue.
   4. *Porphyromonas gingivalis*
      A. *P. gingivalis* is associated with periodontitis.
      B. This organism has the ability to destroy gingival connective and alveolar bone.
      C. *P. gingivalis* also has the ability to enter the junctional epithelium and multiply in that location.

Box 5-1

Pronunciation Guide to Bacterial Tongue Twisters

Name	Pronunciation Guide
Actinobacillus	act-tin-oh-baa-sill-us
Actinomycetemcomitans	act-tin-oh-my-see-tem-comb-ah-tans
Bacteroides	back-tir-roy-deez
forsythus	fore-sigh-thus
(Tannerella forsythensis)	
Fusobacterium	fuse-so-back-tier-EEE-um
Nucleatum	nu-klee-ah-tum
Porphyromonas	pour-fy-roh-mo-nas
Gingivalis	ging-jih-val-lis

http://www.kcom.edu/faculty/chamberlain/website/studio.htm
Dr. Neal Chamberlain's **Bacterial Pathogen Pronunciation Station**—hear Dr. Chamberlain pronounce *Actinobacillus actinomycetemcomitans*.

SECTION 4: SUBGINGIVAL PLAQUE BIOFILM

THREE ZONES OF PLAQUE BIOFILM

1. **Types of Plaque within the Periodontal Pocket.** The subgingival plaque biofilm has three zones: (i) tooth-attached plaque, (ii) epithelial-attached plaque, and (ii) unattached plaque (**Fig. 5-10**).
   A. **Tooth-Attached Plaque**—bacteria that are attached to the tooth surface.
      1. Bacteria attach to an area of the tooth surface that extends from the gingival margin almost to the junctional epithelium at the base of the pocket.
      2. The inner layers are dominated by gram-positive bacteria, but gram-negative cocci and rods are also present.
   B. **Epithelial-Attached Plaque**—bacteria that are attached to the epithelium. (Also known as epithelium-associated plaque and loosely adherent plaque.)
      1. Bacteria are loosely attached to the epithelium of the pocket wall.
      2. The layers closest to the soft tissue wall contain large numbers of motile gram-negative bacteria and spirochetes.
      3. Bacteria from the epithelial-attached plaque can invade the gingival connective tissue and be found within the periodontal connective tissues and on the surface of the alveolar bone.
      4. Research suggests that this type of plaque is the most detrimental to the periodontal tissues.
   C. **Unattached Plaque**—free floating, unattached bacteria.
      1. Bacteria within the pocket environment are not subject to the mechanical forces (saliva, tongue, mastication, toothbrushing) that tend to dislodge bacteria from supragingival tooth surfaces. Thus, attachment to the tooth surface is not as vital to subgingival bacteria and many bacteria are completely unattached to the biofilm matrix.
      2. The bottom of the sulcus or pocket usually has unorganized gram-negative rods and spirochetes separated from the epithelium by a layer of leukocytes (defensive cells).

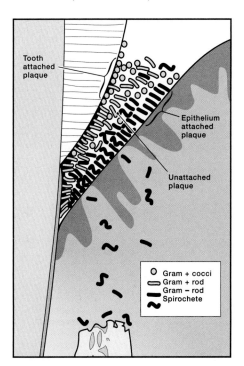

Figure 5-10. Three Zones of Subgingival Plaque Biofilm. Subgingival plaque as three zones (i) tooth-attached plaque, (ii) epithelial-attached plaque, and (iii) unattached—free-floating—plaque.

2. Relationship of Plaque Biofilm to Alveolar Bone
  A. The distance from plaque biofilm to the alveolar bone is never less than 0.5 mm and never greater than 2.7 mm.[13,14]
  B. This consistent distance between the biofilm and the crest of the alveolar bone indicates that the bacteria are capable of causing bone destruction only in alveolar bone located less than 3 mm away from the dental plaque biofilm (**Fig. 5-11**).

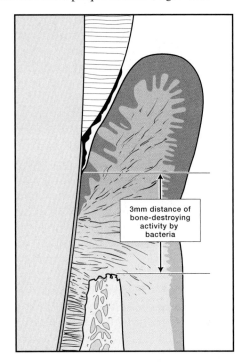

Figure 5-11. Bone-Destroying Activity of Dental Plaque Biofilm. Bacteria are capable of causing bone destruction only in alveolar bone located less than 3 mm away from the dental plaque biofilm.

BACTERIAL VIRULENCE FACTORS

The mechanisms that enable biofilm bacteria to colonize, invade, and damage the tissues of the periodontium are called **virulence factors**. Virulence factors may be structural characteristics of the bacterium itself or substances produced and released into the environment by bacteria (**Fig. 5-12**).

  1. Bacterial Characteristics
    A. Bacterial Invasion
      1. Periodontal pathogens have the ability to actively penetrate the epithelium lining the pocket wall and invade the gingival connective tissue.
      2. Both gram-positive and gram-negative bacteria have been observed in the intercellular spaces of the gingival connective tissue and near the alveolar bone.
        a. Bacteria may invade the gingival connective tissue through ulcerations in the pocket epithelium.
        b. *A. actinomycetemcomitans, P.,* and *T. denticola* have been demonstrated to directly invade host tissue cells.
        c. The presence of bacteria within the tissues makes periodontitis more resistant to treatment.
    B. Endotoxins
      1. Lipopolysaccharide (LPS)—also known as **endotoxin**—is a major component of the cell walls of gram-negative bacteria.
      2. LPS is released only when the structure of the cell wall breaks up and the cell dies. LPS, once released from the cell at death, stimulates host biologic activities that promote tissue damage, including tissue destruction, bone resorption, and the breakdown of collagen fibers.

2. **Bacterial Products**
   A. Exotoxin Production. **Exotoxins** are harmful proteins released from the bacterial cell that act on host cells at a distance. For example, *A. actinomycetemcomitans* produces leukotoxin (LT), an exotoxin that may enable these bacteria to destroy leukocytes in the sulcus or pocket.
   B. Bacterial Enzyme Production. **Bacterial enzymes** are agents that are harmful or destructive to host cells. Enzymes function in a variety of ways to assist the bacteria in invading the tissues. Once released, bacterial enzymes have the ability to:
      1. Increase permeability of the epithelial lining of the sulcus (allowing bacteria to penetrate sulcular epithelium more easily).
      2. Contribute to the breakdown of the collagen fibers in the gingival connective tissue.
      3. Promote apical migration of the junctional epithelium along the root surface.
      4. Cause widening of the intercellular spaces.
      5. Diminish the ability of immunoglobulins and other body proteins to defend the host.

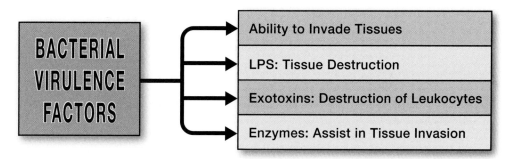

Figure 5-12. Bacterial Virulence Factors. Bacteria have several virulence factors that allow them to colonize, invade, and damage the tissues of the periodontium. LPS, lipopolysaccharides.

CHAPTER SUMMARY STATEMENT

More than 500 bacterial strains have been identified in dental biofilm. Experts agree that most forms of periodontal disease are caused by specific pathogens, particularly gram-negative bacteria. The numbers of bacteria found at a site vary greatly in health, gingivitis, and periodontitis. Periodontitis is associated with large numbers of gram-negative bacteria.

The recognition that dental plaque is a biofilm helps to explain why periodontal diseases have been so difficult to prevent and to treat. Periodontal pathogens within a biofilm environment behave very differently from free-floating bacteria. The protective extracellular slime matrix makes bacteria extremely resistant to antibiotics, antimicrobial agents, and the body's immune system. Mechanical removal is the most effective treatment for the control of dental plaque biofilms.

Bacteria in dental plaque biofilms play a key role in the initiation and progression of periodontal disease. A bacterial infection alone, however, is insufficient to cause periodontal disease. The host response plays a critical role in the tissue destruction seen in periodontitis. Host response in periodontal disease is discussed in Chapter 6. Other contributing risk factors for periodontal disease include local oral conditions, habits, systemic disease, and genetic factors.

SECTION 5: FOCUS ON PATIENTS

CASE 1
You have just completed a thorough cleaning of a tooth surface. Describe what deposits you might expect to form on the tooth surface over the next few days if the patient does absolutely no further cleaning of the tooth surface.

CASE 2
Imagine that you are holding an "interview" of bacteria living in an oral biofilm. How might the bacteria respond to your question about advantages of living in a biofilm?

References

1. Kroes I, Lepp PW, Relman DA. Bacterial diversity within the human subgingival crevice. *Proc Natl Acad Sci USA*. 1999;96:14547–14552.
2. Coghlan A. Slime city. *New Sci.* 1996;2045:32–36.
3. Elder MJ, Stapleton F, Evans E, et al. Biofilm-related infections in ophthalmology. *Eye.*, 1995;9(Pt 1):102–109.
4. Costerton JW, Lewandowski Z, Caldwell DE, et al., Microbial biofilms. *Annu Rev Microbiol.* 1995;49:711–745.
5. Darveau RP, Tanner A, Page RC. The microbial challenge in periodontitis. *Periodontol 2000.* 1997;14:12–32.
6. Page RC, Offenbacher S, Schroeder HE, et al. Advances in the pathogenesis of periodontitis: Summary of developments, clinical implications and future directions. *Periodontol 2000.* 1997;14:216–248.
7. Socransky SS, Haffajee AD. Dental biofilms: Difficult therapeutic targets, *Periodontol 2002.* 2002;28:12–55.
8. Preus HR, Zambon JJ, Dunford RG, et al. The distribution and transmission of A. actinomycetemcomitans in families with established adult periodontitis. *J Periodontol* 1994;65: 2–7.
9. Petit MD, van Steenbergen TJ, Scholtz LM, et al. Epidemiology and transmission of Porphyromonas gingivalis and Actinobacillus actinomycetemcomitans among children and their family members. A report of 4 surveys. *J Clin Periodontol.* 1993;20: 641–650.
10. Petit MD, Van Steenbergen TJ, De Graaf, J, et al. Transmission of Actinobacillus actinomycetemcomitans in families of adult periodontitis patients. *J Periodontal Res.* 1993;28:335–345.
11. Petit MD, van Winkelhoff AJ, van Steenbergen TJ, et al. Porphyromonas endodontalis: prevalence and distribution of restriction enzyme patterns in families. *Oral Microbiol Immunol.* 1993;8:219–224.
12. Petit MD, van Steenbergen AJ, Timmerman MF, et al. Prevalence of periodontitis and suspected periodontal pathogens in families of adult periodontitis patients. *J Clin Periodontol.* 1994;21:76–85.
13. Waerhaug J. The angular bone defect and its relationship to trauma from occlusion and downgrowth of subgingival plaque. *J Clin Periodontol.* 1979;6:61–82.
14. Waerhaug J. The gingival pocket. *Odont Tidsk.* 1952;60(Suppl 1):1–186.

SECTION 6: CHAPTER REVIEW QUESTIONS

1. A single microscopic organism is termed:
   A. Bacteria
   B. Bacterium
   C. Nucleoid
   D. Aerobic

2. Bacteria that have double cell walls and that do not stain purple with crystal violet are called:
   A. Aerobic
   B. Anaerobic
   C. Gram-positive
   D. Gram-negative

3. A well-organized community of bacteria that adheres to surfaces and is embedded in an extracellular slime layer is termed:
   A. Aerobic
   B. Anaerobic
   C. Biofilm
   D. Bacterial microcolony

4. Which structure of a biofilm protects the bacterial microcolonies from systemic antibiotics and the body's immune system?
   A. Dental pellicle
   B. Extracellular slime layer
   C. Fluid channels
   D. Primitive communication system

5. Which structure of a biofilm facilitates the movement of nutrients to the bacteria?
   A. Dental pellicle
   B. Extracellular slime layer
   C. Fluid channels
   D. Primitive communication system

6. Which of the following would be most effective in controlling the bacteria in a dental plaque biofilm?
   A. Systemic antibiotic (an antibiotic pill)
   B. Antimicrobial
   C. Very high doses of an antibiotic
   D. Toothbrush and floss

7. Why is frequent periodontal instrumentation important in the control of dental plaque biofilms located in periodontal pockets?
   A. A toothbrush and floss cannot clean root surfaces within a periodontal pocket
   B. Few patients take the time for self-care at home

8. Which of the following bacterium can be transmitted from one family member to another?
   A. *Actinobacillus actinomycetemcomitans*
   B. *Bacteroides forsythus (Tannerella forsythensis)*
   C. *Fusobacterium nucleatum*
   D. *Porphyromonas gingivalis*

Chapter

6 Host Immune Response

Learning Objectives

- Define the term immune system and name its primary function.
- Define the term inflammation and name two events that can trigger the inflammatory response.
- Name the five classic symptoms of inflammation and explain what events in the tissues result in these classic symptoms.
- Give an example of a type of injury or infection that would result in inflammation in an individual's arm. Describe the symptoms of inflammation that the individual would experience.
- Compare and contrast acute inflammation and chronic inflammation.
- Examine the periodontium of a patient with gingivitis and point out the signs of inflammation that are visible in the tissues.
- Define the term phagocytosis and describe the steps in this process.
- Describe the role of polymorphonuclear leukocytes in the immune system.
- Describe the role of macrophages in the immune system.
- Contrast the terms macrophage and monocyte.
- Describe the role of B lymphocytes in the immune system.
- Describe the role of T lymphocytes in the immune system.
- Describe the three main ways that antibodies participate in the host defense.

- Define the term inflammatory mediator and name three types of mediators.
- List the functions of cytokines in the host response.
- List the functions of prostaglandins in the host response.
- List the functions of matrix metalloproteinases (MMP) in the host response.
- Describe the tissue destruction that can be initiated by the immune mediators secreted by immune cells.
- Define complement system and explain its principal functions in the immune response.
- Describe the changes that occur in the early bacterial accumulation phase of subclinical gingivitis.
- Describe the changes that occur in the plaque overgrowth phase of early gingivitis.
- Describe the changes that occur in the subgingival plaque phase of established gingivitis.
- Describe the changes that occur in the tissue destruction phase of periodontitis.
- Explain the roles that the bacterial component (bacterial infection) and host component play in determining whether gingivitis progresses to periodontitis in an individual.

KEY TERMS

Immune response
Host
Host response
Inflammation
Edema fluid
Edematous
Acute inflammation
Chronic inflammation
Phagocytes
Phagocytosis
Polymorphonuclear
  leukocyte (PMN)
Lysosome

Macrophage
Monocyte
Lymphocyte
B lymphocyte (B cell)
T lymphocyte (T cell)
Immunoglobulins
Cytokines
Interleukin-1
Interleukin-6
Interleukin-8
Tumor necrosis factor
Prostaglandins

Prostaglandins of the E
  series (PGE)
Matrix metalloproteinases
  (MMP)
Complement system
Opsonization of pathogens
Membrane attack complex
Host response to
  periodontal disease
Gingivitis
Periodontitis

SECTION 1: THE BODY'S DEFENSE SYSTEM

The **immune system** is a complex system in the body that is responsible for fighting disease. Its primary function is to identify foreign substances in the body (bacteria, viruses, fungi, or parasites) and develop a defense against them. The prime purpose of the human immune system is to defend the life of the individual (**host**). The way that the body responds to an infection is known as the **host response**.

In the case of periodontal disease, the immune system strives to defend the body against periodontal pathogens. The body's defenses are employed with the purpose of eliminating the invading bacteria, not to preserve the tooth or its supporting periodontal tissues.

This chapter explains the components of the body's immune system as they relate to periodontal disease and how the host response to bacteria results in the breakdown of the gingival connective tissue and the loss of alveolar bone.

THE BODY'S INFLAMMATORY PROCESS

Inflammation is the body's reaction to injury or invasion by disease-producing organisms. The inflammatory response focuses host defense components at the site of the infection to eliminate microorganisms and heal damaged tissue. The clinician should have a general understanding of the inflammatory process to recognize the clinical signs of inflammation in periodontal disease.

1. **Major Events in the Inflammatory Response** (Fig. 6-1)
   A. The inflammatory response is triggered by the invasion of pathogens or tissue injury.
   B. There is an increased blood flow to the tissue that has been infected or injured. This increased blood flow is needed to deliver immune defenders to the site.
   C. Leukocytes and plasma proteins leak from the capillaries into the tissues at the site of infection or injury. This fluid that accumulates in the tissues is termed **edema fluid**. Thus, the swollen tissue is referred to as being **edematous**.
   D. The leukocytes and plasma proteins have a direct role in the defense against invading microorganisms.
   E. *In the periodontium, the inflammatory response can also result in considerable destruction of tissue cells, connective tissue, and bone in the region surrounding the area of inflammation.*

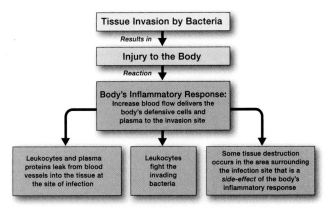

Figure 6-1. Major Events in the Body's Inflammatory Response. Inflammation is the body's response to injury or invasion by disease-producing organisms. This response focuses the body's defense mechanisms at the site of an injury or infection.

2. **Five Classic Symptoms of Inflammation**
   To inflame means "to set on fire," which makes us think of red, heat, and pain. Clinically, there are five classic symptoms of inflammation at the site of infection or injury:
   A. Heat—a localized increase in temperature due to an increased amount of blood at the site.
   B. Redness—the result of increased blood in the area
   C. Swelling—the result of the accumulation of fluid at the site. The leukocytes and plasma that collect at the site cause the swelling (edema) associated with inflammation.
   D. Pain—the result of pressure from edema in the tissue. The excess fluid in the tissues puts pressure on sensitive nerve endings, causing pain.
   E. Loss of function—the result of swelling and pain. For example, inflammation of a finger (swelling and pain) would cause you to favor that finger and not use it in a normal manner.

TWO STAGES OF INFLAMMATION

1. **Acute inflammation** refers to an inflammatory response that begins suddenly and is of short duration (2 weeks or less) (**Fig. 6-2**).
   A. Acute inflammation has the warning signs of heat, redness, swelling, and pain.
   B. If the body succeeds in eliminating all microorganisms, the tissue will heal and the inflammation will cease.
2. **Chronic inflammation** is a long-lived inflammatory response that continues for more than a few weeks.
   A. *The warning signs of inflammation may be absent in chronic inflammation—such as periodontitis—and the problem may go unnoticed by the host (patient). Clinically, pain is often absent.*
   B. Chronic inflammation occurs when the body is unable to eliminate the microorganisms. In this stage, the invading microorganisms are persistent and stimulate an exaggerated response by the host's immune system.
   C. The signs and symptoms of a chronic infection at times may partially or completely disappear during a period of **remission**. The signs and symptoms may recur in all their severity in an active period of disease known as **exacerbation**.

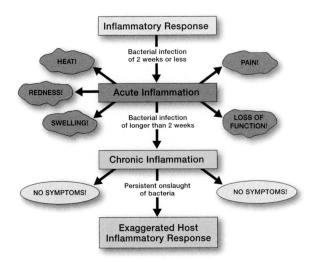

Figure 6-2. Two Stages of Inflammation. Acute inflammation is of short duration, whereas chronic inflammation is a long-lived inflammatory response.

SECTION 2: IMMUNE SYSTEM COMPONENTS

Humans are surrounded by millions of microorganisms, many of which may prove to be deadly. For this reason, the human immune system attempts to control quickly the spread of invading microorganisms. The body recognizes bacteria, viruses, fungi, and parasites as something foreign to itself and responds by (i) sending certain types of cells to the infection site and (ii) producing substances to counteract the foreign invaders. Components of the immune system that play an important role in combating periodontal disease are the (i) cellular defenders (phagocytes, lymphocytes), and (ii) the complement system.

CELLULAR COMPONENTS

1. **Phagocytes. Phagocytes** (literally cell eaters) are leukocytes that can ingest (engulf) and digest microorganisms. The two major types of leukocytes that are active in combating periodontal pathogens are polymorphonuclear leukocytes (PMNs) and macrophages.
   A. **Phagocytosis** is the process by which leukocytes engulf and digest microorganisms.
      1. Steps in Phagocytosis.
         a. First, the external cell wall of a phagocytic cell (such as a neutrophil or macrophage) adheres to the bacterium (**Fig. 6-3**).
         b. Second, the phagocytic cell extends fingerlike projections that surround the bacterium.
         c. Next, the bacterium is surrounded by a phagocytic vesicle called a **phagosome**. Lysosome granules fuse with the vesicle to form a **phagolysosome**. The bacterium is digested within the phagolysosome.
         d. Finally, the phagocytic cell discharges the contents of the phagolysosome into the surrounding tissue.
      2. **Local Tissue Destruction from Phagocytosis**
         a. Lysosomal enzymes and other microbial products are released from the neutrophil after phagocytosis or when the host cell dies.
         b. Once released the lysosomal enzymes cause damage to tissue cells in the same manner that they destroy bacteria.

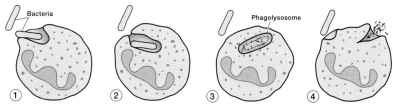

Figure 6-3. Phagocytosis. The steps in phagocytosis, the process by which leukocytes engulf and digest microorganisms.

   B. **PMNs** are leukocytes that play a vital role in combating the pathogenic bacteria responsible for periodontal disease (**Fig. 6-4**).
      1. PMNs also are known as **neutrophils**.
      2. PMNs are phagocytic cells that actively engulf and destroy microorganisms.
      3. The cytoplasm of a PMN contains many granules filled with strong bactericidal and digestive enzymes. These granules (called **lysosomes**) can kill and digest bacterial cells after phagocytosis.
      4. These cells provide the first line of defense against many common microorganisms and are essential for the control of bacterial infections.
      5. The bacteria associated with periodontal disease are most effectively phagocytized by PMNs.
      6. PMNs are short-lived cells that die when they become engorged with the bacteria they phagocytize. The pus formed at sites of inflammation contains many dead and dying PMNs.

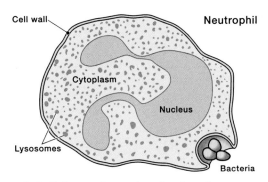

Figure 6-4. Polymorphonuclear Leukocyte.
Polymorphonuclear leukocytes (PMNs) contain lysosomes that
are used to digest bacteria.

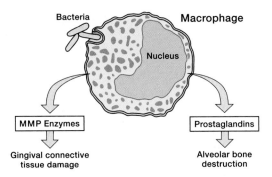

Figure 6-5. Macrophage. These phagocytic cells produce
products that damage the gingival connective tissue and alveolar
bone.

C. **Macrophages** are large leukocytes with one kidney-shaped nucleus and some
   granules (**Fig. 6-5**).
   1. These leukocytes are called **monocytes** when found in the bloodstream and
      macrophages when they are located in the tissues.
   2. Macrophages are highly phagocytic cells that actively engulf and destroy mi-
      croorganisms. Macrophages contain a few granules that are filled with bacteri-
      cidal and digestive enzymes.
   3. Macrophages are slower to arrive at the infection site than PMNs. The slower
      macrophages are often the most numerous cells in chronic inflammation.
   4. These are long-lived cells that play an important role in chronic periodontitis.
2. **Lymphocytes.** Lymphocytes are small white blood cells that play an important role
   in recognizing and controlling foreign invaders. The two main classes of lymphocytes
   are B lymphocytes and T lymphocytes.
   A. B lymphocytes also are known as B cells.
      1. Specialized **B lymphocytes**, known as plasma cells, work chiefly by secreting
         antibodies that neutralize microorganisms. Each B lymphocyte manufactures
         millions of antibodies and pours them into the bloodstream (**Fig. 6-6**).
      2. Antibodies participate in host defense in three main ways:
         1. Neutralize bacteria or bacterial toxins to prevent bacteria from destroying
            host cells.
         2. Coat bacteria making them more susceptible to phagocytosis.
         3. Activate the complement system.
      3. All antibodies have the same overall structure and are known collectively as
         immunoglobulins. The five major classes of immunoglobulin are im-
         munoglobulin M (IgM), immunoglobulin D (IgD), immunoglobulin G (IgG),
         immunoglobulin A (IgA), and immunoglobulin E (IgE).
   B. T lymphocytes
      1. T lymphocytes also are known as T cells.
      2. The main function of the **T lymphocytes** is to intensify the response of other im-
         mune cells—such as B lymphocytes and macrophages—to the bacterial invasion.

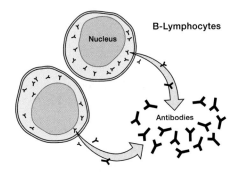

Figure 6-6. B Lymphocytes. B-lymphocytes
secrete antibodies that neutralize microorganisms.

3. **Cellular Compounds.** Immune cells secrete compounds—called **inflammatory mediators**—that activate the body's inflammatory response, Inflammatory mediators of importance in periodontitis are the cytokines, prostaglandins, and matrix metalloproteinases (Table 6-1).

A. **Cytokines** are powerful mediators produced by immune cells that influence the behavior of other cells. The cytokine (literally cell protein) is a molecule that transmits information or signals from one cell to another. When released by host cells, cytokines signal the immune system to send additional phagocytic cells to the site of an infection.

1. Cytokines are produced by many different cells, including PMNs, macrophages, B lymphocytes, epithelial cells, gingival fibroblasts, and osteoblasts in response to microorganisms or tissue injury.

2. Functions of Cytokines

   a. Recruit cells such as PMNs and macrophages to the infection site.

   b. Increase vascular permeability that leads to increased movement of immune cells and complement into the tissues.

   c. *Have the potential to initiate tissue destruction and bone loss in chronic inflammatory diseases, such as periodontitis.*

   d. Cytokines that play an important role in periodontitis include interleukin-1 (IL-1), interleukin-6 (IL-6), interleukin-8 (IL-8), and tumor necrosis factor-α (TNF-α).

B. **Prostaglandins** are a series of powerful inflammatory mediators, of which prostaglandins D, E, F, G, H, and I are the most important biologically. **Prostaglandins of the E series (PGE) play an important role in the bone destruction seen in periodontitis.**

1. Most cells can produce prostaglandins, but PMNs and macrophages are particularly important sources. The major source of PGE in inflamed periodontal tissues is the macrophage, although PMNs and gingival fibroblasts also produce them.

2. Functions of Prostaglandins

   a. Increase the permeability and dilation of the blood vessels, leading to redness and edema of the connective tissue.

   b. Trigger increased osteoclast activity. Osteoclasts are bone-consuming cells that destroy bone.

   c. Promote the overproduction of destructive MMP enzymes.

   d. *Prostaglandins initiate most of the alveolar bone destruction in periodontitis.*

C. **Matrix metalloproteinases (MMP)** are a family of at least 12 different enzymes produced by various cells of the body. These enzymes can act together to break down the connective tissue matrix.

1. MMPs are produced by PMNs, macrophages, gingival fibroblasts, and junctional epithelial cells. PMNs and gingival fibroblasts are the major source of MMPs in periodontitis.

2. MMPs Effects

   a. Under normal, healthy conditions, MMPs facilitate the normal turnover of the periodontal connective tissue matrix.

   b. In the presence of bacterial infection, large amounts of MMPs are released in an attempt to kill the invading bacteria. This overproduction of MMPs results in the breakdown of the connective tissue of the periodontium.

   c. *In the presence of increased MMP levels, extensive collagen destruction occurs in the periodontal tissues.* Collagen provides the structural framework of all periodontal tissues. Without collagen, the tissues of the gingiva, periodontal ligament, and supporting alveolar bone degrade, resulting in gingival recession, pocket formation, and tooth mobility.

Table 6-1. Tissue Destruction by Immune Mediators in Periodontitis

Mediators	Local Effects
Cytokine IL-1	Stimulates osteoclast activity resulting in bone resorption[1–4]
Cytokine IL-6	Stimulates bone resorption[5] Inhibits bone formation[6]
Cytokine IL-8	Stimulates connective tissue destruction[7,8] Stimulates bone resorption[1,3,4,9–11]
Prostaglandin E$_2$	Stimulates MMP secretion[12,13] Stimulates bone resorption[1,14–17]
MMP enzymes	Induce breakdown of collagen matrix in gingiva, periodontal ligament, and alveolar bone[18]

THE COMPLEMENT SYSTEM

In addition to the cellular defenders, the other major component of the immune response is the complement system.

1. **Definition.** The **complement system** is a series of proteins circulating in the blood that work to facilitate phagocytosis or kill bacteria directly by puncturing bacterial cell membranes.
2. **Three Principal Functions of Complement** (Fig. 6-7)
   A. **Recruitment of Phagocytes.** The complement system recruits additional phagocytic cells to the site of the infection.
   B. **Opsonization of Pathogens.** The complement system facilitates the engulfment and destruction of microorganisms by phagocytes. This process, known as **opsonization of pathogens**, is the most important action of the complement system. Complement components coat the surface of the bacterium allowing the phagocytes to recognize, engulf, and destroy the bacterium.
   C. **Destruction of Pathogens.** Components of complement can destroy certain microorganisms directly by forming pores in their cell membranes. To accomplish this task, the complement system creates a protein unit called the **membrane attack complex** that is capable of puncturing the cell membranes of certain bacteria.

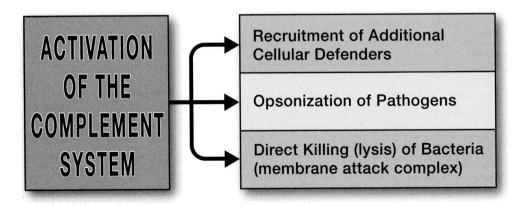

Figure 6-7. Complement System Functions. The three main functions of the complement system are recruitment of phagocytes, opsonization of bacteria, and direct killing of bacteria.

SECTION 3: HOST RESPONSE IN PERIODONTAL DISEASE

INTRODUCTION TO HOST RESPONSE

1. **Role of Bacterial Pathogens**
   A. For many years it was assumed that pathogenic bacteria were the *sole cause* of the tissue destruction seen in periodontal disease.
   B. The presence of pathogenic bacteria, however, does not necessarily mean that an individual will experience periodontitis.
      1. Some persons with abundant bacterial plaque exhibit only mild disease, while others with light bacteria plaque suffer severe disease.
      2. Untreated gingivitis does not always lead to periodontitis, and everyone infected with periodontal pathogens does not experience periodontitis.
2. **Role of the Immune System**
   A. Recent research findings indicate that *it is the body's response to the periodontal pathogens—the actions of the immune system—that is the cause of nearly all the destruction seen in periodontal disease.*
   B. When pathogenic bacteria successfully infect the periodontium, the body responds by mobilizing defensive cells and releasing a series of chemicals to combat them. This body defense mechanism is referred to as the host response.
      1. **Host response in periodontal disease** refers to the body's immune system response to periodontal pathogens invading the tissues of the periodontium.
      2. *It is the body's immune response to the bacteria that actually causes most of the destruction of periodontal tissues.*
         a. The body's immune system causes the tissue destruction in an attempt the stop the bacterial infection.
         b. *It is the complex interaction between periodontal pathogens and host response that determines the onset and severity of periodontal disease.*
2. **Characteristics of the Host Response**
   A. The intensity of the immune response varies considerably from one individual to another.
   B. The local immune response can vary in its intensity from site to site within a patient's mouth.
      1. One site may have active disease and high levels of inflammatory cells and mediators.
      2. A second site in the same mouth may have no active disease and normal levels of inflammatory cells and mediators.
      3. This variation in the intensity of immune response helps explain the episodic and site-specific nature of periodontal disease.
3. **Nature of Immune Response**
   A. The immune system has the primary function of defending the body.
   B. Once set in motion, the activity of the immune system can lead to massive tissue damage in the inflamed area.
   C. Thus, the body's immune response to infection is both protective and destructive.
4. **Microscopic Phases of Periodontal Disease**
   A. Marked changes occur in the periodontium as the result of the body's inflammatory response to bacterial invasion of the junctional epithelium and gingival connective tissue.
   B. *Page et al.*[13] *described the three distinct stages of the microscopic changes in periodontal disease:*
      1. Subclinical gingivitis (Box 6-1)
      2. Gingivitis
         a. Early gingivitis (Box 6-2)
         b. Established gingivitis (Box 6-3)
      3. Periodontitis (Box 6-4)

Box 6-1

Early Bacterial Accumulation Phase: Subclinical Gingivitis

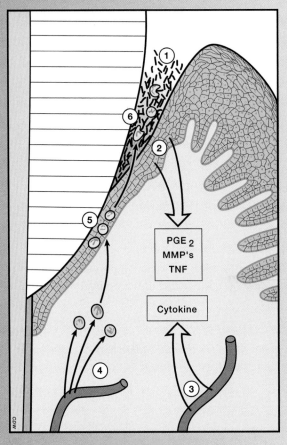

Subclinical Gingivitis—Early Bacterial Accumulation Phase. This first phase is characterized by bacterial colonization near the gingival margin.

1. Bacteria, their metabolic products, and the lipopolysaccharide (LPS) in the cell walls of gram-negative bacteria trigger the body's host response

2. In response to the bacterial challenge, the cells of the junctional epithelium release inflammatory mediators that activate the immune response.

3. Small blood vessels dilate and release cytokines to attract more polymorphonuclear leukocytes (PMNs) to the site.

4. PMNs pass from blood vessels into connective tissue.
   a. The PMNs need to reach the sulcus into order to fight the bacterial infection located there.
   b. As they pass into the gingival connective tissue the PMNs release cytokines. *Cytokines released by the PMNs destroy healthy gingival connective tissue creating a pathway that allows the PMNs to move quickly through the tissue.*
   c. The goal of the PMNs is reach the bacteria in the sulcus and destroy them. The damage to the healthy connective tissue is not a concern. In a healthy body, this tissue destruction will be repaired after the bacterial infection is brought under control.

5. PMNs migrate from connective tissue into junctional epithelium.

6. PMNs migrate into sulcus and phagocytize bacteria. If the bacterial infection is brought under control—through the efforts of the immune system and effective plaque control—the body is able to repair the destruction caused by the immune response.

Box 6-2

Plaque Overgrowth Phase: Early Gingivitis

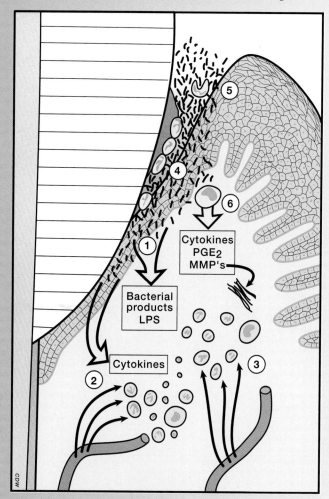

Early Gingivitis—The Plaque Overgrowth Phase.

1. If the bacterial infection is not resolved in the early accumulation phase, the bacteria penetrate through the junctional epithelium into the underlying connective tissue.

2. In response to increased numbers of bacteria, the junctional epithelium cells release inflammatory mediators to attract additional polymorphonuclear leukocytes (PMNs), macrophages, and lymphocytes to the site.

3. Increased permeability of the blood vessels allows large numbers of PMNs to rush to the site.

4. The increasing numbers of PMNs destroy additional healthy gingival connective tissue as they rush toward the bacterial invaders.

4. PMNs form a "wall of cells" between the plaque biofilm and tissue. These PMNs comprise the most important component of the local defense against bacteria.

5. The PMNs phagocytize bacteria in the sulcus in an effort to protect the host tissues from the bacterial challenge.

6. Macrophages release many inflammatory mediators including cytokines, PGE_2, and MMPs. These mediators recruit additional immune cells to the site. If the bacterial infection is brought under control—through the efforts of the immune system and effective plaque control—the body is able to repair the destruction caused by the immune response.

Box 6-3

Subgingival Plaque Phase: Established Gingivitis

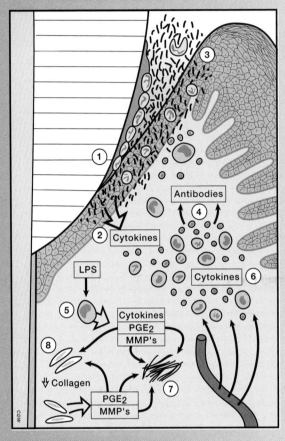

Established Gingivitis—Subgingival Plaque Phase.

1. Subgingival plaque extends into the gingival sulcus, disrupting the coronal-most portion of the junctional epithelium.
2. Macrophages and lymphocytes, recruited to the area, become the most numerous cells in the tissue.
3. Polymorphonuclear leukocytes (PMNs) continue to battle in the sulcus.
4. Lymphocytes produce large quantities of antibodies to assist in the fight against bacteria.
5. The immune system keeps sending more immune cells to fight the bacteria. More toxic chemicals are released and additional healthy connective tissue is destroyed. Macrophages exposed to gram-negative bacteria produce cytokines, prostaglandins of the E series (PGE)$_2$, and MMPs.
6. Cytokines recruit additional macrophages and lymphocytes to the area.
7. PGE$_2$ and the MMPs cause destruction of collagen fibers in the gingival connective tissue.
8. PGE$_2$ stimulates the gingival fibroblasts to produce additional PGE$_2$ and MMPs. If the bacterial infection is brought under control—through the efforts of the immune system and effective plaque control—the body is able to repair the destruction caused by the immune response. In certain susceptible individuals, if the bacterial infection is not controlled, gingivitis progresses to periodontitis. Unfortunately, no one cannot predict when and if gingivitis will progress to periodontitis. Much current research is directed to trying to determine which individuals are at risk for developing periodontitis.

Box 6-4

Tissue Destruction Phase: Periodontitis

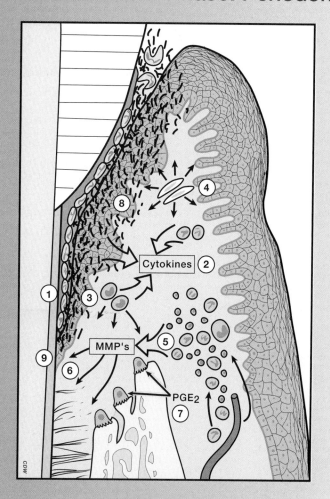

Periodontitis—Tissue Destruction Phase. This phase represents a change from previous phases (in which the host is controlling the bacterial challenge) to a stage in which the bacterial challenge is not well controlled and tissue destruction is evident. The bacteria flourish in the biofilm, protected from host defenses.

1. The plaque biofilm grows laterally and apically along the root surface, and the transition from gingivitis to periodontitis is initiated. This relentless bacterial challenge sets the stage for the tissue destruction of periodontitis.

2. The immune system keeps trying to eliminate the bacteria but the bacteria are not eliminated. As more and more immune cells rush to the site, more tissue is damaged. The tissue destruction caused by the immune response now over-whelms any tissue repair. Tissue destruction becomes the main outcome of the immune system response.

3. Macrophages produce high concentrations of cytokines, PGE$_2$, and MMPs that result in *destruction of connective tissue and alveolar bone*.

4. Gingival fibroblasts shift to a state that favors the *destruction of the gingival connective tissue and periodontal ligament fibers*.

5–6. PMNs and lymphocytes produce MMPs. MMPs cause *destruction of the gingival connective tissue and periodontal ligament fibers*.

7. Osteoclasts, stimulated by PGE$_2$, *destroy the crest of the alveolar bone*.

8–9. The junctional epithelium extends rete ridges into the connective tissue and migrates apically along the tooth root.

CHAPTER SUMMARY STATEMENT

Periodontal disease is a bacterial infection of the periodontium. The presence of pathogenic bacteria, however, does not necessarily mean that an individual will experience periodontitis.

■ Some persons with abundant bacterial plaque exhibit gingivitis, while others with light dental plaque experience severe periodontitis.
■ Untreated gingivitis does not always lead to periodontitis, and everyone infected with periodontal pathogens does not experience periodontitis.

   Additional factors, other than the presence of bacteria, play a significant role in determining why some individuals are more susceptible to periodontal disease than others.

■ When pathogenic bacteria successfully infect the periodontium, the body responds by mobilizing defensive cells and releasing a series of chemicals to combat them.
■ This body defense mechanism is referred to as the host response.
■ *It is the body's immune response to the bacteria that actually causes most of the destruction of periodontal tissues.*

   The microscopic changes in periodontal disease are described as three distinct phases: (i) subclinical gingivitis, (ii) gingivitis, and (iii) periodontitis. For the periodontium to remain healthy, the bacterial infection must be controlled so as not to trigger an exaggerated host immune response.

SECTION 4: FOCUS ON PATIENTS

CASE 1
You suddenly injure your arm by accidentally stabbing it with an ice pick. Within minutes following the injury, you note some changes in the tissues in the area of the injury. What changes in the tissues should you expect if your body responds with a typical inflammatory response?

CASE 2
A patient who has been previously treated for chronic periodontitis and has been followed by your dental team for several years, calls your dental office with a concern. She is scheduled to undergo a liver transplant and has been warned by her physician that the medications she will need will make her more susceptible to infections. She asks if these medications might have an effect on her continuing treatment for periodontitis. How might you respond to her concern?

CASE 3
In reading a dental journal you find an article that describes a new medication that is reported to stop collagen destruction by one of the matrix metalloproteinases (MMPs). If this new medication does indeed block such collagen destruction, what effect might this medication have on a patient with periodontitis?

References

1. Schwartz Z., Goultshin J, Dean DD, et al. Mechanisms of alveolar bone destruction in periodontitis. *Periodontol 2000.* 1997; 14:158–172.
2. Gowen M, Meikle MC, Reynolds JJ. Stimulation of bone resorption in vitro by a non-prostanoid factor released by human monocytes in culture. *Biochim Biophys Acta.* 1983;762:471–474.
3. Qwarnstrom EE, MacFarlane SA, Page RC. Effects of interleukin-1 on fibroblast extracellular matrix, using a 3-dimensional culture system. *J Cell Physiol.* 1989;139:501–508.
4. Stashenko P, Dewhirst FE, Peros WJ, et al. Synergistic interactions between interleukin 1, tumor necrosis factor, and lymphotoxin in bone resorption. *J Immunol.* 1987;138:1464–1468.
5. Roodman GD. Interleukin-6: An osteotropic factor? *J Bone Miner Res.* 1992;7: 475–478.
6. Hughes FJ, Howells GL. Interleukin-6 inhibits bone formation in vitro. *Bone Miner.* 1993;21:21–28.
7. Meikle MC, Atkinson SJ, Ward RV, et al. Gingival fibroblasts degrade type I collagen films when stimulated with tumor necrosis factor and interleukin 1: Evidence that breakdown is mediated by metalloproteinases. *J Periodontal Res.* 1989;24:207–213.
8. Dayer JM, Beutler B, Cerami A. Cachectin/tumor necrosis factor stimulates collagenase and prostaglandin E2 production by human synovial cells and dermal fibroblasts. *J Exp Med.* 1985;162:2163–2168.
9. Bertolini DR, Nedwin GE, Bringman TS, et al. Stimulation of bone resorption and inhibition of bone formation in vitro by human tumour necrosis factors. *Nature.*, 1986;319:516–518.
10. Mundy GR. Inflammatory mediators and the destruction of bone. *J Periodontal Res.* 1991;26(3 Pt 2):213–217.
11. Thomson BM, Mundy GR, Chambers TJ. Tumor necrosis factors alpha and beta induce osteoblastic cells to stimulate osteoclastic bone resorption. *J Immunol.* 1987;138:775–779.
12. Gemmell E, Marshall RI, Seymour GJ. Cytokines and prostaglandins in immune homeostasis and tissue destruction in periodontal disease. *Periodontol 2000.* 1997;14:112–143.
13. Page RC, Offenbacher S, Schroeder HE, et al. Advances in the pathogenesis of periodontitis: Summary of developments, clinical implications and future directions. *Periodontol 2000,* 1997;14:216–248.
14. Dietrich JW, Goodson JM, Raisz LG. Stimulation of bone resorption by various prostaglandins in organ culture. *Prostaglandins.* 1975;10:231–240.
15. Goodson JM, Dewhirst FE, Brunetti A. Prostaglandin E2 levels and human periodontal disease. *Prostaglandins* 1974;6:81–85.
16. Offenbacher S, Farr DH, Goodson JM. Measurement of prostaglandin E in crevicular fluid. *J Clin Periodontol.* 1981;8:359–367.
17. ElAttar TM, Lin Hs. Prostaglandins in gingiva of patients with periodontal disease. *J Periodontol.* 1981;52:16–19.
18. Reynolds JJ,. Meikle MC. Mechanisms of connective tissue matrix destruction in periodontitis. *Periodontol 2000.* 1997;14:144–157.

Suggested Reading

Page RC, Offenbacher S, Schroeder HE, et al. Advances in the pathogenesis of periodontitis: Summary of developments, clinical implications, and future directions. *Periodontol 2000.* 1997;14:216–248.

AQ1

SECTION 5: CHAPTER REVIEW QUESTIONS

1. The primary purpose of the immune system when it responds to a bacterial infection of the periodontium is to:
   A. Defend the life of the host (the individual with the bacterial infection)
   B. Identify the bacterial invaders
   C. Preserve the tooth and its periodontium so that no teeth are lost
   D. Phagocytize bacteria at the site

2. All of the following are classic symptoms of inflammation, EXCEPT:
   A. Loss of function
   B. Bruising
   C. Swelling
   D. Heat

3. In which stage of inflammation is pain a <u>common</u> symptom?
   A. Acute inflammation
   B. Chronic inflammation

4. Which of these immune cells secrete antibodies?
   A. Macrophages
   B. Polymorphonuclear leukocytes
   C. B lymphocytes
   D. T lymphocytes

5. Which of the following is a series of proteins circulating in the bloodstream that facilitate the destruction of bacteria?
   A. Immune mediators
   B. Prostaglandins
   C. Matrix metalloproteinase (MMP) enzymes
   D. Complement system

6. When polymorphonuclear leukocytes (PMNs) rush to the site of infection of the periodontium, they release substances that destroy healthy gingival connective tissue. What is the advance of connective tissue destruction in this instance?
   A. The tissue needs to be destroyed just in case some bacteria are in the tissue.
   B. The connective tissue destruction existed before the PMNs arrived in the tissue.
   C. Tissue destruction allows the blood vessels to dilate.
   D. This creates a pathway for the PMNs to move quickly through the tissue.

7. Which of the following is the cause of nearly all the destruction seen in periodontitis?
   A. Bacteria
   B. Host response

8. The immune mediators secreted by the immune cells are responsible for which of the following tissue destruction seen in periodontitis?
   A. Destruction of gingival connective tissue
   B. Resorption of alveolar bone
   C. Breakdown of periodontal ligament
   D. All of the above

Chapter

7 Local Contributing Factors

Refer to the CD packaged with this book for full color versions of the clinical photographs in this chapter.

Learning Objectives

- Define the terms pathogenicity and local contributing factors.
- Describe two common local contributing factors that can increase plaque retention.
- Explain how local contributing factors can lead to an increased pathogenicity of plaque.
- Describe four local contributing factors that can lead to direct damage to the periodontium.
- In the clinical setting, point out local contributing factors in a patient's oral cavity to your clinical instructor.

KEY TERMS

Disease sites
Local contributing factors
Pathogenicity
Dental calculus
Pellicle
Overhanging restoration
Palatogingival groove
Trauma from occlusion
Primary trauma from
    occlusion

Secondary trauma from
    occlusion
Functional occlusal forces
Parafunctional occlusal
    forces
Clenching
Bruxism
Occlusal adjustment
Food impaction

Tongue thrusting
Mouth breathing
Embrasure space
Encroaching on the
    embrasure space
Prosthesis
Removable prosthesis

SECTION 1: INTRODUCTION TO LOCAL CONTRIBUTING FACTORS

1. Local contributing factors for periodontal disease are oral conditions that increase an individual's susceptibility to periodontal infection in specific sites.
   A. It is critical for the dental team to recognize local contributing factors for periodontal disease. Contributing factors should be eliminated or minimized during the nonsurgical periodontal treatment.
      1. The conditions discussed in this chapter refer to circumstances that favor periodontal breakdown and can contribute to gingivitis or periodontitis in individual sites in the mouth.
      2. In this context, disease sites mean individual teeth or specific surfaces of a tooth that are experiencing periodontal destruction.
      3. Examples of potential local contributing factors include dental calculus, faulty dental restorations, developmental defects, dental decay, patient habits, and trauma from occlusion.
   B. Local contributing factors *do not initiate* either gingivitis or periodontitis but only act to contribute to the disease process previously initiated by bacterial plaque.
      1. Local contributing factors may increase the risk of developing gingivitis or periodontitis.
      2. Local contributing factors may also increase the risk of developing more severe disease when gingivitis or periodontitis are already established.
      3. Local contributing factors should not be confused with the systemic conditions that can affect the periodontium. Systemic contributing factors that can increase a patient's overall susceptibility to periodontal infection are discussed in Chapter 8.
2. **Mechanisms.** Local contributing factors can increase the risk of developing gingivitis or periodontitis through several mechanisms.
   A. There are three mechanisms by which local factors can increase the risk of periodontal disease.
      1. A local factor can increase plaque retention.
      2. A local factor can increase plaque pathogenicity.
         a. Pathogenicity is the ability of a disease-causing agent to produce a disease.
         b. In the dental context, pathogenicity is the ability of the dental plaque biofilm to cause periodontal disease.
      3. A local factor can cause direct damage to the periodontium.
   B. Local contributing factors may increase disease risk through any of these three mechanisms and may also increase the severity of existing gingivitis or periodontitis through these mechanisms.
   C. Table 7-1 summarizes mechanisms for increasing disease risk in local sites, and each of these mechanisms is discussed in detail in the following sections of this chapter.

Table 7-1. Mechanisms for Increasing Disease Risk in Local Sites

Mechanism	Clinical Example
Local factor that increases plaque retention	Rough edge on a restoration harbors plaque and makes it difficult to remove plaque with a brush and floss
Local factor that increases plaque pathogenicity	Calculus, which harbors plaque, allowing it to grow uninhibited for an extended period of time
Local factor that can inflict damage to the periodontium	Heavy occlusal forces on a tooth that far exceed the tooth's normal capacity to adapt

SECTION 2: LOCAL FACTORS THAT INCREASE PLAQUE RETENTION

This section presents local risk factors that can increase plaque retention. Most often these factors include rough or irregular surfaces that *decrease the effectiveness of self-care.*

DENTAL CALCULUS

Dental calculus is the most obvious example of a local environmental factor that can lead to increased plaque retention. **Dental calculus** is mineralized bacterial plaque, covered on its external surface by nonmineralized, living bacterial plaque. Mineralization of plaque can begin from 48 hours up to 2 weeks after plaque formation.

1. **Effects of Calculus on the Periodontium**
    A. The surface of a calculus deposit is irregular and is always covered with disease-causing bacteria. Thus, even calculus that has not built up enough to result in a ledge or irregular tooth contour can lead to plaque retention in the site simply because of the rough nature of the calculus surface and its tendency to harbor bacteria.
    B. As dental calculus deposits build up, they can lead to irregular surfaces, ledges on the teeth, and other alterations of the contours of the teeth (**Fig. 7-1**). All these contour changes can result in areas of plaque retention that are difficult or impossible for a patient to clean.
    C. Since a living layer of bacterial plaque always covers a calculus deposit, dental calculus plays a significant role as a local contributing factor in periodontal disease. Plaque retention in sites with dental calculus can subsequently lead to increased risk for disease in these sites.
    D. It is difficult to bring either gingivitis or periodontitis under control in the presence of dental calculus, and the importance of removing these deposits cannot be overemphasized. The removal of dental calculus is discussed in Chapter 17.

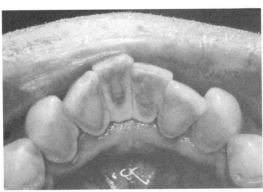
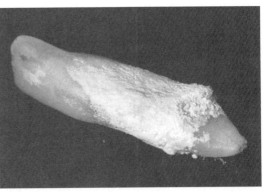

A   **B**

Figure 7-1A and 7-1B. Irregular Surface of Calculus Deposits. A: Heavy calculus deposits on the lingual surfaces of the mandibular anterior teeth. These deposits are so large that they interfere with the patient's plaque control efforts. In addition, calculus deposits harbor living bacteria that are in contact with the gingival tissue. B: Calculus deposit on the crown and root surfaces of an extracted mandibular canine. (Photograph B courtesy of Dr. Don Rolfs, Periodontal Foundations, Wenatchee, WA.)

2. **Composition of Dental Calculus**
    A. Inorganic Portion
        1. The inorganic portion makes up 70% to 90% of the composition of calculus.
        2. This inorganic portion of dental calculus is primarily calcium phosphate.
        3. Dental calculus also contains some calcium carbonate and magnesium phosphate.
        4. The inorganic portion of calculus is similar to the inorganic portion of bone.
    B. Organic Portion
        1. The organic portion makes up 10% to 30% of the composition of calculus.

    2. Components of the organic portion include materials derived from plaque, derived from dead epithelial cells, and derived from dead white blood cells.

3. Types of Dental Calculus

  A. Crystalline Forms of Dental Calculus. As calculus ages on a tooth surface, the inorganic component changes through several different crystalline forms.

    1. Newly formed calculus appears as a crystalline form called brushite.

    2. In deposits less than 6 months old, the crystalline form is primarily octocalcium phosphate.

    3. In mature deposits that are more than 6 months old, the crystalline form is primarily hydroxyapatite.

  B. Location of Calculus Deposits

    1. Supragingival Deposits—calculus deposits located coronal to (above) the gingival margin. Other terms that have been used to refer to deposits above the gingival margin are supramarginal calculus and salivary calculus.

      a. Distribution—supragingival deposits usually are found in localized areas of the dentition, such as lingual surfaces of mandibular anteriors, facial surfaces of maxillary molars, and on teeth that are crowded or in malocclusion.

      b. Shape—supragingival deposits most often are irregular, large deposits.

    2. Subgingival Deposits—calculus deposits located apical to (below) the gingival margin. Other terms that have been used for deposits below the gingival margin are submarginal calculus or serumal calculus.

      a. Distribution—subgingival deposits may be localized in certain areas or generalized throughout the mouth.

      b. Shape—subgingival deposits are most often flattened. The shape of the deposit may be guided by pressure of the pocket wall against the deposit.

  C. Modes of Attachment to Tooth Surfaces. Dental calculus attaches to tooth surfaces through several modes; different attachment mechanisms can exist in the same calculus deposit.

    1. Attachment by Means of Pellicle

      a. The **pellicle** is a thin, bacteria-free membrane that forms on the surface of the tooth during the late stages of eruption.

      b. This mode of attachment occurs most commonly on enamel tooth surfaces.

      c. Calculus deposits are removed easily because the attachment is on the surface of the pellicle (and not locked into the tooth surface).

    2. Attachment to Irregularities in the Tooth Surface

      a. Tooth irregularities include cracks—tiny openings left where periodontal ligament fibers are detached—and grooves in cemental surfaces as the result of overinstrumentation during previous calculus removal procedures.

      b. Complete calculus removal is difficult since deposits lie sheltered in these tooth defects.

    3. Attachment by Direct Contact of the Calcified Component and the Tooth Surface

      a. In this mode of attachment, the matrix of the calculus deposit is interlocked with the inorganic crystals of the tooth.

      b. Deposits, firmly interlocked in the tooth surface, are difficult to remove.

TOOTH MORPHOLOGY

1. Poorly Contoured Restorations

  A. When a dentist places a restoration, it is not always possible to contour the restoration perfectly smoothly with the existing tooth structure. This condition is referred to as an **overhanging restoration** or overhang (**Fig. 7-2**).

  B. Because of difficulty in access to tooth surfaces protected by an overhang, it is often impossible for a patient to remove plaque effectively from the tooth surface adjacent to an overhang. This leads to plaque retention in the site and can subsequently lead to increased severity of either gingivitis or periodontitis in the site.

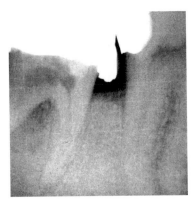

Figure 7-2. Radiographic Evidence of a Poorly Contoured Restoration. Note that the restoration on the molar tooth is not smoothly contoured with the tooth surface and would lead to plaque retention in this area. (Courtesy of Dr. Don Rolfs, Periodontal Foundations, Wenatchee, WA.)

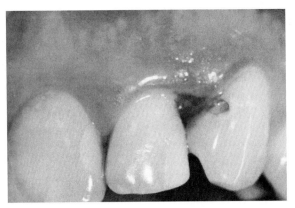

Figure 7-3. Untreated Decay. Note that this untreated tooth decay leaves an actual hole in the tooth surface that harbors periodontal pathogens. (Courtesy of Dr. Don Rolfs, Periodontal Foundations, Wenatchee, WA.)

2. **Untreated Tooth Decay.** Untreated tooth decay is another example of a local contributing factor that can increase plaque retention. Since tooth decay can result in defects in tooth structure (dental cavities), these defects can also act as protected environments for bacteria that cause gingivitis and periodontitis to live and grow undisturbed (Fig. 7-3).

3. **Tooth Grooves or Concavities**
   A. Naturally occurring developmental grooves and concavities frequently lead to difficulty in plaque control in the site and can be a local contributing factor for gingivitis and periodontitis.
   B. During development of some incisor teeth, a groove forms on the palatal surface of the tooth. This groove is a developmental defect called a **palatogingival groove**. Plaque retention is common in a palatogingival groove since the groove is difficult to clean (Fig. 7-4).
   C. Some tooth root surfaces have naturally occurring concavities that can lead to plaque retention when those root surfaces become exposed through attachment loss caused by periodontitis (Fig. 7-5).

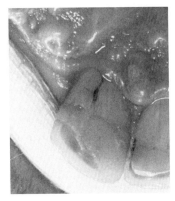

Figure 7-4. Palatogingival Groove. The palatogingival groove on this maxillary lateral incisor can result in plaque retention in the site.

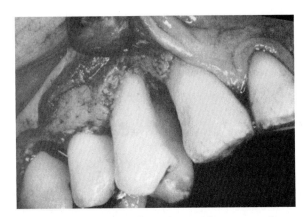

Figure 7-5. Root Concavity. The mesial root concavity on a maxillary first premolar. This photograph was taken during a periodontal surgical procedure designed to allow better visualization and treatment of the root concavity.

SECTION 3: LOCAL FACTORS THAT INCREASE PLAQUE PATHOGENICITY

Section 2 examined local contributing factors that can result in plaque retention and an increase in the mass of plaque at a given site. Section 3 looks at how local contributing factors may result in increased plaque pathogenicity. Plaque pathogenicity relates to the character of the plaque rather than simply an increase in the amount of plaque.

UNDISTURBED PLAQUE GROWTH

1. **Plaque Maturation**
   A. Plaque allowed to grow undisturbed is said to mature. As plaque matures, it becomes colonized with large numbers of disease-causing bacteria.
   B. Starting with a perfectly clean tooth surface, plaque bacteria accumulate in a predictable pattern on any tooth surface not being cleaned by the patient. This predictable pattern for plaque development is briefly outlined below.
      1. Immediately after cleaning, salivary proteins attach to the tooth surface and form the pellicle.
      2. Within the first 2 days, the tooth surface covered by pellicle becomes colonized with gram-positive facultative cocci. These bacteria can cause gingivitis but do not cause periodontitis.
      3. Over the next week, other bacteria enter the plaque. These new bacteria can cause periodontitis.
         a. The bacteria in this early stage of plaque development include some gram-negative anaerobic cocci and gram-negative rods.
         b. In addition, at this stage there are *Fusobacterium* sp. and *Prevotella intermedia*.
      4. Later, other bacteria including *Porphyromonas gingivalis* colonize the plaque. This bacterium is also associated with causing periodontitis.
2. **Increased Plaque Pathogenicity**
   A. Pathogenicity is the ability of the bacteria in the dental plaque biofilm to produce periodontal disease.
      1. Plaque left undisturbed and allowed to mature is eventually colonized by bacteria known to cause periodontitis.
      2. A mature plaque biofilm is more pathogenic than the plaque that first developed on the tooth surface (Fig. 7-6).
   B. Increased plaque pathogenicity is closely related to some of the factors discussed under increased plaque retention. The factors discussed in Section 1 cannot only allow an increase in the amount of plaque, they can also allow plaque to mature and increase in pathogenicity.

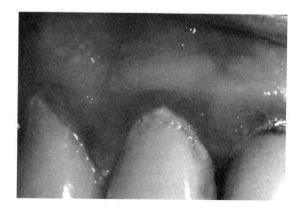

Figure 7-6. Mature Dental Plaque. Note the thick dental plaque at the gingival margin of the lateral incisor in this photograph. This plaque has been present for several weeks and is more pathogenic than a less mature plaque biofilm.

SECTION 4: LOCAL FACTORS THAT CAUSE DIRECT DAMAGE

Section 4 considers a few of the local risk factors that may cause direct damage to the periodontium. These factors also may alter the progress of periodontitis at individual sites. Some local contributing factors that can directly damage the periodontium include occlusal forces, food impaction, patient habits, and faulty restorations or appliances.

DIRECT DAMAGE FROM OCCLUSAL FORCES

1. **Trauma from Occlusion**
   A. Definition
      Direct damage to the periodontium can result from heavy occlusal forces on the teeth. When excessive occlusal forces cause damage to the periodontium, this is referred to as **trauma from occlusion**. When trauma from occlusion occurs, alveolar bone resorption can result, allowing for more rapid destruction by any existing periodontitis (**Fig. 7-7**).
   B. Signs and Symptoms of Trauma from Occlusion
      1. Clinical Signs and Symptoms
         a. Tooth mobility
         b. Sensitivity to pressure
         c. Migration of teeth
      2. Radiographic Signs of Trauma from Occlusion
         a. Enlarged, funnel-shaped periodontal ligament space
         b. Alveolar bone resorption

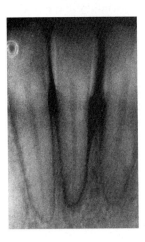

Figure 7-7. Radiographic Evidence of Trauma from Occlusion. Note the absence of alveolar bone along the lateral root surfaces on the mandibular right central incisor (center tooth). The alveolar bone has been destroyed because of the pressures resulting from trauma from occlusion.

   C. Types of Occlusal Trauma
      Trauma from occlusion has been classified as either primary trauma from occlusion or secondary trauma from occlusion.
      1. **Primary trauma from occlusion** is defined as excessive occlusal forces on a healthy periodontium.
         a. Examples of causes of primary trauma from occlusion include placement of a high restoration or insertion of a fixed bridge or partial denture that places excessive force on the abutment teeth
         b. The changes seen in primary occlusal trauma include a wider periodontal ligament space, tooth mobility, and even pain. These changes are reversible if the trauma is removed.
      2. **Secondary trauma from occlusion** is defined as normal occlusal forces on an unhealthy periodontium previously weakened by periodontitis.

a. Secondary trauma from occlusion occurs to a tooth in which the surrounding periodontium has experienced apical migration of the junctional epithelium and loss of connective tissue attachment. In this type of trauma, the periodontium was unhealthy prior to experiencing excessive occlusal forces.

b. A tooth with an unhealthy, inflamed periodontium that is subjected to excessive occlusal forces may experience rapid bone loss and pocket formation (**Fig. 7-8**).

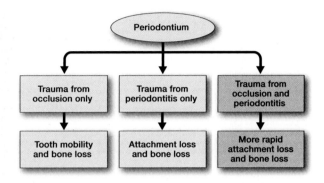

Figure 7-8. Possible Effects of Trauma from Occlusion. The combination of trauma from occlusion with periodontitis can result in more rapid attachment loss and more rapid alveolar bone loss.

2. **Parafunctional Occlusal Forces.** The two types of occlusal forces produced by the muscles of mastication are functional and parafunctional occlusal forces.
   A. **Functional occlusal forces** are the normal forces produced during the act of chewing food.
   B. **Parafunctional occlusal forces** result from tooth-to-tooth contact made when not in the act of eating.
      1. Examples of these parafunctional habits are clenching of the teeth together as a release of nervous tension or grinding the teeth together for the same release. These parafunctional habits can occur without the person having conscious knowledge of the habit. Some individuals exhibit these habits while asleep.
         a. **Clenching** is the continuous or intermittent forceful closure of the maxillary teeth against the mandibular teeth.
         b. **Bruxism** is forceful grinding of the teeth.
      2. Parafunctional habits can exert excessive force on the teeth and to the periodontium.
      3. There are several clinical therapies that can be used by a dentist to help control the damage from trauma from occlusion. When the trauma is a result of a faulty bite (referred to as a faulty occlusion), the dentist can make minor adjustments in the bite to minimize the damaging forces. This procedure is called an **occlusal adjustment**. When the trauma is a result of bruxism, the dentist can fabricate an acrylic appliance known as a night guard appliance that can protect the teeth during part of each day.

DIRECT DAMAGE DUE TO FOOD IMPACTION

1. **Definition. Food impaction** refers to forcing food (such as pieces of tough meat) between teeth during chewing, trapping the food in the interdental area.
2. **Effect of Food Impaction**
   A. Food forced into a tooth sulcus can strip the gingival tissues away from the tooth surface and contribute to periodontal breakdown.
   B. Food impaction not only damages the gingival tissues directly, but can also lead to alterations in gingival contour that result in interdental areas that are difficult for patients to clean (**Fig. 7-9**).

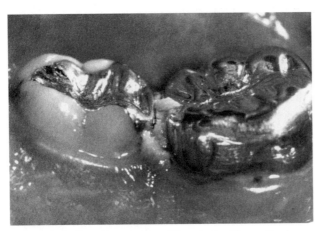

Figure 7-9. Food Impaction. Note the food impaction between the two molar teeth. (Courtesy of Dr. Don Rolfs, Periodontal Foundations, Wenatchee, WA.)

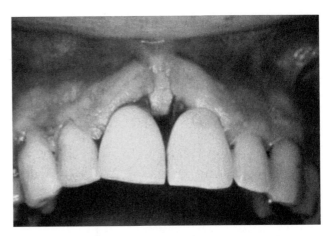

Figure 7-10. Misuse of Toothpick. The interdental papilla between the two central incisors has been destroyed by the patient's habit of repeatedly forcing a toothpick between the teeth.

DIRECT DAMAGE FROM PATIENT HABITS

1. **Description.** Patient habits such as tongue thrusting, mouth breathing, or the improper use of toothpicks and other interdental aids can cause direct damage to the periodontium.
2. **Improper use.** Improper use of interdental aids can result in direct damage to the gingival tissues causing loss of the physiological contours of the tissues (**Fig. 7-10**).
3. **Tongue thrusting** is the application of forceful pressure against the anterior teeth with the tongue.
   A. Tongue thrusting is often the result of an abnormal tongue positioning during the initial stage of swallowing.
   B. This oral habit exerts excessive lateral pressure against the teeth and may be traumatic to the periodontium (**Fig. 7-11**).
   C. **Mouth breathing** is the process of inhaling and exhaling air primarily through the mouth, rather than the nose, and often occurs while the patient is sleeping. Mouth breathing has a tendency to dry out the gingival tissues in the anterior region of the mouth.

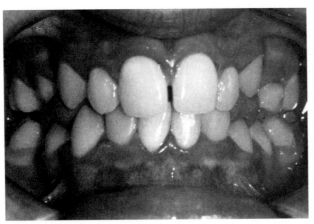
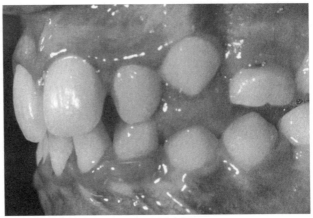

A   **B**

Figure 7-11A and 7-11B. Tongue Thrust. A: Facial view of a patient with a tongue thrust. Note that the patient applies lateral pressure with her tongue against the anterior teeth. **B:** Side view of the tongue thrust. The tongue is visible in the canine region of the mouth as the patient presses her tongue forward when swallowing. (Courtesy of Dr. Don Rolfs, Periodontal Foundations, Wenatchee, WA.)

DIRECT DAMAGE DUE TO FAULTY RESTORATIONS AND APPLIANCES

1. **Faulty Crown Design.** A **crown** is a metal, ceramic, or ceramic-bonded-to-metal covering for a badly damaged tooth. Placing a crown on a damaged tooth is a common mechanism used to preserve the life of the tooth.
   A. Crowns can sometimes be placed inappropriately when tooth structure is minimal. There can be direct damage to the periodontium when the edges of a crown—called margins—are placed below the gingival margin and too near the alveolar bone.
   B. *A crown margin that is closer than 2 mm to the crest of the alveolar bone can result in resorption of alveolar bone* (**Fig. 7-12**).

2. **Improperly Contoured Restoration**
   A. Bulky crowns or restorations can result in inadequate space between the teeth to accommodate the interdental papilla.
   B. The open space apical to the contact area of two adjacent teeth is referred to as an **embrasure space.** In health, the embrasure space is filled by an interdental papilla.
   C. Bulky crowns reduce the embrasure space so that inadequate space exists between the teeth to accommodate the interdental papilla. In this situation, the bulky crowns are described as **encroaching upon the embrasure space** (**Fig. 7-13**).

3. **Faulty Removable Prosthesis**
   A. A **prosthesis** is an appliance used to replace missing teeth.
      1. A **removable prosthesis** is one that the patient can remove for cleaning and before going to bed. A removable prosthesis is commonly called a removable denture.
      2. A removable prosthesis should be differentiated from a fixed prosthesis. A fixed prosthesis is a prosthesis that is cemented to the teeth (fixed bridge).
   B. A damaged or poorly fitting removable prosthesis can impinge on gingival tissue and favor plaque accumulation and thus hasten the progress of periodontitis (**Fig. 7-14**).

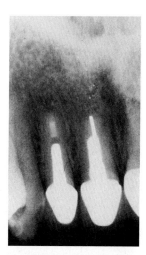

Figure 7-12. Direct Damage to the Periodontium. This radiograph reveals a crown with a margin that is approximately 1 mm from the alveolar bone. This distance is too close to bone to allow for normal soft tissue attachment to the tooth.

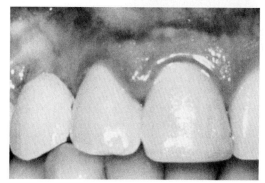

Figure 7-13. Bulky Crown Encroaching on Interdental Space.
The crowns shown here are so bulky in contour that they fill the embrasure space leaving no room for the papilla. Note the papilla between the central and lateral incisors appears enlarged because it is being pushed from between the teeth.

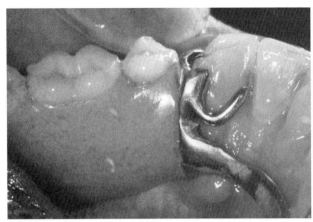
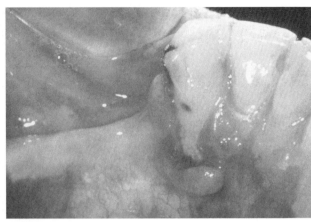

A   B

Figure 7-14A and 7-14B. Tissue Damage by a Poorly Fitting Removable Prosthesis. A: A photograph showing a removable prosthesis (lower partial denture) that replaces the extracted posterior teeth. B: With the prosthesis removed, the tissue damage to the mandibular canine is revealed. Gingival recession on the canine is due in part to the clasp of the faulty prosthesis impinging upon the gingival tissue. (Courtesy of Dr. Don Rolfs, Periodontal Foundations, Wenatchee, WA.)

CHAPTER SUMMARY STATEMENT

Local contributing factors can (i) increase the risk of developing gingivitis or periodontitis or (ii) increase the risk of developing more severe disease when gingivitis or periodontitis are already established. The three mechanisms in which local factors can increase the risk of periodontal disease are by (i) increasing plaque retention, (ii) increasing plaque pathogenicity, and (iii) causing direct damage to the periodontium. As will be discussed in Chapter 12, the dental team must identify these local contributing factors during a clinical assessment so that any local contributing factors can be eliminated or minimized during the nonsurgical periodontal treatment.

SECTION 5: FOCUS ON PATIENTS

CASE 1
Examination of a patient reveals gingivitis. In addition, the patient has generalized calculus deposits and numerous restorations with overhangs. What steps might be necessary to bring the gingivitis under control in this patient?

CASE 2
In a dental hygiene journal you find an article that refers to mature dental plaque. How might the author be expected to define mature dental plaque?

CASE 3
Examination of a patient reveals periodontitis. The patient also has a severe tooth clenching habit. Explain how the tooth clenching habit could be related to the progress of the periodontitis.

SECTION 6: CHAPTER REVIEW QUESTIONS

1. Calculus is considered a local risk factor because
   A. The surface of calculus is irregular and provides a handy place for bacteria to grow undisturbed
   B. The bacteria derive many of their needed nutrients from the hard calculus deposits
   C. The surface of calculus can damage the adjacent soft tissue through direct trauma
   D. It is the primary cause of periodontal disease

2. Which of the following is NOT a mechanism for attachment of calculus to a tooth surface?
   A. Attachment by means of pellicle
   B. Attachment to the blood clots that can form on the tooth
   C. Attachment to irregularities that occur in the surface of a tooth
   D. Attachment by direct contact of the calcified component and the tooth surface

3. The term overhanging restoration refers to restorations (or fillings) that:
   A. Are accidentally placed on the wrong tooth
   B. Are not perfectly smooth with the adjacent tooth surface
   C. Contain grooves or concavities in the surface of the restoration
   D. Cover the entire anatomical crown of the tooth

4. Pathogenicity of plaque refers to
   A. The ability of plaque to contribute to tooth staining
   B. The likelihood that the patient will be able to detect the plaque
   C. Damage to the periodontium from occlusal forces
   D. Disease causing potential of the plaque

5. Parafunctional occlusal forces are forces placed on the teeth that
   A. Occur only during the act of chewing food
   B. Occur from repeated use of chewing gum
   C. Result from tooth to tooth contact other than during chewing food
   D. Can be detected only after occlusal adjustment

6. Which of the following can result in direct damage to the periodontium?
   A. Failure to remove plaque from the surfaces of teeth
   B. A dental prosthesis that impinges on the gingiva
   C. Way too many soft foods in the diet
   D. Both (a) and (b)

Chapter

8 Systemic Contributing Factors

Refer to the CD packaged with this book for full color versions of the clinical photographs in this chapter.

Learning Objectives

- Define and give examples of the term contributing risk factors.
- For a patient in your care with periodontitis, explain to your clinical instructor the factors that may have contributed to your patient's periodontitis.
- Discuss the importance of smoking as a risk factor for periodontitis.
- Define the terms type 1 diabetes, type 2 diabetes, and gestational diabetes.
- Discuss the implications of diabetes on the periodontium.
- Define the term osteoporosis and discuss the link between skeletal osteoporosis and alveolar bone loss in the jaw.
- Discuss how hormone alterations may affect the periodontium.
- Define the term pregnancy-associated pyogenic granuloma.

- Explain how abnormalities of polymorphonuclear leukocytes may affect the body's response to periodontal pathogens.
- Describe the genetic and physical characteristics of Down syndrome.
- Discuss the implications of Down syndrome on the periodontium.
- Describe three types of periodontal disease associated with HIV infection.
- Define the term gingival hyperplasia.
- Name three medications that can cause gingival enlargement.
- Define the term biologic equilibrium and discuss factors that can disrupt the balance between health and disease in the periodontium.

KEY TERMS

Contributing risk factors
Diabetes
Osteoporosis
Pregnancy tumor
Pregnancy-associated pyogenic granuloma
Polymorphonuclear
  leukocytes
Neutrophils
Down syndrome
Acquired immunodeficiency syndrome
  (AIDS)

Necrotizing ulcerative gingivitis (NUG)
Necrotizing ulcerative
  periodontitis (NUP)
Linear gingival erythema (LGE)
Gingival hyperplasia
Phenytoin
Cyclosporine
Nifedipine
Biologic equilibrium
Risk assessment

SECTION 1: SYSTEMIC CONDITIONS AS CONTRIBUTING FACTORS

INTRODUCTION TO SYSTEMIC CONTRIBUTING FACTORS

1. **Major Risk Factors for Periodontal Disease**
   A. Research studies have clearly demonstrated that periodontal disease is a bacterial infection of the periodontium and that bacteria are the primary etiologic agents in periodontal disease.
   B. Most of the tissue destruction seen in periodontal disease is caused by the host response to bacterial infection of the periodontium.
2. **Contributing Factors for Periodontal Disease**
   A. Contributing risk factors are factors that increase an individual's susceptibility to periodontitis by modifying or amplifying the host response to the bacterial infection.
   B. Contributing factors play a role in determining an individual's susceptibility to periodontal disease (Box 8-1).
   C. Two broad categories of contributing risk factors for periodontal disease are systemic and local contributing factors. Systemic contributing factors are discussed in this chapter. Chapter 7 discusses local contributing factors.
   D. Systemic contributing factors for periodontal disease are conditions, habits, or diseases that increase an individual's susceptibility to periodontal infection. Proven periodontal risk factors include:
      1. Tobacco use
      2. Diabetes mellitus
      3. Osteoporosis
      4. Hormone alteration
      5. Psychosocial stress
      6. Genetic influences
      7. Acquired immunodeficiency syndrome (AIDS)
      8. Systemic medications

Box 8-1

Important Concepts About Periodontal Disease

- Periodontal disease is a bacterial infection of the periodontium.
- The host responds to the bacterial invaders by mobilizing its defensive cells and releasing chemicals.
- This host response is responsible for most of the tissue destruction seen in periodontitis.
- Everyone who is infected with periodontal pathogens does not experience periodontitis; some only experience gingivitis.
- Additional contributing factors such as systemic conditions and local factors play a role in determining an individual's susceptibility to periodontal disease.

TOBACCO USE

1. **Smoking as a Risk Factor for Periodontitis**
   A. Smoking appears to be one of the most important risk factors in the development and progression of periodontal disease.
      1. *In smokers*, smoking might be a more significant risk factor for periodontal disease progression than poor plaque control.
         a. Smokers are 2.6 to 6 times more likely to exhibit periodontal destruction than nonsmokers.[1]
         b. Smokers are 12 to 14 times more likely than non-smokers to have severe loss of attachment.[2]
         c. Among periodontally healthy subjects, heavy smokers are 18 times more likely to be infected by periodontal pathogens than nonsmokers.[3]
         d. Smokers lose more teeth than nonsmokers. Only about 20% of people older than 65 years of age who have never smoked are toothless, whereas 41.3% of daily smokers older than 65 are toothless.
         e. Smoking is strongly associated with aggressive periodontal destruction in young adults. Smokers in the 19- to 30-year range were 3.8 times more likely to have periodontitis compared to persons who never smoked.[4]
         f. Tobacco smoking may play an important role in the development of forms of periodontitis that does not respond to treatment despite excellent patient compliance and appropriate periodontal therapy.[5]
      2. *The knowledge that smoking is a significant risk factor suggests that in smokers, smoking cessation counseling might prevent more periodontal disease than daily plaque control self-care.*
   B. Smoking may be responsible for more than half of the cases of periodontal disease among adults in the United States.
      1. The National Health and Nutrition Examination Survey (NHANES III) was conducted on large segments of the U.S. population between 1988 and 1994. Nearly 40,000 people were interviewed and had medical and dental examinations for this survey. Smokers made up 28% of the study group.
      2. Evaluation of the NHANES III data found that smokers and former heavy smokers accounted for 53% of the periodontitis cases.[6]
   C. The extent of periodontal disease is directly related to the number of cigarettes smoked and the number of years of smoking. The more a person smokes and the longer a person smokes, the more disease that individual will have. As the number of cigarettes smoked increases, the number of healthy sextants decreases.
2. **Effects of Smoking on the Periodontium**
   A. Gingival inflammation and gingival bleeding, two of the cardinal signs of periodontal disease, are often reduced or absent in smokers. *For this reason, great care should be taken in performing periodontal screening and examination of smokers. In smokers, the lack of bleeding on probing does not indicate healthy tissue as it does in nonsmokers.*
   B. The gingival tissue of smokers tends to be fibrotic with thickened rolled margins and a pale pinkish color.
   C. Smokers exhibit no differences in plaque levels but have considerably more calculus than nonsmokers.
   D. One in three smokers exhibits increased melanin pigmentation on the surface of the gingiva, usually on the attached gingiva of the lower anterior teeth.

DIABETES MELLITUS

1. Diabetes is a disease in which the body does not produce or properly use insulin. Insulin is a hormone that is needed to convert sugar, starches, and other food into energy that the body uses to sustain life

2. **Types of Diabetes**
   A. Type 1 diabetes (previously called insulin-dependent diabetes mellitus or juvenile-onset diabetes)
      1. Type 1 diabetes is caused by damage to the pancreas. The pancreas is an organ (located near the stomach) that produces insulin. Insulin is a hormone that allows the body cells to take in the glucose that they need. Without insulin, the glucose stays in the bloodstream instead of going into the cells. The glucose builds up in the blood, resulting in diabetes.
      2. This type accounts for approximately 5% to 10% of all diagnosed cases of diabetes.
      3. Treatment of type 1 diabetes includes a carefully calculated diet, exercise, home blood glucose testing several times per day, and multiple daily insulin injections to replace the insulin hormone that the pancreas no longer makes.
   B. Type 2 diabetes (previously called non–insulin-dependent diabetes mellitus [NIDDM] or adult onset diabetes)
      1. Type 2 diabetes occurs when (i) the body does not make enough insulin hormone and/or (ii) the body cells ignore the insulin and fail to use it to help bring glucose into the cells.
      2. This type is the most common form of diabetes, accounting for approximately 90% to 95% of all diagnosed cases of diabetes.
      3. Treatment of type 2 diabetes includes diet control, exercise, home glucose testing, oral medication, and/or insulin. Approximately 40% of people with type 2 diabetes require insulin injections.
   C. Gestational Diabetes
      1. Gestational diabetes is a form of diabetes that occurs during pregnancy in women who have never had diabetes before pregnancy. Gestational diabetes starts when a woman's body is not able to make and use all the insulin it needs for pregnancy. This type of diabetes usually disappears when the pregnancy is over.
      2. This type affects about 4% of all pregnant women, about 135,000 cases in the United States each year.
      3. Persons at risk for gestational diabetes include women who are 25 years or older; were overweight before becoming pregnant; have a family history of diabetes; and are Hispanic, African American, Native American, Asian American, or Pacific Islander.

3. **Diabetes and Risk of Periodontitis.** Individuals with *undiagnosed or uncontrolled diabetes* are more likely to have periodontal disease than people without diabetes, probably because these individuals are more susceptible to contracting infections.
   A. Incidence of Periodontitis
      1. Patients with *well-controlled diabetes* have no more periodontal disease than persons without diabetes. Diabetes is **well controlled** if the blood glucose levels are stabilized within the recommended range. Blood glucose levels are discussed in Chapter 14.
      2. Individuals with *undiagnosed or poorly controlled diabetes* are at greater risk for severe periodontitis than are persons with controlled diabetes and nondiabetic individuals. In fact, periodontal disease is considered a complication of uncontrolled diabetes.
   B. Effects of Increased Glucose Blood Levels on the Periodontium
      1. An individual with uncontrolled or poorly controlled blood glucose levels has an increased risk for developing acute periodontal abscesses, more extensive attachment loss, and a much greater risk of progressive bone loss.
      2. Increased glucose content has been demonstrated in the gingival crevicular fluid of diabetic patients. Since many bacteria thrive on sugars, this glucose-rich crevicular fluid may result in altered bacterial composition within the plaque microcolonies and influence the development of periodontal disease.

3. Several studies have shown that gingivitis is more severe in children with diabetes than in those without the disease.

C. Implications of Diabetes for the Periodontium
   1. The rate of development of periodontal disease in diabetic subjects is 2 to 3 times greater than that observed in nondiabetic patients.
   2. The response of well-controlled diabetics to nonsurgical periodontal therapy, including periodontal debridement of tooth surfaces, appears to be similar to that of nondiabetic individuals.
   3. Patients with poorly controlled diabetes have a poorer response to nonsurgical and surgical periodontal therapy, more rapid recurrence of deep pockets, and a less favorable long-term response to treatment.
   4. A diabetic who smokes, and who is age 45 or older, is 20 times more likely than a nondiabetic, nonsmoking individual to experience severe periodontitis.

D. Oral Manifestations of Diabetes
   1. Reduced salivary flow and burning tongue are common complaints of patients with uncontrolled diabetes.
   2. Xerostomia can encourage the growth of *Candida albicans* and the development of candidiasis.
   3. Dental healthcare professionals should suspect undiagnosed diabetes as a likely cause of burning tongue and refer the patient to a physician for follow-up care.

OSTEOPOROSIS

1. **Osteoporosis** is a disorder characterized by the loss of bone mineral, occurring most frequently in postmenopausal women, in sedentary or bedridden individuals, and in patients receiving long-term steroid therapy.
   A. Postmenopausal osteoporosis is a disorder caused by the cessation of estrogen production and is characterized by bone fractures.
   B. Osteoporosis affects more than 20 million people in the United States, most of whom are women, and results in nearly 2 million bone fractures per year.

2. **Osteoporosis and the Risk of Periodontitis**
   A. There may be a link between skeletal osteoporosis and alveolar bone loss in the jaw. Preliminary studies report significant correlations between mandibular bone mineral density and hipbone mineral density.
   B. In and of itself, osteoporosis does not initiate tissue destruction; however, it may aggravate the progression of periodontal disease. Loss of density of the alveolar bone may exacerbate the bone resorption seen in periodontitis.
   C. In the case of postmenopausal osteoporosis, hormone replacement therapy (HRT) within 5 years of menopause may lessen inflammation and slow the progression of alveolar bone loss, thus helping to protect the teeth.[7]

HORMONE ALTERATION

Levels of sex hormones vary during various periods of life, most strikingly during puberty, pregnancy, and menopause. Some studies indicate that changes in hormone levels may have an effect on the periodontium.

1. **Puberty**
   A. Increased levels of sex hormones during puberty cause increased blood circulation to the gingival tissues and may cause an increased sensitivity to local irritants, such as bacterial plaque, resulting in pubertal gingivitis.
   B. Pubertal gingivitis occurs equally in girls and boys. The tendency for plaque-induced gingivitis decreases as the young person progresses through puberty.
   C. The dental hygienist should explain the importance of thorough plaque control and its role in the prevention of plaque-induced gingivitis during puberty.

2. **Pregnancy**
   A. Inflammation of the gingiva increases in pregnant women in the presence of small amounts of bacterial plaque.
      1. In most cases, increased gingival inflammation only occurs in patients who had evidence of gingivitis before becoming pregnant.
      2. If the patient has healthy gingiva prior to pregnancy and maintains good plaque control throughout pregnancy, she should remain free of gingival inflammation.
      3. The likelihood of gingival inflammation increases in the second month when the circulating hormones related to pregnancy rise in the blood, increasing sensitivity to bacterial plaque and other local irritants.
      4. The incidence of gingival inflammation is highest in the eighth month when the levels of circulating hormones are at their peak.
   B. Oral Manifestations of Inflammation of the Periodontium
      1. The gingival tissue may be edematous and dark red, with bulbous interdental papillae.
      2. In some cases, a gingival papilla can react so strongly to bacterial plaque that a large lump, called a **pregnancy tumor**, may form on the interdental gingiva or on the gingival margin (**Fig. 8-1**). Another, more precise term for a pregnancy tumor is a **pregnancy-associated pyogenic granuloma**.
         a. These growths are noncancerous and are generally not painful.
         b. If the growth persists after delivery, it can be surgically removed.
   C. Since oral contraceptives contain synthetic hormones, women who use oral contraceptives may experience plaque-induced gingivitis. Problems with gingival inflammation do not occur as frequently now as in the past, since modern oral contraceptive medications contain lower doses of synthetic hormones.
   D. Dental hygienist should stress the importance of thorough plaque control and its role in the prevention of plaque-induced gingivitis during pregnancy and when using oral contraceptive medications.

3. **Menopause and Postmenopause**
   A. Decreased levels of circulating hormones in women who are menopausal or postmenopausal may result in oral changes, such as dry mouth, burning sensations, or altered taste.
   B. In addition, as mentioned previously in the Osteoporosis section, alveolar bone loss may be exacerbated by lower estrogen levels.

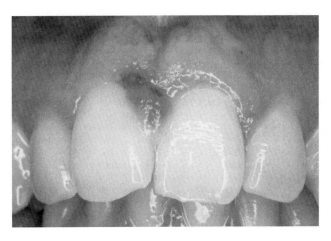

Figure 8-1. Pregnancy-Associated Pyogenic Granuloma.
In pregnancy, the gingiva can react strongly to the presence of plaque. A large lump may form on the interdental gingiva.

PSYCHOSOCIAL STRESS

1. The connection between stress and periodontal disease may involve stress-related changes in behavior such as:
   A. Neglect of plaque control self-care
   B. Changes in diet

    C. An increase in smoking

    D. Increase in other habits like bruxism.

2. Meticulous plaque control is critical to successful treatment of stress-related periodontal disease.

3. High levels of financial stress and poor coping abilities may double the likelihood of developing periodontal disease.[8]

    A. Subjects who reported high levels of financial strain and poor coping skills had higher levels of attachment loss and alveolar bone loss than those with low levels of financial strain.

    B. Subjects who dealt with their financial problems in an active and practical way, however, had no more risk of severe periodontal disease than those without money problems.

4. Evidence strongly suggests that a periodontal condition known as necrotizing ulcerative gingivitis (NUG) has a stress-related component to its etiology (**Fig. 8-2**).

    A. NUG is most often seen in young adults under stress, such as college students at examination time and soldiers on the front line.

    B. Smoking is an additional risk factor for NUG, because most patients who experience NUG are smokers.

    C. Necrotizing periodontal diseases are discussed further in Chapter 11.

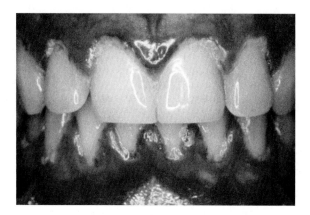

Figure 8-2. Necrotizing Ulcerative Gingivitis. Stress is a contributing factor in the development of this painful gingival disease.

GENETIC INFLUENCE

Considerable evidence suggests that there is some genetic basis for certain periodontal diseases. Certain rare severe genetic disorders are considered to be risk factors for periodontitis because individuals with these genetic disorders often exhibit severe periodontal disease. In addition, genetic variations—such as variation in the expression of inflammatory cytokines—may increase the likelihood of developing severe periodontitis.

1. **The Role of Genetics and Heredity in Periodontitis**

    A. Observations that successive generations of some families had severe periodontal disease lead to the supposition that periodontal disease may have a genetic component.

        1. *Current research seems to indicate that certain individuals have a genetically determined immune response that makes them more susceptible to periodontal disease.*[9–12]

        2. Studies with twins indicate that heredity plays a large role in periodontal susceptibility. Genetic influences may account for perhaps as much as 50% of the risk for periodontitis.

        3. The most rapid disease progression is seen in a relatively small number of persons in who periodontitis starts at a young age. There is some evidence that these individuals have some genetic susceptibility to periodontitis.[13–15]

B. The interleukin-1 genotype has been identified as a specific genetic marker that may put an individual at risk for periodontitis.[16]

1. This relationship has only been demonstrated in nonsmokers.
2. This genetic factor does not seem to be as strong a risk factor for periodontitis as smoking.

C. Epidemiological studies of individuals with and without periodontitis are needed before the genetic contribution to periodontitis can be clarified.

2. **Abnormalities of Polymorphonuclear Leukocytes (PMNs). Polymorphonuclear leukocytes** are immune cells that play a vital role in combating the pathogenic bacteria responsible for periodontal disease. PMNs are also known as **neutrophils.**

A. Hereditary abnormalities in PMN function or cell number can lead to overwhelming systemic bacterial infection and are often associated with increased susceptibility to severe periodontal destruction.

1. PMNs, the most abundant type of white blood cells present in the peripheral blood, play a critical role in host defense against pathogenic bacteria.
2. Individuals with defective PMN production or function have increased susceptibility to recurrent bacterial infections.
3. Persons with PMN abnormalities often suffer ulcerations of the oral mucosa, gingivitis, and/or periodontitis.

B. Inherited Systemic Diseases in which PMN Function Is Compromised

1. Systemic diseases in which PMN function is compromised include Chédiak-Higashi syndrome, Down syndrome (trisomy 21), leukocyte adhesion deficiency syndrome, Job syndrome, Papillon-Lefèvre syndrome, Crohn's disease, acute monocytic leukemia, as well as cyclic and chronic neutropenia.
2. Major genetic disorders, fortunately, are quite rare.
   a. Dental hygienists are unlikely to encounter patients with most of these severe genetic disorders outside a hospital dentistry setting.
   b. Persons with Down syndrome, however, frequently are treated in general and periodontal dental offices.

3. **Down Syndrome**

A. Down syndrome is one of the most common birth defects. Usually, children born with the condition have some degree of mental retardation, as well as characteristic physical features. Many of these children also have other health problems.

1. Normally, the nucleus of each cell contains 46 chromosomes. In Down syndrome, however, the nucleus contains 47 chromosomes. Most cases of Down syndrome occur because there are three copies of the 21st chromosome. For this reason, Down syndrome is also referred to as trisomy 21.
2. More than 350,000 people in the United States have Down syndrome.
3. Due to advances in medical treatment, 80% of adults with Down syndrome reach age 55, and many live longer. As the mortality rate associated with Down syndrome decreases, the prevalence of adults with Down syndrome in our society will increase. More and more dental healthcare providers will interact with individuals with this condition, increasing the need for education and acceptance.

B. Physical Characteristics. Among the most common physical traits of infants with Down syndrome are:

1. Flat facial profile with a small nose with a depressed nasal bridge
2. Upward slant to the eyes and small skin folds on the inner corners of the eyes
3. Protruding tongue and an open mouth

C. Medical and Developmental Problems

1. Children with Down syndrome are at increased risk for congenital heart defects, increased susceptibility to infection, respiratory problems, gastrointestinal abnormalities, and childhood leukemia.
2. Abnormal PMN function is seen in about half of all patients with Down syndrome.
3. Most individuals with Down syndrome have some level of mental retardation with IQs in the mild to moderate range of mental retardation. Those who

receive good medical care and experience a supportive social environment can attend school, hold jobs, and participate in decisions that affect them. Some live with family or friends, and some live independently.

   D. Implications for the Periodontium
      1. It is widely known that individuals with Down syndrome often develop severe, aggressive periodontitis. The prevalence of periodontal disease ranges from 60% to 100% of young adults under 30 years of age with Down syndrome.[17,18]
      2. A recent study indicates that periodontal pathogens colonize the gingival tissues in the very early childhood years of children with Down syndrome.[19]

ACQUIRED IMMUNODEFICIENCY SYNDROME

1. Acquired immunodeficiency syndrome (AIDS) is a communicable disease caused by the human immunodeficiency virus (HIV).
2. **Implications for the Periodontium**
   A. Necrotizing ulcerative gingivitis (NUG) in HIV-positive individuals is a form of gingivitis that involves tissue necrosis that is limited to the gingivitis.
   B. Necrotizing ulcerative periodontitis (NUP) in HIV-positive individuals is a severe form of periodontitis that involves tissue necrosis of the gingival tissues combined with loss of attachment and alveolar bone loss (**Fig. 8-3**).
      1. NUP is an indication of severe immune suppression.
      2. This condition is characterized by severe pain, loosening of teeth, bleeding, fetid odor, ulcerated gingival papillae and rapid loss of bone and soft tissue. Patients often refer to their pain as "deep jaw pain."
   C. Linear Gingival Erythema (LGE) in HIV-positive individuals, a periodontal disease, presents as a red band along the gingival margin, which may or may not be accompanied by occasional bleeding and discomfort.
      1. LGE is characterized by a 2 to 3 mm marginal band of intense gingival erythema (redness) with areas of redness that may extend beyond the mucogingival line.
      2. LGE is seen most frequently in association with anterior teeth, but commonly extends to the posterior teeth.
      3. LGE can also present on attached and nonattached gingiva as petechialike patches (patches of tiny red or purplish spots on the tissue).
      4. LGE does not respond to periodontal instrumentation and daily plaque control.

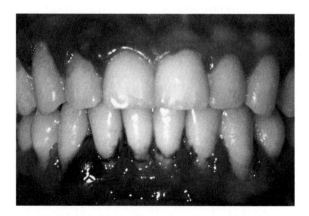

Figure 8-3. NUP in an HIV-Positive Individual. This HIV-positive individual exhibits a severe form of necrotizing ulcerative periodontitis with tissue necrosis of the gingival tissues combined with loss of attachment. Clinical signs are notably visible on the mandibular anterior sextant.

SYSTEMIC MEDICATIONS WITH PERIODONTAL SIDE EFFECTS

A number of medications used to treat systemic diseases can cause oral complications. Effects of medications can modify oral hygiene habits, plaque composition, size of gingival tissues, level of bone, and salivary flow. Educating patients about the oral side effects of taking medication is critical to reducing the medication-related risks of periodontal disease. Commonly prescribed medications that can affect the periodontium are summarized in Table 8-1.

1. **Effects of Oral Medications**
   A. Alteration of Plaque Composition
      1. Cough drops, cough syrups, tonics, vitamins, and other medications that contain sugar add significantly to the alteration of plaque pH and composition.
      2. Sugar is metabolized by bacteria to form acid, causing enamel to demineralize. The demineralized areas are rough and act as attachment sites for bacteria, keeping bacterial plaque against tissues and eventually resulting in inflammation of the gingiva.
   B. Effect on Gingival Tissues
      1. The most dramatic medication-related change seen in the gingiva is an overgrowth of the gingival tissues known as gingival hyperplasia. Gingival hyperplasia is an enlargement of the gingiva due to an increase in the number of cells.
      2. Gingival enlargement is a possible side effect of anticonvulsants, immunosuppressants, and calcium channel blockers. These three classes of medications influence gingival fibroblasts to overproduce collagen matrix when stimulated by gingival inflammation.[20]
   C. Effect on Salivary Flow
      1. Adequate saliva flow is necessary for the maintenance of healthy oral tissues. The ability of saliva to limit the growth of pathogens is a major determinant of systemic and oral health.
         a. The physical flow the saliva helps to dislodge microbes from the teeth and mucosa surfaces. Saliva can also cause bacteria to clump together so that they can be swallowed before they become firmly attached.
         b. Saliva is rich in antimicrobial components. Certain molecules in saliva can directly kill or inhibit a variety of microbes.
         c. Saliva contains molecules that help to repair and regenerate the oral tissues.
      2. More than 400 over-the-counter and prescription drugs have xerostomia as a possible side effect.[21] Antihypertensives, narcotic analgesics, tranquilizers, diuretics, antimetabolites, antihistamines, sedatives, and high doses of certain vitamins are examples of medications that decrease saliva flow.
2. **Medications Associated with Gingival Enlargement.** More than 20 medications have been shown to have the potential to induce gingival enlargement. The three major classes of medications associated with gingival enlargement are anticonvulsants, immunosuppressives, and calcium channel blocking agents.

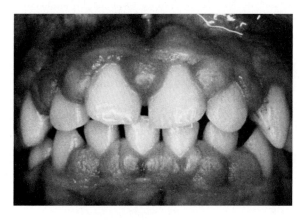

Figure 8-4. Phenytoin-Associated Gingivitis. Overgrowth of the gingiva is one of the most common side effects of phenytoin (Dilantin).

   A. Phenytoin
      1. Phenytoin (FEN-i-toyn) is an anticonvulsant medication used to control convulsions or seizures in the treatment of epilepsy. Phenytoin is marketed under various trade names including Dilantin 4, Dilantin Kapseals 4, and Phenytoin. Phenytoin is among the 20 most-prescribed drugs in the world.

2. Overgrowth of the gingiva is one of the most common side effects of phenytoin (Fig. 8-4). It has been estimated that 40% to 50% of the millions of individuals who take phenytoin will develop gingival overgrowth to some extent. Overgrowths appear to be more common in children and young adults.
3. Gingival overgrowth begins with enlargement of the interdental papillae.
    a. The interdental papillae overgrow, forming firm triangular tissue masses that protrude from the interdental area.
    b. Gradually the enlarged papillae may fuse mesially and distally and partially cover the anatomic crown with marginal gingiva. Overgrowths are most commonly seen on the facial aspect of the anterior teeth.
    c. In the presence of good plaque control, the enlarged tissue is pink in color and firm and rubbery in consistency. In the presence of poor plaque control, the tissue appears red, edematous, and spongy.

B. Cyclosporine
1. Cyclosporine (SIGH-kloe-spor-een) belongs to the group of medicines known as immunosuppressive agents. It is used to reduce the body's immune response in patients who receive organ (kidney, liver, or heart) transplants. When a patient receives an organ transplant, the body will try to reject the transplanted organ. Cyclosporine works by preventing this response.
2. The incidence of cyclosporine-associated gingival overgrowth affects approximately 25% of patients taking the medication.
3. The clinical appearance of cyclosporine-associated gingival overgrowth resembles that of phenytoin-associated gingival enlargement.
4. Patients receiving cyclosporine are usually medically compromised, requiring close consultation with the patient's physician to assure safe management of the patient's periodontal condition.

C. Nifedipine
1. Nifedipine (nye-FED-I-peen), one type of calcium channel blocker, is used as a coronary vasodilator in the treatment of hypertension, angina, and cardiac arrhythmias. Calcium channel blockers are a class of drugs that block the influx of calcium ions through cardiac and vascular smooth muscle cell membranes. This results in the dilation of the main coronary and systemic arteries.
2. Approximately 38% of patients taking nifedipine experience gingival enlargement.
3. The clinical appearance of nifedipine-associated gingival overgrowth resembles that of phenytoin-associated gingival enlargement.
4. Surgical elimination of the tissue overgrowth is often required. Unfortunately, the gingival overgrowth is likely to recur within 1 to 2 years even in the presence of good plaque control, especially if the patient is younger than 25. If plaque control is inadequate, the regrowth will occur rapidly. The patient should be advised of the likelihood of the recurrence of the gingival overgrowth following surgery.

Table 8-1. Effects of Commonly Prescribed Medications on Periodontium

Medication Class	Generic Name (Brand Name)	Effect on Periodontium
Antibiotic	Tetracycline (Achromycin)	Inhibits alveolar bone loss
Anticonvulsant	Phenytoin (Dilantin)	Gingival overgrowth
Antianxiety agents	Alprazolam (Xanax)	Decreased plaque formation
Antihypertensive	Enalapril (Vasotec)	Increased gingival inflammation
Calcium blocker	Nifedipine (Procardia)	Gingival overgrowth
Immunosuppressive	Cyclosporine (Sandimmune)	Gingival overgrowth
Nonsteroidal anti-inflammatory (NSAID)	Ibuprofen (Advil, Midol, Nuprin)	Inhibits alveolar bone loss

SECTION 2: BALANCE BETWEEN PERIODONTAL HEALTH AND DISEASE

BIOLOGIC EQUILIBRIUM

1. **Equilibrium Between Health and Disease.** The human body is continually working to maintain a state of balance in the internal environment of the body, known as **biologic equilibrium.**
   A. Periodontal Health
      1. In the oral cavity, most of the time, things are in a state of balance between the bacterial plaque and the host.
      2. For the periodontium to remain healthy, the bacterial challenge must be contained at a level that can be tolerated by the host.
      3. The situation can be thought of as a balance scale, with the disease-promoting factors on one side of the scale and the health-promoting factors on the other. As long as the two sides of the scale are in balance, there will be no disease progression.
   B. Periodontal Disease
      1. The intermittent pattern of disease activity seen in periodontitis is believed to result from the changing balance between the pathogenic bacteria and the host's inflammatory and immune responses.
      2. This balance also can be affected by other risk factors, such as local or systemic variables.
         a. Local Risk Factors
            1) Local risk factors can increase the weight of the disease-promoting factors, tipping the balance scale toward disease progression (Fig. 8-5).
            2) If the bacterial challenge increases, for example, the scale will tip toward disease.
2. Systemic and Acquired Risk Factors. Changes in the host environment such as illness, medications, diet, stress, or smoking can disturb the balance, tipping the scale toward disease progression (Fig. 8-6).

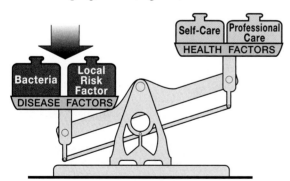

Figure 8-5. **Local Contributing Factor.** A new restoration has a large interproximal overhang. The patient's self-care efforts are no longer sufficient to control the bacteria in the localized area near the overhang. Plaque accumulates at the site.

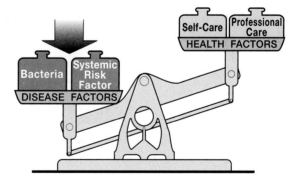

Figure 8-6. **Systemic Contributing Factor.** A new systemic health problem, such as undiagnosed diabetes, is added to the disease-promoting factors. The scale will tip toward disease since the disease-promoting factors now outweigh the health-promoting factors.

RESTORING BALANCE

When active periodontal disease sites are present in the mouth, the goal is to return the oral cavity to a state of biologic equilibrium.

1. **Inadequate Self-Care**
   There are many patients who are unable or unwilling to perform the self-care necessary to control bacterial plaque. For these patients, it is necessary to increase the

frequency of professional care to compensate for the inadequate level of patient self-care. A professional care at frequent intervals can be effective in restoring the balance between health and disease (**Fig. 8-7**).

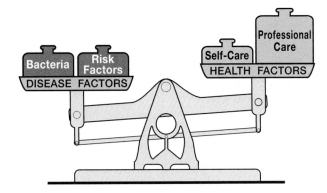

Figure 8-7. Frequent Professional Care. An individual who is unwilling or unable to obtain adequate plaque control on a daily basis. More frequent periodontal instrumentation can help to control the development of mature plaque biofilms.

2. **Differences in Host Response**

   Experienced dental hygienists will attest to the fact that major differences exist in the way that individuals respond to the plaque biofilm. Even with inadequate plaque control, *most* patients will never progress from gingivitis to periodontitis. *Some* patients with inadequate plaque control will experience the shift from gingivitis to periodontitis.

   A. Inadequate Plaque Control and Gingivitis. Many patients return to the dental office year after year with generalized bacterial plaque. These patients exhibit gingivitis and yet, year after year, show no clinical signs of progression to periodontitis. For some reason, gingivitis never progresses to periodontitis in these individuals.

      1. It is possible that such individuals benefit from immune systems that are especially effective in controlling periodontal pathogens.

      2. Perhaps these individuals have no systemic or acquired factors that add stress to the biologic equilibrium. Basically, if an individual's immune system can effectively deal with a mouthful of periodontal pathogens, there will be no destructive periodontal disease (**Fig. 8-8**).

   B. Inadequate Self-Care and Periodontitis. In a few individuals, gingivitis progresses to periodontitis. It is theorized that such individuals may possess systemic risk factors (such as genetic variables or systemic disease) that significantly increase their susceptibility to periodontitis (**Fig. 8-9**).

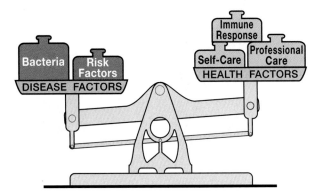

Figure 8-8. Gingivitis in the Presence of Plaque Biofilms. In individuals with a low susceptibility to periodontitis, gingivitis may never progress to periodontitis.

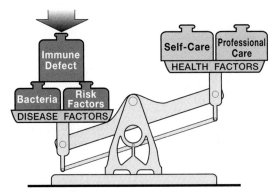

Figure 8-9. Periodontitis in the Presence of Plaque Biofilm. In a few susceptible individuals, gingivitis progresses to periodontitis.

3. **Local Contributing Factors**

   A. Eliminate a Local Risk Factor (**Fig. 8-10**). It is possible to totally eliminate a local risk factor in many cases. A faulty restoration is a good example of a local factor that can be corrected, restoring the balance between local disease-promoting and health-promoting factors at the site.

Chapter 8 Systemic Contributing Factors

Chapter 8 Systemic Contributing Factors **129**

B. Compensate for a Local Risk Factor. In other cases, it is possible to compensate for a local risk factor by improving the patient's self-care and/or increasing the frequency of professional care. For example, the patient may need to use tufted dental floss to clean around the abutment teeth of a fixed bridge. This situation can be compared to adding more weight on the health side of the balance scale to equal or exceed the weight on the disease side of the scale.

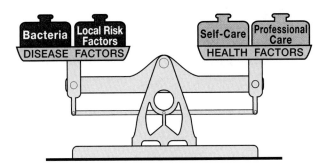

Figure 8-10. Eliminate a Local Contributing Factor.
Replacing a faulty restoration will restore the balance between health and disease. The patient's self-care efforts are now able to disrupt the dental plaque that forms on the restoration.

4. Systemic Contributing Factors
   A. Control a Systemic Risk Factor/Eliminate an Acquired Risk Factor (**Fig. 8-11**). Certain systemic or acquired risk factors are possible to control or eliminate if the patient is willing to do so. For example, the individual can work with a physician to keep diabetes well controlled. A smoker may decide to stop smoking. In both cases the individual has made a change that is health promoting, both systemically and for the periodontium.
   B. Compensate for Systemic Risk Factors
   1. In the case of a systemic risk factor that cannot be controlled, it is necessary to add weight to the health-side of the scale. Maintaining good self-care while increasing the frequency of professional care can restore the balance between health and disease.
   2. Some individuals have genetic risk factors, such as abnormal neutrophil function, that cause them to be susceptible to severe periodontitis. At the present time, we are unable to eliminate or control genetic risk factors. It is possible, however, to assist the patient in maintaining health by increasing the extent of professional care. Frequent professional care will increase the weight on the health-side of the scale (**Fig. 8-12**).

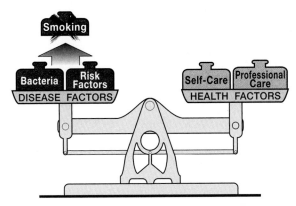

Figure 8-11. Eliminating a Systemic Risk Factor.
Smoking cessation, combined with adequate self-care and professional care, restores the balance.

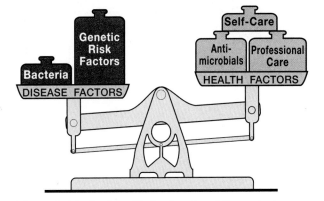

Figure 8-12. Assist with Professional Care. At the present time, there are some risk factors that cannot be eliminated or controlled. Professional care can help slow disease progression.

QUESTIONNAIRES FOR PERIODONTAL RISK ASSESSMENT

1. **Introduction to Periodontal Risk Assessment**
    A. Many factors interact to determine a patient's susceptibility to periodontal disease (Box 8-2).
    B. Risk assessment for dentistry has been defined as the identification of risk factors to determine which patients are more or less likely to prevent or control their dental disease.
    C. It is becoming possible to consider an individual's risk factors for periodontal disease (systemic disease, genetic information, personal habits, and characteristics) and to classify patients into high- or low-risk groups.
2. **Risk Assessment Tools**
    A. The development of genetically based tests will facilitate risk assessment and improve the ability of dental healthcare providers to customize treatment.
    B. Risk assessment questionnaires are practical tools that can be helpful in identifying individuals who are at high-risk for periodontal disease. Figures 8-13 and 8-14 are examples of a 2-page periodontal risk questionnaire that can be used to elicit the presence of common periodontal risk factors. Dental hygienists can use this type of questionnaire to initiate discussion with patients about periodontal risk factors.

Box 8-2

Susceptibility to Periodontal Disease

1. Periodontal disease is a bacterial infection of the periodontium.
    - The presence of pathogenic bacteria, however, does not necessarily mean that an individual will experience periodontitis.
    - Some persons with abundant bacterial plaque exhibit only gingivitis, while others with light plaque experience severe periodontitis.
2. It is the host's immune response to the bacterial pathogens that causes most of the tissue destruction seen in periodontal disease.
3. Additional factors, other than the presence of bacteria, play a significant role in determining why some individuals are more susceptible to periodontitis than others. Contributing factors such as systemic disease, smoking, and genetic influences can "play a significant role in determining the onset and progression of periodontal disease.

PERIODONTAL ASSESSMENT QUESTIONNAIRE FOR _____

TOBACCO USE

Tobacco use is the most significant risk factor for gum disease.

Do you now or have you ever used the following?

	Amount per day?	How many years?	If you quit, what year?
☐ Cigarette	_____	_____	_____
☐ Cigar	_____	_____	_____
☐ Pipe	_____	_____	_____
☐ Chew	_____	_____	_____
☐ Snuff	_____	_____	_____

HEART ATTACK AND STROKE

Untreated gum disease can increase your risk for heart attack and stroke.

Do you have any other risk factors for heart disease or stroke?

☐ Family history of heart disease   ☐ Tobacco use
☐ High cholesterol   ☐ High blood pressure

If you have any of these other risk factors it is especially important for you to always keep your gums as healthy and inflammation free as possible to reduce your overall risk for heart attack and stroke.

MEDICATIONS

A side effect of some medications can cause changes in your gums.

Have you ever taken any of the following medications?

☐ Dilantin anti-seizure medication

☐ Calcium channel blocker blood pressure medicine
  (such as Procardia, Cardizem, Norvasc, Verapamil, etc.)

☐ Cyclosporin immunosuppresant therapy

GENETIC

The tendency for gum disease to develop can be inherited.

Has anyone on your side of the family had gum problems? (e.g., your mother, father, or siblings)

☐ Yes

☐ No

CONTAGIOUS

The bacteria which cause gum disease may be spread to other family members.

Has anyone in your immediate family been tested or treated for gum problems? If so, whom?

☐ Spouse

☐ Children

FEMALES

Females can be at increased risk for gum disease at different points in their life.

The following can adversely affect your gums. Please check all that apply

☐ Pregnant   ☐ Nursing   ☐ Osteoporosis
☐ Taking birth control pills
☐ Taking hormone supplements
☐ Infrequent care during previous pregnancies

over

Figure 8-13. Side 1 of Periodontal Risk Questionnaire. Risk assessment questionnaires are practical tools that can be helpful in identifying individuals who have a high susceptibility to periodontitis. Side 1 of a risk assessment questionnaire is shown here. See Figure 8-14 for side 2 of this questionnaire. (Used by permission of Douglas W. Schutte, DMD, and Timothy G. Donley, DDS, MSD, Program of Dental Hygiene, Western Kentucky University, Bowling Green, KY.)

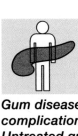

DIABETES

Gum disease is a common complication of diabetes. Untreated gum disease makes it harder for diabetes to control their blood sugar.

If you *ARE* diabetic...

For how many years? _____

Is your diabetes well controlled? ☐ Yes ☐ No

Who is your physician for diabetes? _____

If you *ARE NOT* diabetic...

Any family history of diabetes? ☐ Yes ☐ No

Have you had any of these warning signs of diabetes?

☐ Frequent urination   ☐ Excessive thirst
☐ Excessive hunger   ☐ Tingling or numbness in extremities
☐ Weakness and fatigue   ☐ Slow healing of cuts
☐ Unexplained weight loss   ☐ Any change of vision

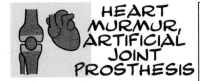

HEART MURMUR, ARTIFICIAL JOINT PROSTHESIS

With the slightest amount of gum inflammation, bacteria from the mouth can enter the bloodstream and cause a serious infection of the heart muscle or your artificial joint.

Do you have a heart murmur or artificial joint?
☐ Yes ☐ No

If so, does your physician recommend antibiotics prior to dental visits? ☐ Yes ☐ No

Name of physician: _____

It is especially important in your case to always keep your gums as healthy and inflammation-free as possible to reduce the chance of bacterial infection originating in the mouth.

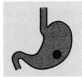

GASTRIC ULCERS

When your gums are inflamed, bacteria from the mouth can travel to the gut and cause ulcers to become active.

Have you been treated for ulcers?
☐ Yes ☐ No

Is the ulcer active now?
☐ Yes ☐ No

Ulcers are caused by bacteria. If you have been treated for ulcers you should make sure your gums are as inflammation-free as possible.

ALL PATIENTS PLEASE COMPLETE THE FOLLOWING:

Have you noticed any of the following signs of gum disease?

☐ Bleeding gums during toothbrushing   ☐ Pus between the teeth and gums
☐ Red, swollen, or tender gums   ☐ Loose or separating teeth
☐ Gums that have pulled away from the teeth   ☐ Change in the way your teeth fit together
☐ Persistent bad breath   ☐ Food catching between teeth

Is it important to you to keep your teeth as long as possible? ☐ Yes ☐ No
Any particular reason why missing teeth have not been replaced?

_____

Do you like the appearance of your smile? ☐ Yes ☐ No
Do you like the color of your teeth? ☐ Yes ☐ No
Do your teeth keep you from eating any specific food? ☐ Yes ☐ No

Figure 8-14. Side 2 of Periodontal Risk Questionnaire. Side 2 of a risk assessment questionnaire. (Used by permission of Douglas W. Schutte, DMD, and Timothy G. Donley, DDS, MSD, Program of Dental Hygiene, Western Kentucky University, Bowling Green, Kentucky.)

CHAPTER SUMMARY STATEMENT

Periodontal disease is a bacterial infection of the periodontium. The presence of pathogenic bacteria, however, does not necessarily mean that an individual will experience periodontitis.

- Additional factors play a role in determining why some individuals are more susceptible to periodontitis than others.
- Contributing factors are factors that increase an individual's susceptibility to periodontitis by modifying the host response to bacterial infection.
- Contributing factors such as systemic disease, smoking, and genetic factors can play a significant role in determining the onset and progression of periodontitis.

In the oral cavity, most of the time, things are in a state of balance between the bacterial plaque and the host.

- For the periodontium to remain healthy, the bacterial challenge must be contained at a level that can be tolerated by the host.
- The situation can be thought of as a balance scale, with the disease-promoting factors on one side of the scale and the health-promoting factors on the other.
- As long as the two sides of the scale are in balance, there will be no disease progression.
- The intermittent pattern of disease activity seen in periodontitis is believed to result from the changing balance between the pathogenic bacteria and the host's inflammatory and immune responses.

Daily plaque control by the patient and routine professional care are the best methods for prevention of periodontal disease. Other risk factors must be evaluated, however, to develop the best treatment plan for each individual. In addition, dental healthcare providers should provide tobacco cessation and other health promotion programs that contribute to both overall and periodontal health.

SECTION 3: FOCUS ON PATIENTS

CASE 1

A new patient with severe chronic periodontitis has a history of smoking one to two packs of cigarettes each day. The patient informs you that he will do "anything" to save his teeth, but that he cannot quit smoking. What counsel would you provide this patient about the effect of the smoking habit on the likelihood of long-term control of his periodontitis?

CASE 2

A new patient in your practice with mild (slight) chronic periodontitis has very poor plaque control. The patient is a nonsmoker. You have recently learned that the results of the patient's test for the interleukin-1 (IL-1) genotype are positive. What counsel would you provide this patient about the significance of the positive test for IL-1 genotype?

CASE 3

The parents of a young patient currently being treated by your dental team inform you that following a lengthy illness, their daughter has recently been diagnosed by her physician with a neutrophil defect. Neutrophils are also known as polymorphonuclear leukocytes. They inquire about any dental implications of this diagnosis. How might you respond to this inquiry?

References

1. Stoltenberg JL, Osborn JB, Pihlstrom BL, et al. Association between cigarette smoking, bacterial pathogens, and periodontal status. *J Periodontol.* 1993;64:1225–1230.

2. Grossi SG, Genco RJ, Machtei EE, et al. Assessment of risk for periodontal disease. II. Risk indicators for alveolar bone loss. *J Periodontol.* 1995;66:23–29.

3. Shiloah J, Patters MR, Waring MB. The prevalence of pathogenic periodontal microflora in healthy young adult smokers. *J Periodontol.* 2000;71:562–567.

4. Haber J, Wattles J, Crowley M, et al. Evidence for cigarette smoking as a major risk factor for periodontitis. *J Periodontol.* 1993;64:16–23.

5. MacFarlane GD, Herzberg MC, Wolff LF, et al. Refractory periodontitis associated with abnormal polymorphonuclear leukocyte phagocytosis and cigarette smoking. *J Periodontol.* 1992;63:908–913.

6. Tomar SL, Asma S. Smoking-attributable periodontitis in the United States: Findings from NHANES III. National Health and Nutrition Examination Survey. *J Periodontol.* 2000;71:743–751.

7. Reinhardt RA, Payne JB, Maze CA, et al. Influence of estrogen and osteopenia/osteoporosis on clinical periodontitis in postmenopausal women. *J Periodontol.* 1999;70:823–828.

8. Genco RJ, Ho AW, Grossi SG, et al. Relationship of stress, distress and inadequate coping behaviors to periodontal disease. *J Periodontol.* 1999;70:711–723.

9. Fredriksson M., Gustafsson A, Asman B, et al. Hyper-reactive peripheral neutrophils in adult periodontitis: Generation of chemiluminescence and intracellular hydrogen peroxide after in vitro priming and FcgammaR-stimulation. *J Clin Periodontol.*, 1998;25:394–398.

10. Fredriksson, M., Gustaffson AK, Bergstrom AG, et al. Constitutionally hyperreactive neutrophils in periodontitis. *J Periodontol.* 2003;74:219–224.

11. Michalowicz BS, Diehl SR, Gunsolley JC, et al. Evidence of a substantial genetic basis for risk of adult periodontitis. *J Periodontol.* 2000;71:1699–1707.

12. Michalowicz BS, Wolff LR, Klump D, et al. Periodontal bacteria in adult twins. *J Periodontol.* 1999;70:263–273.

13. Thomson WM, Edwards SJ, Dobson-Le DP, et al. IL-1 genotype and adult periodontitis among young New Zealanders. *J Dent Res.* 2001;80:1700–1703.

14. Parkhill JM, Henning BJ, Chapple IL, et al. Association of Interleukin-1 gene polymorphisms with early on-set periodontitis. *J Clin Periodontol.* 2000;27:682–689.

15. Columbo AP, Eftimiadi C, Haffajee AD, et al. Serum IgG2 level, Gm (23) allotype and FcgammaRIIa and FcgammaRIIIb receptors in refractory periodontal disease. *J Clin Periodonto.* 1998;25:464–474.

16. Kornman KS, di Giovine FS. Genetic variations in cytokine expression: A risk factor for severity of adult periodontitis. *Ann Periodontol.* 1998;3:327–338.

17. Barnett ML, Press KD, Friedman D, et al. The prevalence of periodontitis and dental caries in a Down's syndrome population. *J Periodontol.* 1986;57:288–293.

18. Izumi Y, Sugiyama S, Shinozuko O, et al. Defective neutrophil chemotaxis in Down's syndrome patients and its relationship to periodontal destruction. *J Periodontol.* 1989;60:238–242.

19. Amano A, Kishima T, Kimura S, et al. Periodontopathic bacteria in children with Down syndrome. *J Periodontol.* 2000;71:249–255.

20. Kinane DF. Periodontitis modified by systemic factors. *Ann Periodontol.* 1999;4(1)(:54–64.

21. Sreebny LM, Schwartz SS. A reference guide to drugs and dry mouth—2nd edition. *Gerodontology.* 1997;14:33–47.

SECTION 4: CHAPTER REVIEW QUESTIONS

1. Factors that increase an individual's susceptibility to periodontitis by modifying the host response to bacterial infection are called:
   A. Contributing factors
   B. Genetic influences
   C. Neutrophils
   D. Biologic equilibrium

2. In smokers, smoking cessation might prevent more periodontal disease than daily plaque control.
   A. True
   B. False

3. Smoking may be responsible for more than half of the cases of periodontal disease among adults in the United States.
   A. True
   B. False

4. Gingival inflammation and bleeding usually is very pronounced in smokers.
   A. True
   B. False

5. Which of the following individuals is MOST likely to have periodontitis?
   A. An individual with well controlled diabetes
   B. An individual who does not have diabetes
   C. An individual with poorly controlled diabetes

6. Levels of sex hormones may have an effect on the periodontium.
   A. True
   B. False

7. ALL pregnant women develop gingivitis.
   A. True
   B. False

8. Certain individuals have a genetically determined immune response that predisposes them to periodontal disease.
   A. True
   B. False

9. Abnormalities in PMN function can lead to overwhelming systemic bacterial infection and increased susceptibility to severe periodontal destruction.
   A. True
   B. False

10. Individuals with Down syndrome rarely develop periodontitis.
    A. True
    B. False

11. Which of the following medications commonly cause gingival hyperplasia?
    A. Tetracycline (Achromycin)
    B. Ibuprofen (Advil, Midol, Nuprin)
    C. Phenytoin (Dilantin)
    D. Alprazolam (Xanax)

9 Classification of Periodontal Diseases and Conditions

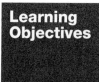

Learning Objectives

- Describe the American Academy of Periodontology Classification of Periodontal Diseases and Conditions.
- Compare and contrast the terms periodontal disease, gingivitis, and periodontitis.

KEY TERMS

Classification
Gingivitis

Periodontitis
Periodontal disease

American Academy of
Periodontology (AAP)

SECTION 1: INTRODUCTION TO DISEASE CLASSIFICATION

Periodontal disease is a broad term used to refer to a bacterial infection of the periodontium, just as heart disease is a general term. There are many different diseases of the heart, such as coronary artery disease, congestive heart failure, valvular disease, rheumatic heart disease, and infectious endocarditis. As with heart disease, there are many specific periodontal diseases that affect the gingival tissues, periodontal connective tissues, and/or the supporting alveolar bone.

This chapter outlines a periodontal disease classification adopted in 1999 at the International Workshop for a Classification of Periodontal Diseases and Conditions. Gingival diseases are discussed in detail in Chapter 10. The types of periodontitis are presented in detail in Chapter 11.

MAJOR DIAGNOSTIC CATEGORIES OF PERIODONTAL DISEASE

Periodontal diseases are divided into types or **classifications** based on their specific bacterial etiology, development, and clinical manifestations.
1. **Diagnostic Categories of Periodontal Disease.** The two basic diagnostic categories of periodontal disease are (i) gingivitis and (ii) periodontitis (**Fig. 9-1**). It is important to recognize the differences among health, gingivitis, and periodontitis (**Fig. 9-2**).

Figure 9-1. Periodontal Disease. There are two major categories of periodontal disease: (i) gingivitis and (ii) periodontitis.

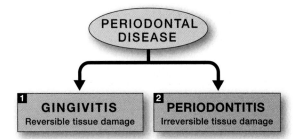

A. **Gingivitis** is a bacterial infection that is confined to the gingiva. It results in damage to the gingival tissues that is reversible.
B. **Periodontitis** is a bacterial infection of all parts of the periodontium including the gingiva, periodontal ligament, bone, and cementum. It results in irreversible destruction to the tissues of the periodontium.
C. It is important to recognize the differences among health, gingivitis, and periodontitis (Fig. 9-2).

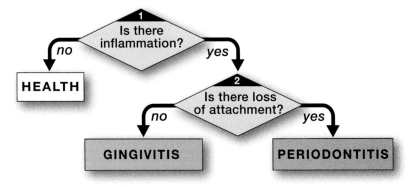

Figure 9-2. Decision Tree. Is it health, gingivitis, or periodontitis?

2. Terminology: *Periodontal Disease* **Versus** *Periodontitis*

   A. Many beginning clinicians confuse the meaning of the terms *periodontal disease* and *periodontitis*. Often these terms are used interchangeably, as if they mean the same thing. They do not.

   B. Periodontal disease refers to a bacterial infection of the periodontium.

   1. Periodontal disease that is limited to an inflammation of the gingival tissues is called gingivitis (Box 9-1).

   2. Periodontal disease that involves all the structures of the periodontium is called periodontitis (Box 9-2).

   C. It is important to understand that the terms *periodontal disease* and *periodontitis* are not identical in their meaning and not interchangeable in their use.

   1. When a dental hygienist says to the dentist, "My patient has periodontal disease," the hygienist is conveying the general information that the patient has gingivitis and/or periodontitis.

   2. When the hygienist says, "My patient has periodontitis," the hygienist is conveying the specific information that the patient has a bacterial infection that involves all tissues of the periodontium including the periodontal ligament, cementum, and alveolar bone.

PURPOSES OF CLASSIFICATION SYSTEMS

A periodontal classification system provides information necessary in:

   1. Communicating clinical findings accurately to other dental healthcare providers and to dental insurance providers.

   2. Presenting information to the patient about his or her disease.

   3. Formulating individualized treatment plans.

   4. Predicting treatment outcomes.

Box 9-1

Gingivitis

- Tissue usually red or reddish-blue
- Gingival margin is swollen and rounded
- Interdental papillae are bulbous and swollen
- Bleeding upon gentle probing
- Probing depths may be greater than 3 mm due to swelling of the tissues
- No apical migration of the junctional epithelium or bone loss
- Gingivitis may persist for years without ever progressing to periodontitis

---

Box 9-2

Periodontitis

- Tissue may appear pale pink (firm, rigid tissue) or bright red, purplish-red (spongy tissue)
- Gingival margin may be swollen or fibrotic
- Interdental papillae may not fill the interdental embrasure space
- Bleeding upon gentle probing; pus may be visible
- Probing depths are 4 mm or greater due to apical migration of the junctional epithelium
- There is loss of alveolar bone

SECTION 2: AMERICAN ACADEMY OF PERIODONTOLOGY CLASSIFICATION SYSTEM FOR PERIODONTAL DISEASES

In 1999, an international workshop adopted a new classification system for periodontal diseases and conditions developed by the American Academy of Periodontology (AAP) (Box 9-3).[1]

Box 9-3

AAP Classification of Periodontal Diseases and Conditions

I. Gingival Diseases
  A. Dental plaque-induced gingival diseases*
  1. Gingivitis associated with dental plaque only
      a. Without other local contributing factors
      b. With local contributing factors
  2. Gingival diseases modified by systemic factors
      a. Associated with the endocrine system
          1) Puberty-associated gingivitis
          2) Menstrual cycle-associated gingivitis
          3) Pregnancy-associated
              a) Gingivitis
              b) Pyogenic granuloma
          4) Diabetes mellitus-associated gingivitis
      b. Associated with blood dyscrasias
          1) Leukemia-associated gingivitis
          2) Other
  3. Gingival diseases modified by medications
      a. Drug-influenced gingival diseases
          1) Drug-influenced gingival enlargements
          2) Drug-influenced gingivitis
              a) Oral contraceptive-associated gingivitis
              b) Other
  4. Gingival diseases modified by malnutrition
      a. Ascorbic acid-deficiency gingivitis
      b. Other
  B. Nonplaque-induced gingival lesions
  1. Gingival diseases of specific bacterial origin
      a. *Neisseria gonorrhea*-associated lesions
      b. *Treponema pallidum*-associated lesions
      c. Streptococcal species-associated lesions
      d. Other
  2. Gingival diseases of viral origin
      a. Herpesvirus infections
          1) Primary herpetic gingivostomatitis
          2) Recurrent oral herpes
          3) Varicella zoster infections
      b. Other
  3. Gingival diseases of fungal origin
      a. *Candida*-species infections
          1) Generalized gingival candidosis
      b. Linear gingival erythema
      c. Histoplasmosis
      d. Other
  4. Gingival lesions of genetic origin
      a. Hereditary gingival fibromatosis
      b. Other

  5. Gingival manifestations of systemic conditions
      a. Mucocutaneous disorders
          1) Lichen planus
          2) Pemphigoid
          3) Pemphigus vulgaris
          4) Erythema multiforme
          5) Lupus erythematosus
          6) Drug-induced
          7) Other
      b. Allergic reactions
          1) Dental restorative materials
              a) Mercury
              b) Nickel
              c) Acrylic
              d) Other
          2) Reactions attributable to
              a) Toothpastes/dentifrices
              b) Mouthrinses/mouthwashes
              c) Chewing gum additives
              d) Foods and additives
          3) Other
  6. Traumatic lesions (factitious, iatrogenic, accidental)
      a. Chemical injury
      b. Physical injury
      c. Thermal injury
  7. Foreign body reactions
  8. Not otherwise specified (NOS)
II. Chronic Periodontitis†
  A. Localized
  B. Generalized
III. Aggressive Periodontitis†
  A. Localized
  B. Generalized
IV. Periodontitis as a Manifestation of Systemic Diseases
  A. Associated with hematological disorders
      1. Acquired neutropenia
      2. Leukemias
      3. Other
  B. Associated with genetic disorders
      1. Familial and cyclic neutropenia
      2. Down syndrome
      3. Leukocyte adhesion deficiency syndromes
      4. Papillon-Lefèvre syndrome
      5. Chediak-Higashi syndrome

(continued)

Box 9-3 (continued)

6. Histiocytosis syndromes
7. Glycogen storage disease
8. Infantile genetic agranulocytosis
9. Cohen syndrome
10. Ehlers-Danlos syndrome (Types IV and VIII)
11. Hypophosphatasia
12. Other
C. Not otherwise specified (NOS)
V. Necrotizing Periodontal Diseases
   A. Necrotizing ulcerative gingivitis (NUG
   B. Necrotizing ulcerative periodontitis (NUP)
VI. Abscesses of the Periodontium
   A. Gingival abscess
   B. Periodontal abscess
   C. Pericoronal abscess
VII. Periodontitis Associated with Endodontic Lesions
   A. Combined periodontic-endodontic lesions
VIII. Developmental or Acquired Deformities and Conditions
   A. Localized tooth-related factors that modify or predispose to plaque-induced gingival diseases or periodontitis
      1. Tooth anatomic factors
      2. Dental restorations/appliances
      3. Root fractures
      4. Cervical root resorption and cemental tears

B. Mucogingival deformities and conditions around teeth
   1. Gingival/soft tissue recession
      a. Facial or lingual surfaces
      b. Interproximal (papillary)
   2. Lack of keratinized gingiva
   3. Decreased vestibular depth
   4. Aberrant frenum/muscle position
   5. Gingival excess
      a. Pseudopocket
      b. Inconsistent gingival margin
      c. Excessive gingival display
      d. Gingival enlargement
   6. Abnormal color
C. Mucogingival deformities and conditions on edentulous ridges
   1. Vertical and/or horizontal ridge deficiency
   2. Lack of gingiva/keratinized tissue
   3. Gingival/soft tissue enlargement
   4. Aberrant frenum/muscle position
   5. Decreased vestibular depth
   6. Abnormal color
D. Occlusal trauma
   1. Primary occlusal trauma
   2. Secondary occlusal trauma

*Can occur on a periodontium with no attachment loss or on a periodontium with attachment loss that is not progressing.
†Can be further classified on the basis of extent and severity.
Used by permission from 1999 International Workshop for a Classification of Periodontal Diseases and Conditions. Papers. Oak Brook, Illinois, October 30–November 2, 1999. *Ann Periodontol.* 1999;4:2, 3.

GINGIVAL DISEASES

Gingival diseases usually involve inflammation of the gingival tissues, most often in response to bacterial plaque. Gingival diseases have been subdivided into two major categories: (i) dental plaque-induced gingival diseases and (ii) nonplaque-induced gingival lesions.

1. **Dental Plaque-Induced Gingival Diseases**
   A. Definition. **Plaque-induced gingival diseases** are periodontal diseases involving inflammation of the gingiva in response to bacteria located at the gingival margin.
   B. There are four main types of plaque-induced gingival diseases.
      1. **Gingivitis associated with dental plaque only**—the most common form is gingivitis resulting from dental plaque only.
      2. **Gingival diseases modified by systemic factors**—gingival diseases with contributing systemic factors.
      3. **Gingival diseases modified by medications**—medication-induced gingival diseases.
      4. **Gingival diseases modified by malnutrition**—gingival diseases with malnutrition as a contributing factor.
   C. Disease Progression. Gingivitis may persist for years without ever progressing to periodontitis.
2. **Nonplaque-induced gingival lesions.**
   A. A small percentage of gingivitis is not caused by bacterial plaque.
   B. Nonplaque-induced gingivitis can result from such varied causes as viral infections, fungal infections, dermatologic (skin) diseases, allergic reactions, or mechanical trauma.

PERIODONTITIS

1. **Types of Periodontitis.** Periodontitis has been subdivided into seven major categories (Box 9-1):
   (1) Chronic periodontitis
   (2) Aggressive periodontitis
   (3) Periodontitis as a manifestation of systemic disease
   (4) Necrotizing periodontal diseases
   (5) Abscesses of the periodontium
   (6) Periodontitis associated with endodontic lesions
   (7) Developmental or acquired deformities and conditions

2. **Chronic Periodontitis (Most Common Form of Periodontitis)**
   A. Definition. **Chronic periodontitis**—the most common form of periodontitis—is a bacterial infection within the supporting tissues of the teeth. The disease is characterized by destruction of the periodontal ligament fibers and alveolar bone, and by pocket formation and/or gingival recession. This type of periodontitis was previously known as adult periodontitis.
   B. Clinical Features
      1. Chronic periodontitis is most prevalent in adults but may occur in both the primary and adult dentitions.
      2. The disease usually progresses (worsens) at a slow to moderate rate, but there may be short periods of rapid disease progression.
      3. The amount of tissue destruction is consistent with the presence of local etiologic factors.
      4. Bacterial plaque and subgingival calculus are frequent findings.
      5. The disease can be modified by and/or associated with systemic disease.
      6. Other factors, such as smoking, can be predisposing factors.
      7. Chronic periodontitis can be further classified on the basis of extent and severity.

3. **Aggressive Periodontitis (Highly Destructive Form of Periodontitis)**
   A. Definition. **Aggressive periodontitis** is characterized by a rapid loss of attachment and a less predictable response to periodontal therapy (than chronic periodontitis). Aggressive periodontitis affects individuals who otherwise are clinically healthy. This type of periodontitis was previously known as early-onset periodontitis.
      1. Localized aggressive periodontitis was formerly known as localized juvenile periodontitis.
      2. Generalized aggressive periodontitis was formerly known as generalized juvenile periodontitis.
   B. Clinical Features
      1. Aggressive periodontitis is less common than chronic periodontitis and may occur in both the primary and adult dentitions.
      2. The disease usually progresses at a rapid rate.
      3. The amount of tissue destruction may be inconsistent with the presence of local etiologic factors. Rapid disease progression can occur in the presence of relatively small amounts of bacterial plaque exhibited by the patient.
      4. The disease can be modified by and/or associated with immune deficiencies and other genetic factors.

4. **Periodontitis as a Manifestation of Systemic Diseases.** **Periodontitis as a manifestation of systemic diseases** is a group of periodontal diseases that are associated with (i) hematologic disorders, such as leukemia or acquired neutropenia, and (ii) genetic disorders, such as Down syndrome or leukocyte adhesion deficiency syndrome.

5. **Necrotizing Periodontal Diseases.** **Necrotizing periodontal diseases** are a unique type of periodontal disease that involve tissue necrosis (localized tissue death) that is limited to the gingival tissues (necrotizing ulcerative gingivitis) or tissue necrosis of the gingival tissues combined with loss of attachment and alveolar bone loss (necrotizing ulcerative periodontitis).

6. **Abscesses of the Periodontium**
   A. **A periodontal abscess** is a localized collection of pus that forms in a circumscribed area of the periodontal tissues.
   B. Periodontal abscesses are a common feature of moderate or advanced periodontitis.

7. **Periodontitis Associated with Endodontic Lesions**
   A. Endodontic Lesion. A tooth can be affected by **pulpal disease**—the infection or death of the tissues that comprise the pulp of the tooth. Pulpal disease can result in bone loss around the apex of the tooth. Pulpal disease in a tooth usually requires **endodontic treatment** (a root canal) to save the tooth.
   B. In some patients, periodontitis and pulpal disease can be related. Sometimes periodontitis is so severe that it affects the apex of the tooth or one of the accessory openings into the pulp chamber that occur in some teeth. When this occurs, the bacterial infection of the periodontium can lead to infection of the dental pulp.
   C. In advanced stages of pulpal disease, the pulpal disease can result in periodontal destruction by spreading of the infection from the dental pulp to the periodontal ligament and alveolar bone.
   D. A tooth can be affected by both periodontal disease and pulpal disease at the same time. When periodontitis and bone loss caused by pulpal disease affect the same tooth so severely that they become combined into one lesion, the condition usually is referred to as a **combined periodontal-endodontic lesion**.

8. **Developmental or Acquired Deformities and Conditions.** This category includes conditions that exist around the teeth that may predispose the periodontium to disease such as anatomic features of the teeth, root abnormalities, dental restorations, mucogingival deformities (such as soft tissue recession), and occlusal trauma.

CHAPTER SUMMARY STATEMENT

The two basic diagnostic categories of periodontal disease are (i) gingivitis and (ii) periodontitis. It is important to be thoroughly familiar with the terms periodontal disease, gingivitis, and periodontitis and the precise definition of each term. There are many specific periodontal diseases that have been subdivided into classifications. Periodontal disease classifications assist the dental hygienist in communicating with other dental healthcare providers, patients, and dental insurance providers.

Reference

1. 1999 International Workshop for a Classification of Periodontal Diseases and Conditions. Papers. Oak Brook, Illinois, October 30-November 2, 1999. *Ann Periodontol.* 1999;4:1–112.

Suggested Readings

Parameters of care. American Academy of Periodontology. *J Periodontol.* 2000;71(Suppl 5): i–ii, 847–883.

American Academy of Periodontology. *Current Procedural Terminology for Periodontics and Insurance Reporting Manual.* 8th ed. Chicago: American Academy of Periodontology; 2000.

American Academy of Periodontology. *Glossary of Periodontal Terms.* 4th ed. Chicago: American Academy of Periodontology; 2001.

SECTION 3: CHAPTER REVIEW QUESTIONS

1. Which of the following are periodontal diseases?
   A. Gingivitis
   B. Periodontitis
   C. Both (a) and (b)

2. Which of the following is a classification of periodontal disease that is described as a bacterial infection of all parts of the periodontium?
   A. Gingivitis
   B. Periodontitis
   C. Periodontal disease

3. Which of the following are periodontal diseases?
   A. Dental plaque-induced gingival diseases
   B. Gingival disease modified by medications
   C. Chronic periodontitis
   D. All of the above

4. Which of the following is a classification of periodontal disease that is described as periodontal disease with a rapid loss of attachment and a less predictable response to periodontal therapy?
   A. Chronic periodontitis
   B. Aggressive periodontitis
   C. Periodontitis as a manifestation of systemic disease
   D. Necrotizing periodontal diseases

5. Which of the following is a classification of periodontal disease that is described as a group of periodontal diseases that are associated with hematologic disorders and genetic disorders?
   A. Chronic periodontitis
   B. Aggressive periodontitis
   C. Periodontitis as a manifestation of systemic disease
   D. Necrotizing periodontal diseases

6. Which of the following is a classification of periodontal disease that is described as a unique type of periodontal disease that involves tissue necrosis of the gingival tissues combined with loss of attachment and alveolar bone loss?
   A. Chronic periodontitis
   B. Aggressive periodontitis
   C. Periodontitis as a manifestation of systemic disease
   D. Necrotizing periodontal diseases

7. Which of the following is a classification of periodontal disease that is described as the most common form of periodontal disease due to inflammation of only the gingiva in response to bacteria located at the gingival margin?
   A. Gingivitis associated with dental plaque only
   B. Gingival diseases modified by medications
   C. Chronic periodontitis
   D. Aggressive periodontitis

chapter

10 Gingival Diseases

Refer to the CD packaged with this book for full color versions of the clinical photographs in this chapter.

Learning Objectives

- Describe characteristics of the gingiva in health.
- List clinical signs of gingival inflammation.
- Explain the difference in color between acute and chronic inflammation.
- Differentiate between bulbous, blunted, and cratered papilla.
- Write a description of gingival inflammation that includes descriptors of duration, extent, and distribution of inflammation.
- Name and define the two major subdivisions of gingival disease.
- Compare and contrast dental plaque-induced gingival diseases and nonplaque-induced gingival lesions.
- For a patient with plaque-induced gingivitis, point out to your clinical instructor the signs of inflammation present in the patient's mouth.
- List systemic factors that will modify gingival disease.

- Theorize why the use of certain medications and malnutrition can modify gingival disease.
- Formulate a treatment plan for primary herpetic gingivostomatitis.
- Describe clinical manifestations of an allergic reaction to toothpaste or mouthwash.
- Identify etiology of nonplaque-induced gingival lesions.

KEY TERMS

Gingivitis
Stippling
Bulbous papilla
Blunted papilla
Cratered papilla
Acute gingivitis
Chronic gingivitis
Localized inflammation
Generalized inflammation
Papillary inflammation
Marginal inflammation
Diffuse inflammation
Dental plaque-induced gingival diseases
Plaque-induced gingivitis

Gingivitis on a periodontium with no attachment loss
Gingivitis on a reduced but stable periodontium
Peri-implant gingivitis
Gingival diseases with modifying factors
Gingival diseases modified by systemic factors
Gingival diseases associated with hormone fluctuations
Gingival diseases modified by medications
Gingival disease modified by malnutrition
Nonplaque-induced gingivitis
Primary herpetic gingivostomatitis

SECTION 1: GINGIVAL TISSUES

Gingival diseases are the mildest and most common form of periodontal disease. **Gingivitis** is an inflammation of the gingiva causing the tissue to become red and swollen, to bleed easily, and often to become slightly tender. These changes result from plaque biofilm accumulation along the gingival margins and the host's inflammatory response to the bacterial products. Gingivitis is reversible with professional treatment, good patient self-care, and the removal of local factors (such as a faulty dental restoration). This chapter begins with a review of the signs of healthy gingival tissue, followed by a discussion of the common types of gingival disease.

CHARACTERISTICS OF THE GINGIVA IN HEALTH

A key component of the periodontal assessment is an accurate gingival description. To describe diseased periodontal tissues, it is important to know what healthy tissues look like. This section reviews the characteristics of the gingiva in health and disease. Healthy gingival tissue is free of inflammation and has not been altered by disease or trauma (**Fig. 10-1**).

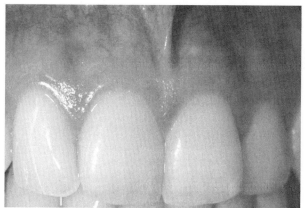
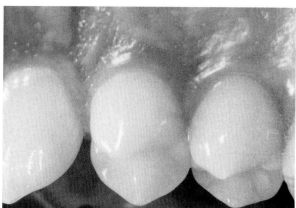

A   B

Figure 10-1. Healthy Gingiva. A: This tissue on the facial aspect of the maxillary anteriors exhibits all the characteristics of health, including a tapered margin slightly coronal to the cementoenamel junction (CEJ) and pointed papillae that completely fill the space between the teeth. **B:** This tissue on the lingual aspect of the maxillary premolar region shows healthy tissue with a slightly rounded gingival margin and papillae that completely fill the space between the teeth. (Photos courtesy of Dr. Don Rolfs, Periodontal Foundations, Wenatchee, WA.)

1. **Color**
    A. The gingival tissue should appear uniformly pink.
        1. The shade of pink will be lighter in blondes with fair complexions and darker in brunettes with dark complexions.
        2. The pink gingiva is easily distinguished from the darker alveolar mucosa.
    B. Healthy tissue also can be pigmented. The pigmented areas of the attached gingiva may range from light brown to black.
2. **Size.** In health, the gingival tissue lies snugly around the tooth and firmly against the alveolar bone.
3. **Shape**
    A. The gingival margin meets the tooth with a tapered, flat, or slightly rounded edge and follows the curvature of the tooth to create scalloped contours.
    B. Papillae come to a point and fill the space between teeth.
    C. Teeth with a diastema (no contact between adjacent teeth) or large spaces between teeth will have flat papillae.

4. **Consistency**
   A. The attached gingiva is firmly connected to the underlying cementum and alveolar bone.
   B. The tissue is resilient (elastic). If gentle pressure is applied to the gingiva with the side of a probe, the tissue resists compression and springs back almost immediately.
   C. The attached gingiva will not pull away from the tooth when air is blown into the sulcus.
5. **Surface Texture**
   A. In health, the surface of the attached gingiva is firm and may have a dimpled appearance similar to the skin of an orange peel.
   B. This dimpled appearance is known as **stippling**. The presence of stippling is best viewed by drying the tissue with compressed air.
   C. Healthy tissue may or may not exhibit a stippled appearance as the presence of stippling varies greatly from individual to individual.
6. **Position of Gingival Margin.** In a healthy mouth, the gingival margin is at or slightly coronal to (above) the CEJ.
7. **Bleeding.** Healthy tissue does not bleed.
8. **Exudate.** There is no exudate (discharge of pus) in healthy gingival tissue.

Table 10-1. Characteristics of Healthy Tissue versus Gingivitis

	Healthy Tissue	**Gingivitis**
Color	Uniform pink color Pigmentation may be present	Acute: Bright red Chronic: Purplish-red

Shape	Marginal gingiva:
	    Meets the tooth in a tapered
	    or slightly rounded edge
	Interdental papillae:
	    Pointed papilla fills the space
	    between the teeth
		Marginal gingiva:
		    Meets the tooth in a rolled,
		    thickened edge
		Interdental papillae:
		    Bulbous
		    Blunted
		    Cratered

Consistency	Firm
	Resilient under compression
		Acute inflammation:
		    Spongy, flaccid
		    Indents easily when pressed
		    lightly
		    Compressed air will deflect the
		    tissue

Texture	Smooth and/or stippled	Acute inflammation:
		    Very shiny
		    Stretched appearance

Margin	Gingival margin at the CEJ	Coronal to the CEJ
Bleeding	No bleeding upon probing	Spontaneous bleeding upon probing
Exudate	No exudate upon pressure	Pus may be visible upon pressure

CEJ, cementoenamel junction.

CHARACTERISTICS OF THE GINGIVA IN DISEASE

The bacterial plaque biofilm at the gingival margin stimulates the host immune response. The inflammatory response to the bacteria results in clinical changes in the gingival tissue involving the free and attached gingiva as well as the papillae (**Table 10-1**).

1. **Tissue Color in Gingivitis**
   A. Acute Inflammation of the Gingiva. Increased blood flow to the gingival tissue causes the tissue to appear bright red.
   B. Chronic Inflammation of the Gingiva. In chronic gingivitis, the gingival tissue may appear bluish-red or purplish-red.
2. **Tissue Size in Gingivitis**
   A. The increase in tissue fluid causes enlargement of the marginal and interproximal gingival tissues.
   B. The change can be localized to a few areas or affect the whole mouth.
3. **Tissue Consistency in Gingivitis**
   A. The tissue is swollen (edematous tissue), soft, spongy, and non-elastic.
   B. When pressure is applied to the gingiva with the side of a probe, the tissue is easily compressed and will retain an imprint of the probe for several seconds.
   C. When air is blown into the sulcus, the tissue is flaccid (loose, flabby), the gingival margin and papillae are readily deflected by the air away from the neck of the tooth.
4. **Tissue Shape in Gingivitis**
   A. In diseased tissue, the free gingiva is no longer flat but rather rolled and thickened as a result of edema (fluid) at the neck of the tooth.
   B. Papillae may be bulbous, blunted, or cratered (**Figs. 10-2, 10-3, and 10-4**).
      1. **Bulbous**—papilla is enlarged and appears to bulge out of the interproximal space.
      2. **Blunted**—papilla is flat and does not fill the interproximal space.
      3. **Cratered**—papilla appears to have been scooped out leaving a concave depression in the midproximal area. Cratered papillae are associated with necrotizing ulcerative gingivitis.

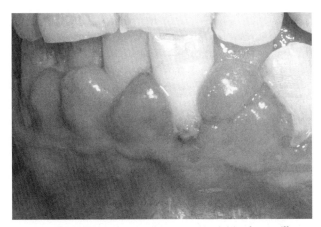

Figure 10-2. Bulbous Papillae. In gingivitis, the papillae may be enlarged and appear to bulge out of the interproximal space. (Courtesy of Dr. Don Rolfs, Periodontal Foundations, Wenatchee, WA.)

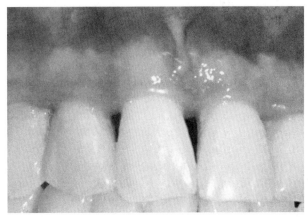

Figure 10-3. Blunted Papillae. In gingivitis, the papillae may be blunted and missing. (Courtesy of Dr. Don Rolfs, Periodontal Foundations, Wenatchee, WA.)

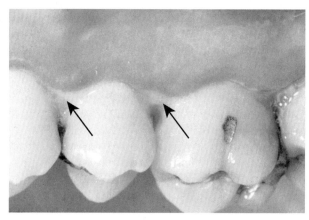

Figure 10-4. Cratered Papillae. In necrotizing ulcerative gingivitis, the papillae may have a concave appearance in the mid-proximal area. Such papillae are referred to as cratered papillae. (Courtesy of Dr. Don Rolfs, Periodontal Foundations, Wenatchee, WA.)

5. **Surface Texture in Gingivitis**
   A. The increase in fluid from the body's inflammatory response causes the gingival tissues to appear smooth and very shiny.
   B. The tissue almost has a stretched appearance that resembles plastic wrap that has been pulled tightly.
6. **Position of Margin in Gingivitis**
   A. In gingivitis, the position of the gingival margin may move more coronally (further above the CEJ).
   B. This change in the position of the gingival margin is due to tissue swelling and enlargement.
7. **Presence of Bleeding in Gingivitis**
   A. In diseased tissue, the sulcus lining becomes ulcerated and the blood vessels become engorged.
   B. When the gingival tissues are disturbed by probing or instrumentation, they can bleed easily.

DESCRIBING GINGIVAL INFLAMMATION

1. **Duration of Gingivitis**
   A. **Acute gingivitis**—gingivitis of a short duration, after which professional care and patient self-care returns the gingiva to a healthy state.
   B. **Chronic gingivitis**—long-lasting gingivitis; gingivitis may exist for years without ever progressing to periodontitis.
2. **Extent of Inflammation**
   A. **Localized gingivitis**—inflammation confined to the gingival tissue of a single tooth or group of teeth.
   B. **Generalized gingivitis**—inflammation of the gingival tissue of all or most of the mouth.
3. **Distribution of Inflammation**
   A. **Papillary**—inflammation of the interdental papilla only.
   B. **Marginal**—inflammation of the gingival margin and papilla.
   C. **Diffuse**—inflammation of the gingival margin, papilla, and attached gingiva.
4. **Use of Descriptive Terminology.** Descriptive terms may be combined to create a verbal picture of the gingiva, such as:
   - Localized marginal inflammation in the mandibular anterior sextant
   - Localized papillary inflammation on the maxillary right canine
   - Generalized marginal inflammation
   - Generalized diffuse inflammation, etc.

SECTION 2: CLASSIFICATION OF GINGIVAL DISEASES

As discussed in Chapter 9, the two major subdivisions of gingival disease are (i) dental plaque-induced gingival diseases and (ii) nonplaque-induced gingival lesions (**Fig. 10-5**). Certain characteristics must be present for a periodontal disease to be classified as a gingival disease (**Box 10-1**).

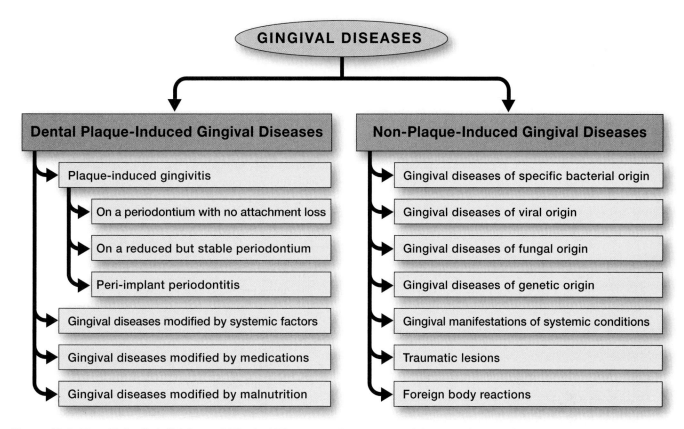

Figure 10-5. Two Major Subdivisions of Gingival Diseases. The two major subdivisions of gingival diseases are (i) dental plaque-induced gingival diseases and (ii) nonplaque-induced gingival lesions. These two major subdivisions are further subdivided into types.

Box 10-1

Characteristics Common to All Gingival Diseases

1. Signs of symptoms of inflammation that are confined to the gingiva
2. The presence of dental plaque biofilm to initiate and/or aggravate the inflammation
3. Clinical signs of inflammation (enlarged gingival contours, color transition to a red and/or bluish-red hue, elevated sulcular temperature, bleeding upon stimulation, increased crevicular fluid flow)
4. Inflammation that is reversible with plaque removal
5. A possible role in the initiation of periodontitis if gingivitis is left untreated

SECTION 3: DENTAL PLAQUE-INDUCED GINGIVAL DISEASES

Dental plaque-induced gingival diseases are periodontal diseases involving inflammation of the gingiva in response to bacteria located at the gingival margin. There are two main subdivisions of dental plaque-induced gingival diseases: (i) plaque-induced gingivitis and (ii) gingival diseases with modifying factors. Treatment is very effective at reversing tissue damage and returning the tissues to health.

PLAQUE-INDUCED GINGIVITIS

1. **Plaque-induced gingivitis** is gingival inflammation of a periodontium resulting from dental plaque (**Box 10-2**).
   A. Plaque-induced gingivitis is by far the most common type of periodontal disease and is characterized clinically by red, swollen, tender gums that bleed easily.
   B. Criteria. Plaque-induced gingivitis must be associated with *stable* attachment levels. Plaque-induced gingivitis can occur:
      1. On a periodontium with no attachment loss. In other words, plaque-induced gingivitis can occur on a tooth that has never experienced periodontitis.
      2. On a periodontium with attachment loss that is not progressing (worsening). In other words, plaque-induced gingivitis could also occur on a tooth that has experienced bone loss at a previous time but the periodontitis is controlled and there is no additional bone loss or loss of attachment at the present time.

Box 10-2

Plaque-Induced Gingivitis

- Most common form of periodontal disease
- Plaque present at the gingival margin
- Gingival redness; tenderness
- Swollen, rolled margins
- Increase in sulcular temperature
- Bleeding upon probing
- No attachment loss or bone loss
- Condition reversible with plaque removal

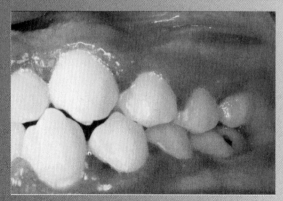

Figure 10-6A. Plaque-Induced Gingivitis. Plaque-induced gingivitis in this patient has resulted in a rolled gingival margin and enlarged papillae.

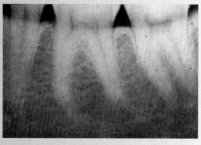

Figure 6B. Radiograph Reveals No Bone Loss. The dental radiographs of an individual with plaque-induced gingivitis do not reveal any changes in either the alveolar bone height or the character of the alveolar bone.

3. **Gingivitis on a Periodontium with No Attachment Loss.** This type of plaque-induced gingivitis occurs on a periodontium that has no attachment loss. In this instance, there is not now, nor has there been, destruction of periodontal fibers or alveolar bone.

4. **Gingivitis on a Reduced but Stable Periodontium.**
   A. This type of plaque-induced gingivitis occurs in patients who have been successfully treated for periodontitis but who afterward develop gingivitis.
   B. In this instance, there is loss of attachment and alveolar bone *(due to previous destruction of fibers and bone)*, but at this time the periodontium is not undergoing any additional attachment loss (**Box 10-3**).

5. **Peri-implant gingivitis** is plaque-induced gingivitis that occurs in the gingival tissues surrounding a dental implant (**Box 10-4**).

Box 10-3

Plaque-Induced Gingivitis on a Reduced but Stable Periodontium

- Pre-existing attachment loss or bone loss
- Plaque present at gingival margin
- Disease begins at the gingival margin
- Gingival redness
- Swollen, rolled margins
- Increase in sulcular temperature
- Bleeding upon probing
- Reversible with plaque removal

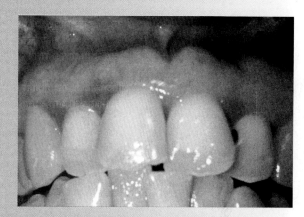

Figure 10-7. Plaque-Induced Gingivitis with Previous Attachment Loss. The teeth pictured here experienced periodontitis several years ago. There has been no additional bone loss since that time. Currently, plaque-induced gingivitis is present, however, probing depths reveal no additional bone loss.

Box 10-4

Peri-Implant Gingivitis

- Gingival inflammation around a dental implant
- Plaque present at gingival margin
- Change in gingival color
- Change in gingival contour
- Bleeding upon probing
- Gingivitis is reversible with good daily plaque control

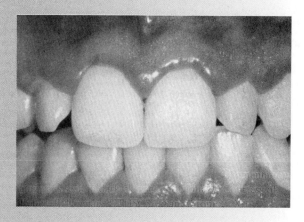

Figure 10-8. Peri-Implant Gingivitis. Peri-implant gingivitis around an implant-supported crown on the left central incisor.

GINGIVAL DISEASES WITH MODIFYING FACTORS

The category, **gingival diseases with modifying factors**, is composed of the less common types of plaque-induced gingivitis. There are three main subcategories of gingival diseases with modifying factors: (i) gingival diseases modified by systemic factors, (ii) gingival diseases modified by medications, and (iii) gingival diseases modified by malnutrition.

1. **Gingival Diseases Modified by Systemic Factors.** In this form of gingival disease, plaque initiates the disease; then, specific systemic factors found in the host will modify the disease process.

   A. **Gingival diseases associated with the endocrine system and fluctuations in sex hormones**
      1. *Puberty-associated gingivitis*—an exaggerated inflammatory response of the gingiva to a relatively small amount of dental plaque and hormones during puberty.
      2. *Menstrual cycle-associated gingivitis*—an exaggerated inflammatory response of the gingiva to dental plaque and hormones before ovulation.
      3. *Oral contraceptive-associated gingivitis*—an exaggerated inflammatory response of the gingiva to dental plaque and oral contraceptives.
      4. *Pregnancy-associated gingivitis*—an exaggerated inflammatory response of the gingiva to dental plaque and hormone changes usually occurring during the second and third trimesters of pregnancy.
      5. *Pregnancy-associated pyogenic granuloma (pregnancy tumor)*—a localized, mushroom-shaped gingival mass projecting from the gingival margin or more commonly from a gingival papilla during pregnancy (**Box 10-5**).

Box 10-5

Pregnancy-Associated Pyogenic Granuloma

- Exaggerated inflammatory response to an irritation
- Can occur anytime during pregnancy
- More common in maxilla and interproximally
- Protuberant mushroom-like mass
- Mass bleeds easily if disturbed
- Growths are non cancerous
- Growths usually are not painful
- Growth regresses after giving birth

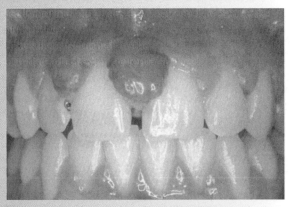

Figure 10-9. Pregnancy-Associated Pyogenic Granuloma. This mushroom-like mass of the gingiva bleeds easily if disturbed.

   B. **Gingival diseases associated with systemic diseases**, such as diabetes–associated gingivitis and leukemia-associated gingivitis
      1. *Diabetes-associated gingivitis*—an inflammatory response of the gingiva to dental plaque that is aggravated by poorly controlled blood glucose levels.
      2. *Leukemia-associated gingivitis*—an exaggerated inflammatory response of the gingiva to plaque resulting in increased bleeding and enlargement. Oral lesions are usually the first clinical signs of leukemia; therefore, dental healthcare providers are quite often the first to suspect that a patient may have leukemia.
      3. *Blood dyscrasias-associated gingivitis*—gingivitis associated with abnormal function or number of blood cells.

2. **Gingival Diseases Modified by Medications**
   A. *Drug-influenced gingivitis*—exaggerated inflammatory response of the gingiva to dental plaque and a systemic medication.
   B. *Drug-influenced gingival enlargement*—enlargement of the gingiva resulting from systemic medications, most commonly anticonvulsants, calcium channel blockers, and immunosuppressants. Plaque accumulation is not necessary for the initiation of gingival enlargement but it will exacerbate the gingival disease. Meticulous plaque control can reduce but will not eliminate gingival overgrowth (**Box 10-6**).
3. **Gingival Diseases Modified by Malnutrition.** Even with our adequate food supply in North America, infants from low socioeconomic families, institutionalized elderly, and alcoholics are all at risk for vitamin deficiencies.
   A. *Ascorbic acid-deficiency gingivitis*—inflammatory response of the gingiva to dental plaque aggravated by chronically low ascorbic acid (vitamin C) levels. Ascorbic acid-deficiency gingivitis manifests as bright red, swollen, ulcerated gingival tissue that bleeds with the slightest provocation.
   B. Other. Specific nutrient deficiencies can exacerbate the response of gingival tissues to plaque. In animal studies, a deficiency in vitamin A, a deficiency in the B-complex vitamins, and starvation have all had an effect on gingival tissues. Vitamin A helps maintain healthy sulcular epithelium. B-complex vitamins help maintain healthy mucosal tissues. Starvation eliminates all nutrients necessary for healthy periodontium.

Box 10-6

Drug-Influenced Gingival Enlargement

- Occurs in individuals taking phenytoin, cyclosporine A, or certain calcium channel blockers
- Onset within 3 months of taking medication
- Exaggerated inflammatory response in relation to the plaque present
- Good daily plaque control limit the severity of lesion
- Higher prevalence in children
- Change in gingival contour, size, and color
- Gingiva in anterior sextants most commonly affected, however, can occur in posterior sextants
- Gingival enlargement first observed at the interdental papilla
- Increased crevicular fluid flow
- Bleeding upon probing
- No attachment loss

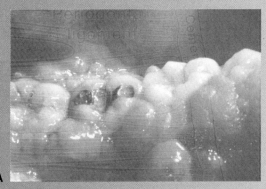
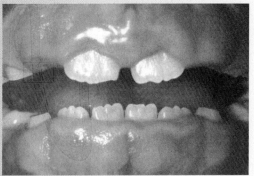

A   B

Figure 10-10. Drug-Induced Gingival Enlargement. A: Gingival changes seen in cyclosporine-induced gingival enlargement. B: Massive-tissue overgrowth may be seen in phenytoin-induced gingival enlargement.

SECTION 4: NONPLAQUE-INDUCED GINGIVAL LESIONS

A small percentage of gingival disease is not caused by bacterial plaque and does not disappear after plaque removal. *It should be emphasized, however, that the presence of dental plaque could increase the severity of the gingival inflammation in nonplaque-induced lesions.* **Nonplaque-induced gingivitis** can result from such varied causes as:

- Viral or fungal infections
- Dermatological (skin) diseases
- Allergic reactions
- Mechanical trauma

Two of these that might be seen in the dental office, primary herpetic gingivostomatitis and allergic reactions, are the most common.

1. **Primary Herpetic Gingivostomatitis**—initial oral infection of the herpes simplex virus characterized by redness and multiple vesicles that easily rupture to form painful ulcers (**Box 10-7**).
    A. Disease Characteristics
       1. The infection usually affects young children (younger than age 10) but may affect young adults (ages 15 to 25).
       2. A significant problem in patients with primary herpetic gingivostomatitis is the pain caused by the mouth ulcers that make eating and drinking difficult.
       3. Primary herpetic gingivostomatitis is a contagious disease that usually regresses spontaneously within 10 to 20 days without scarring.
    B. Clinical Manifestations
       1. Fiery red marginal gingiva, widespread inflammation of the marginal and attached gingiva
       2. Small clusters of vesicles rapidly erupt throughout the mouth; later, these vesicles burst, forming yellowish ulcers that are surrounded by a red halo
       3. Headache, swollen lymph nodes, and sore throat are usually present
       4. Because this condition is a viral infection, there may be a low-grade fever usually not above 101°F.

Box 10-7

Primary Herpetic Gingivostomatitis

- Initial oral infection of the herpes simplex virus
- Most common in children and young adults
- Fiery red marginal gingiva
- Swollen interdental papillae that bleed easily
- Yellowish ulcers surrounded by red halo on gingiva, buccal and labial mucosa, palate, tongue, and lips
- Headache, fever, swollen lymph nodes, sore throat usually present
- Because it is painful for the patient to eat or drink, dehydration is a primary concern.

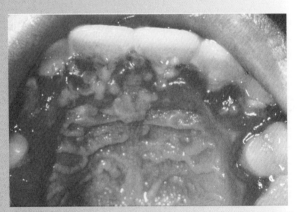

Figure 10-11. Primary Herpetic Gingivostomatitis. Primary herpetic gingivostomatitis is seen on the palate of this patient. View this figure on the CD and note the fiery red gingival margins and ulcers surrounded by red halos.

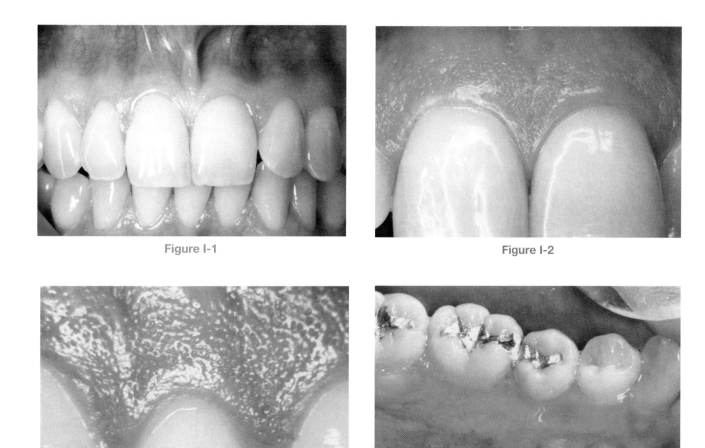

Figure I-1

Figure I-2

Figure I-3

Figure I-4

Figure I-1. Periodontal Health. Periodontal health showing coral pink gingiva and the normal scalloped contours of the gingiva. Note the distinct difference in appearance between the keratinized gingiva and the nonkeratinized alveolar mucosa.

Figure I-2. Periodontal Health. Periodontal health showing a close up view of free gingival margin and free gingival groove.

Figure I-3. Periodontal Health. Periodontal health showing stippling of the gingiva. (Courtesy of Dr. Robert P. Langlais)

Figure I-4. Periodontal Health. Periodontal health on the lingual surface of mandible showing coral pink gingiva with normal gingival contours. (Courtesy of Dr. Robert P. Langlais)

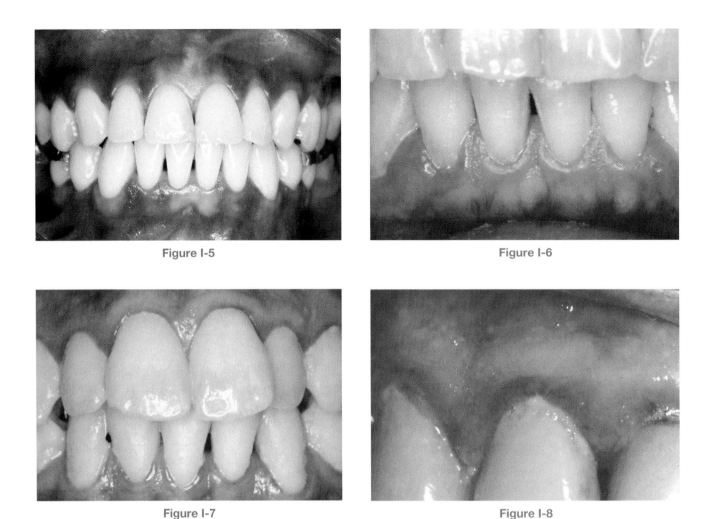

Figure I-5

Figure I-6

Figure I-7

Figure I-8

Figure I-5. Pigmentation of Gingiva. Pigmentation of the gingiva showing how the gingiva can vary in color in some patients.

Figure I-6. Plaque-Induced Gingivitis. Slight plaque-induced gingivitis. Note the very early edema of gingival margins and papillae.

Figure I-7. Plaque-Induced Gingivitis. Slight plaque-induced gingivitis. Note the very early erythema (redness) of gingival margin.

Figure I-8. Plaque-Induced Gingivitis. Moderate plaque-induced gingivitis. Note the redness of the gingival margins and papillae and the plaque and calculus on teeth.

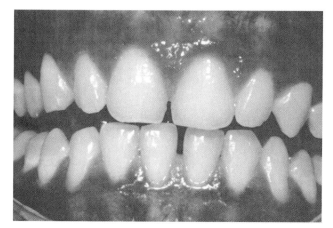

Figure I-9

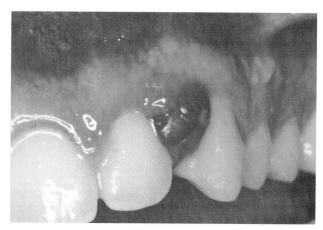

Figure I-10

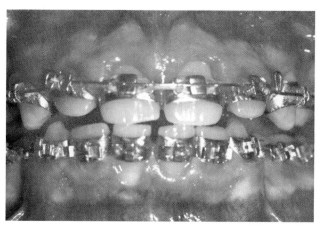

Figure I-11

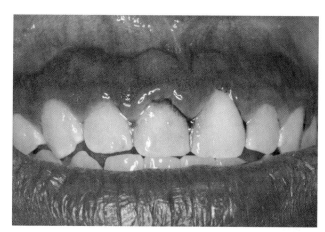

Figure I-12

Figure I-9. Gingivitis from an Allergic Reaction. Gingival changes in a patient with an allergy to a toothpaste ingredient. (Courtesy of Dr. Robert P. Langlais)

Figure I-10. Pregnancy-Associated Gingivitis. Pregnancy-associated gingivitis. This patient exhibits heavy plaque. (Courtesy of Dr. John S. Dozier)

Figure I-11. Plaque-Induced Gingivitis. Gingivitis associated with poor daily plaque control around metal orthodontic appliances (braces). (Courtesy of Dr. Don Rolfs)

Figure I-12. Plaque-Induced Gingivitis. The clinical signs of gingivitis may be less obvious in a patient with pigmentation of the gingiva. Bleeding is an obvious clinical sign, however, in the patient shown in this example. (Courtesy of Dr. Robert J. Foster)

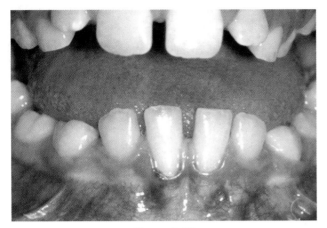

Figure I-13

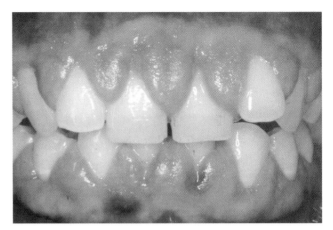

Figure I-14

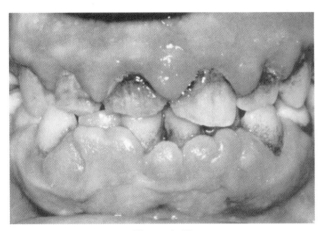

Figure I-15

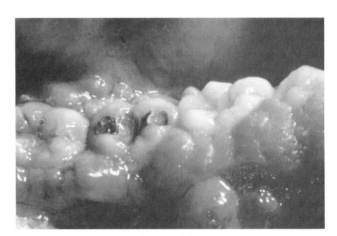

Figure I-16

Figure I-13. Plaque-Induced Gingivitis. Gingivitis on a mixed dentition. (Courtesy of Dr. Don Rolfs)

Figure I-14. Gingival Disease Modified by Medications. Gingival enlargement in a patient taking phenytoin for a seizure disorder. (Courtesy of Dr. John S. Dozier)

Figure I-15. Gingival Disease Modified by Medications. Pronounced gingival enlargement in a patient taking the medication phenytoin for a seizure disorder. (Courtesy of Dr. Robert P. Langlais)

Figure I-16. Gingival Disease Modified by Medications. Gingival enlargement in a patient taking cyclosporine (an immunosuppressive medication). (Courtesy of Dr. Robert P. Langlais)

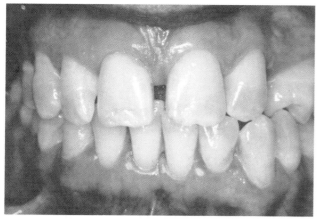

Figure I-17

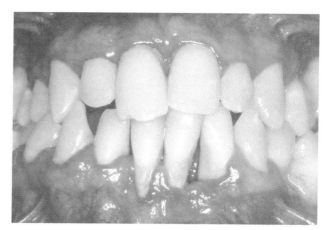

Figure I-18

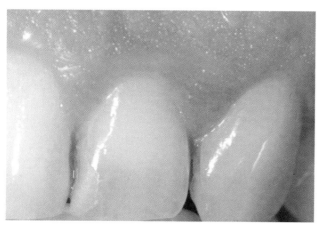

Figure I-19

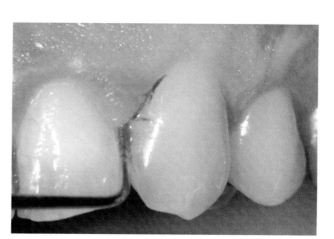

Figure I-20

Figure I-17. Chronic Periodontitis. Chronic periodontitis showing minimal changes in the appearance of the gingiva. It is important to remember that the tissue appearance cannot be relied upon to be a good indicator of the presence or severity of periodontitis.

Figure I-18. Chronic Periodontitis. Chronic periodontitis showing pronounced changes in the appearance of the gingiva. Compare this photograph to the one for Figure I-17. (Courtesy of Dr. John S. Dozier)

Figure I-19. Health or Disease? The clinical appearance of the tissue in this photograph suggests health. In Figure I-20, however, use of a periodontal probe reveals the presence of pocketing. (Courtesy of Dr. Don Rolfs)

Figure I-20. Health or Disease, continued from Figure I-19. The tissue shown in Figure I-19 has no clinical signs of disease. When assessed with a probe, however, a deep pocket 7 mm in depth reveals bone loss on the mesio-facial of the canine. This example underscores the importance of a thorough periodontal assessment of all patients.

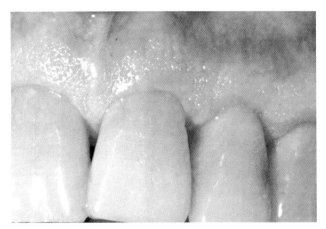

Figure I-21

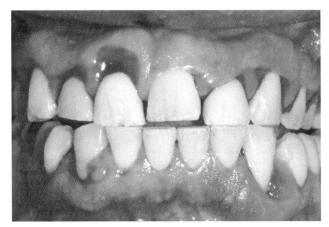

Figure I-22

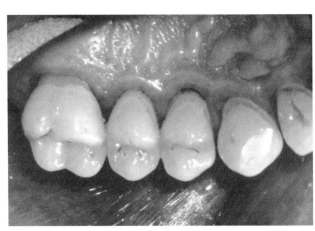

Figure I-23

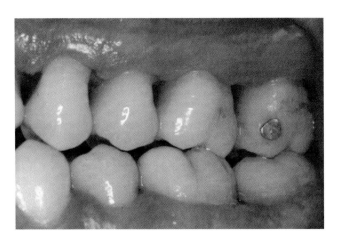

Figure I-24

Figure I-21. Tissue Health or Disease? This individual received periodontal treatment for chronic periodontitis several years ago. The assessment at today's appointment reveals meticulous patient self-care and no additional attachment loss since beginning periodontal maintenance several years ago. Therefore, this tissue is considered healthy. The attachment loss is simply an indicator of previous periodontal disease. (Courtesy of Dr. Don Rolfs)

Figure I-22. Chronic Periodontitis. Chronic periodontitis showing pronounced changes in the appearance of the gingiva.

Figure I-23. Chronic Periodontitis. Palatal gingiva in a patient with chronic periodontitis. Note the calculus deposits on the tooth surfaces and the rolled gingival margins. Clinical signs on the lingual aspect usually are not as evident as those seen on the facial aspect of the gingiva.

Figure I-24. Chronic Periodontitis. Chronic periodontitis showing blunting of the interdental papillae and gingival recession.

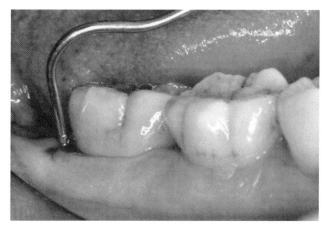

Figure I-25

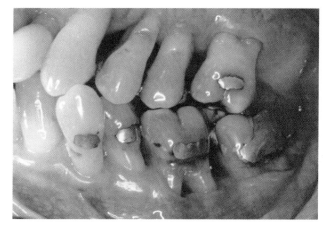

Figure I-26

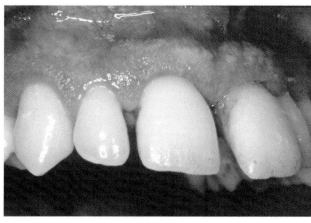

Figure I-27

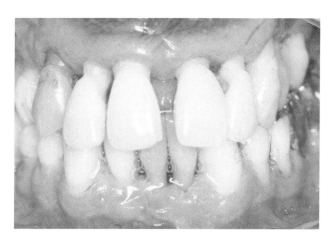

Figure I-28

Figure I-25. Chronic Periodontitis. Chronic periodontitis with probe inserted in a pocket showing attachment loss.

Figure I-26. Aggressive Periodontitis. Aggressive periodontitis in a patient with good plaque control. In aggressive periodontitis, the disease severity typically seems exaggerated given the amount of bacterial plaque.

Figure I-27. Chronic Periodontitis. An example of chronic periodontitis showing firm, nodular (fibrotic) tissue.

Figure I-28. Aggressive Periodontitis. An example of aggressive periodontitis with continued disease progression despite good daily self-care by the patient. (Courtesy of Dr. John S. Dozier)

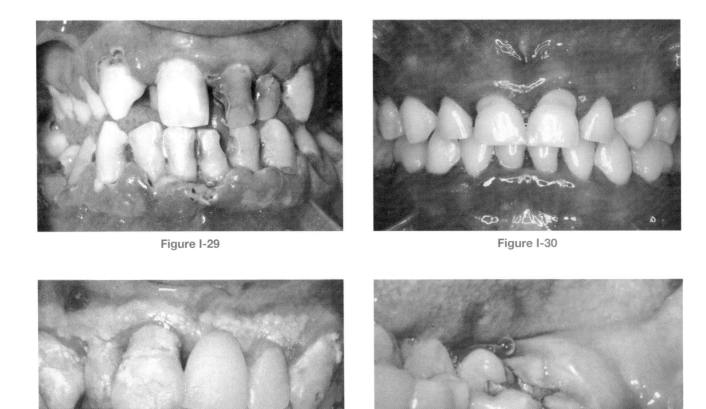

Figure I-29

Figure I-30

Figure I-31

Figure I-32

Figure I-29. Necrotizing Ulcerative Periodontitis. Necrotizing ulcerative periodontitis. (Courtesy of Dr. Don Rolfs)

Figure I-30 Periodontitis Associated with Immune Dysfunction. Periodontitis in a 5-year-old child associated with immune dysfunction.

Figure I-31. Aggressive Periodontitis. Aggressive periodontitis in a 20-year-old male.

Figure I-32. Pericoronitis. Pericoronitis around a third molar tooth. **Pericoronitis** is an infection in the soft tissue surrounding the crown of a partially erupted tooth. Pericoronitis is most frequently seen around third molar teeth, since these teeth often do not have space to erupt fully. A flap of gingival tissue can cover a portion of the crown of a partially erupted tooth and it is an infection under this flap of tissue that is referred to as pericoronitis. (Courtesy of Dr. Robert P. Langlais)

  C. Treatment
    1. If the temperature is below 101°F:
      a. Encourage the intake of fluids to prevent dehydration that can result from fever. Athletic drinks, such as Gatorade, can be consumed to replenish electrolytes lost due to dehydration.
      b. A dietary replacement drink, such as Ensure, can be a good source of nutrition since eating will be difficult. The patient may be able to eat foods processed in a blender.
      c. Counsel the patient that adequate intake of fluids is important. Since eating and drinking are painful, dehydration is a major concern with these individuals.
      d. An antimicrobial mouthwash like Listerine or Peridex should be recommended to prevent a secondary infection.
    2. If the temperature is above 101°F:
      a. Continue with steps 1, 2, and 3 listed above.
      b. A temperature of 102°F or above means that the patient has become septic with oral bacteria that have entered the bloodstream through the open sores on the gingiva and mucosa. This secondary infection usually will respond to penicillin-V, 500 mg, 4 tablets daily, 2 hours after meals, for 7 to 10 days. If the patient is allergic to penicillin, erythromycin can be prescribed.
      c. Counsel the patient that adequate intake of fluids is important. Since eating and drinking are painful, dehydration is a major concern with these individuals.

2. Allergic Reactions to Toothpastes and Mouthwashes—Allergic reactions can occur to ingredients in toothpastes and mouthwashes. These reactions are usually the result of an additive in the product.
  A. Occurrence
    1. Allergic reactions to toothpastes or mouthwashes occur most commonly in patients who have a history of allergic conditions such as hay fever, allergic skin rashes, and asthma.
    2. Allergic patients seem to be particularly sensitive to the flavoring agents and additives in tartar-control toothpastes. The most secret part of the formulation of toothpastes and mouthwashes is the flavoring agent, and this is usually the most allergenic component (**Box 10-8**).

Box 10-8

Allergic Reaction to Tarter Control Toothpaste

- Allergic reaction to additive in toothpaste
- Most common in individuals with a history of allergy (hay fever, asthma, hives)
- Fiery red gingivitis
- Ulcerations may be present
- Tissue sloughing of buccal and labial mucosa
- Cheilitis (painful fissures at the corners of the mouth)
- Discontinue use of suspected product

Cheilitis (painful fissures at the corners of the mouth)

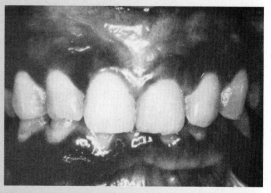

Figure 10-12. Allergic Reaction. Clinical signs of allergic reactions in the gingival tissues include redness extending from the gingival margin to the mucogingival junction. View a color version of this photo on the CD.

B. Recognition and Treatment of Allergic Reaction

1. The hygienist might suspect this problem in a patient with good plaque control who previously has had healthy gingiva (especially if the patient has a history of allergies). Inquire if the patient is using a new toothpaste or mouthwash.
2. Change brands of toothpaste or mouthwash. Cessation of the allergen-containing toothpaste or mouthwash should result in a resolution of the gingivitis.
3. If necessary, the diagnosis of allergic response can be confirmed by a biopsy with a diagnosis of plasma cell gingivitis.
4. When the manufacturer becomes aware of allergic reactions, the flavoring agent or additive causing the problem is usually altered. For this reason, the patient sometimes can switch back to the original product (after 6 to 12 months) and use it without problem.

3. Other Nonplaque-Induced Gingival Lesions

If you would like to learn more about the other nonplaque-induced gingival lesions, an excellent reference is the *1999 International Workshop for a Classification of Periodontal Diseases and Conditions* published by the American Academy of Periodontology (see Suggested Readings).

A. *Gingival diseases of specific bacterial origin*—a bacterial infection of the gingiva by a bacterium that is not a common component of the bacterial plaque biofilm.
B. *Gingival diseases of fungal origin*—white, red, or ulcerative lesions associated with immunocompromised patients, human immunodeficiency (HIV)-positive individuals, and individuals who use inhaled steroid medications to control respiratory problems (such as asthma and emphysema).
C. *Linear gingival erythema*—a gingival manifestation of immunosuppression characterized by a distinct red band limited to the free gingiva (**Box 10-9**).
D. *Gingival manifestations of mucocutaneous disorders*—oral manifestations of skin disorders characterized by erosions of the mucous membranes, vesicles, ulcers, and tissue sloughing. The lesions may be red, white, or striated in appearance.
E. *Traumatic lesions*—these are self-inflicted (factitious) and accidental injuries, or injuries that occur during dental treatment (iatrogenic injuries). The lesions may be abrasions, ulcerations, and burns.

Box 10-9

Linear Gingival Erythema

- Associated with HIV disease
- Plaque present at gingival margin
- Redness of the free and attached gingiva
- Spontaneous gingival bleeding
- Usually does not respond to therapy

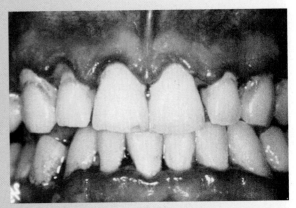

Figure 10-13. Linear Gingival Erythema. This patient has linear gingival erythema associated with HIV infection. View a color version on the CD.

CHAPTER SUMMARY STATEMENT

Gingival diseases are the mildest form of periodontal disease. Plaque-induced gingivitis is the most common of the periodontal diseases. Clinically, plaque-induced gingivitis is characterized by gingiva that is red, swollen, bleeds easily, and is slightly tender. Plaque-induced gingivitis may be modified by systemic factors, medications, or malnutrition. Nonplaque-induced gingival lesions are a group of uncommon gingival lesions that are not caused by bacterial plaque. Nonplaque-induced gingivitis can result from such diverse causes as infection, skin diseases, allergic reactions, or trauma.

Suggested Reading

1999 International Workshop for a Classification of Periodontal Diseases and Conditions. Papers. Oak Brook, Illinois, October 30-November 2, 1999. *Ann Periodontol.* 1999;4: 1–112.

SECTION 5: FOCUS ON PATIENTS

CASE 1

A patient new to your dental team has been appointed to you for a dental prophylaxis. The patient's periodontal diagnosis is generalized moderate plaque-induced gingivitis. During your discussion with the patient, he asks if there is some way he can tell at home if he has gingivitis. How might you reply to this patient's question?

CASE 2

You are scheduled to do a dental prophylaxis on a patient with a diagnosis of localized severe plaque-induced gingivitis. At the time of the appointment the patient informs you that she has just received notice that laboratory results indicate that she is pregnant. How might this pregnancy alter the periodontal diagnosis?

CASE 3

A patient who has been cared for by your dental team suddenly exhibits poor self-care with quite a bit of plaque accumulation. This is unusual for this patient. Discussions reveal that the patient is having difficulty with brushing and flossing due to soreness of the mouth. Examination reveals numerous small mucosal ulcers. Further discussions reveal that the patient has been experiencing this soreness since she began using tartar control toothpaste. How might your dental team manage this patient's diminished effectiveness of self-care?

CASE 4

Your patient is a 12-year-old male, who in spite of good oral hygiene practices, presents with generalized marginal redness and bleeding upon probing. His demonstration of tooth brushing and flossing indicates high dexterity and ability to remove bacterial plaque and in talking with his mother, she confirms that he practices daily oral hygiene. How would you explain the presence of gingival disease to this patient and what would you recommend to improve his gingival health?

SECTION 6: CHAPTER REVIEW QUESTIONS

1. A papilla that is enlarged and appears to bulge out of the interproximal space is called:
   A. Bulbous
   B. Blunted
   C. Cratered
   D. Scooped

2. Papilla that appears to have been scooped out leaving a concave depression in the mid-proximal area is called:
   A. Bulbous
   B. Blunted
   C. Cratered
   D. Scooped

3. In gingivitis, the position of the gingival margin is:
   A. Coronal to the CEJ
   B. Apical to the CEJ
   C. May be coronal or apical to the CEJ

4. A person's complexion can determine the shade of pink in healthy tissues.
   A. True
   B. False

5. If gingival tissues are healthy they will ALWAYS have a stippled appearance.
   A. True
   B. False

6. Gingivitis that has existed for years without progressing to periodontitis is termed:
   A. Localized gingivitis
   B. Generalized gingivitis
   C. Acute gingivitis
   D. Chronic gingivitis

7. Gingivitis in which the inflammation affects only one group of teeth is termed:
   A. Localized gingivitis
   B. Generalized gingivitis
   C. Acute gingivitis
   D. Chronic gingivitis

8. Red gingival tissues with multiple vesicles that easily rupture to form painful ulcers is defined as:
   A. Ascorbic acid deficiency gingivitis
   B. Primary herpetic gingivostomatitis
   C. Diabetes-associated gingivitis
   D. Leukemia-associated gingivitis

9. Which of the following is not a clinical manifestation of an allergic reaction to toothpaste?
   A. Fiery red edematous gingivitis
   B. Tissue sloughing of the buccal and labial mucosa
   C. Cheilitis
   D. Headache, swollen lymph nodes, and sore throat

Chapter

11 Periodontitis

Refer to the CD packaged with this book for full color versions of the clinical photographs in this chapter.

Learning Objectives

■ Name and define the three major categories of periodontitis.
■ Compare and contrast chronic periodontitis and aggressive periodontitis.
■ In the clinical setting, explain to your patient the signs and symptoms of chronic periodontal disease.
■ In a clinical setting for a patient with chronic periodontitis, describe to your clinical instructor the clinical signs of disease present in the patient's mouth.
■ List systemic factors that may be contributing factors to periodontitis.

- In the clinical setting, formulate an initial care plan for a patient with chronic periodontitis and explain it to your clinical instructor.
- Define and describe the clinical signs of recurrent chronic periodontitis.
- Define and describe the clinical signs of refractory chronic periodontitis.
- Discuss the differences between ideal and reasonable treatment goals for aggressive periodontitis.
- Given the clinical and radiographic features for a patient with a history of aggressive periodontitis, determine if the disease is localized or generalized aggressive periodontitis.
- Describe the impact of polymorphonuclear leukocyte (PMN; neutrophil) dysfunction on the periodontium.
- Describe the tissue destruction that occurs in necrotizing periodontal diseases.

KEY TERMS

Periodontitis
Chronic periodontitis
Peri-implantitis
Extent
Severity
Slight to moderate tissue destruction
Advanced tissue destruction
Disease progression
Localized chronic periodontitis
Generalized chronic periodontitis
Recurrent periodontitis

Refractory periodontitis
Aggressive periodontitis
Localized aggressive periodontitis
Generalized aggressive periodontitis
Necrotizing periodontal diseases
Necrotizing ulcerative gingivitis
Necrotizing ulcerative periodontitis
Gingival necrosis
Pseudomembrane
Secondary occlusal trauma

SECTION 1: CLASSIFICATION OF PERIODONTITIS

Periodontitis is a bacterial infection that affects all parts of the periodontium including the gingiva, periodontal ligament, bone, and cementum. It is the result of a complex interaction between the plaque biofilm that accumulates on tooth surfaces and the body's efforts to fight this infection. Periodontitis is the number one cause of tooth loss in adults and is particularly prevalent in smokers and those with modifying factors such as undiagnosed or poorly controlled diabetes mellitus. There are also some individuals who are genetically predisposed to developing this disease.

Periodontitis has been subdivided into three major categories: (i) chronic periodontitis, (ii) aggressive periodontitis, and (iii) less common types of periodontitis. Each major category has two or more subcategories. Refer to Figure 11-1 for a complete list of disease categories and subcategories.

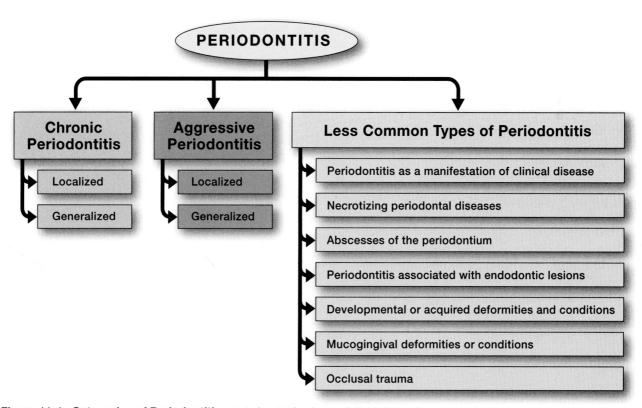

Figure 11-1. Categories of Periodontitis. Periodontitis has been subdivided into three major categories. Each of the three major categories has two or more subcategories.

SECTION 2: CHRONIC PERIODONTITIS—THE MOST COMMON FORM

CHARACTERISTICS OF CHRONIC PERIODONTITIS

1. **Chronic periodontitis** is a bacterial infection resulting in inflammation within the supporting tissues of the teeth, progressive destruction of the periodontal ligament, and loss of supporting alveolar bone. This is the most frequently occurring form of periodontitis.
2. **Alternative Terminology.** Chronic periodontitis was previously known as adult periodontitis. The name adult periodontitis, however, is inaccurate as this type of periodontitis can occur in individuals of any age: children, adolescents, and adults.
3. **Patient Education: The Warning Signs of Chronic Periodontitis**
    A. The warning signs of periodontitis are red or swollen gingiva, bleeding during brushing, a bad taste in the mouth, persistent bad breath, sensitive teeth, loose teeth, and pus around teeth and gingiva.
    B. Pain usually is not a symptom of periodontitis. This absence of pain may explain why periodontitis is often advanced before the patient seeks treatment and why a patient may avoid treatment even after receiving a diagnosis of periodontitis.
    C. Tools such as oral health self-evaluations distributed at health fairs or other events can be helpful in increasing the public's awareness of the signs and symptoms of periodontal disease (Box 11-1).
4. **Clinical Appearance of Chronic Periodontitis**
    A. The gingival tissue may appear bright red or purplish.
        1. In such cases, the clinical signs of chronic periodontitis are very evident at the initial examination of the oral cavity.
        2. An example of chronic periodontitis exhibiting this type of appearance is shown in **Box 11-2.**
    B. The gingival tissue may be pale pink and have an almost normal-looking appearance.
        1. *The appearance of the tissues is not a reliable indicator of the presence or severity of periodontitis.*
        2. At first glance, an inexperienced clinician may mistake the clinical appearance of chronic periodontitis for one of health. Closer examination will reveal firm, rigid (fibrotic) tissue and the presence of pocketing. Chronic periodontitis exhibiting this type of appearance is shown in Box 11-2.

Box 11-1

Patient Self-Evaluation Quiz

Do you have periodontal disease?

1. Do your gums ever bleed when you brush your teeth or when you chew hard food?
2. Do your gums ever feel swollen or tender?
3. Do you have constant bad breath or a bad taste in your mouth?
4. Are your gums pulling back from your teeth or do your teeth look longer than they did before?
5. Is there a change in the way your teeth fit together when you bite or have you noticed any spaces developing between your teeth?
6. Is there any pus between your teeth?
7. Are any of your teeth loose?

If you answered "**Yes**" to any of these questions, you should schedule a check-up with your dentist and help to save your teeth.

Box 11-2

Chronic Periodontitis

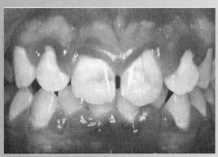

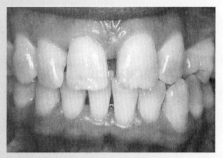

Figure 11-2A. Highly Visible Changes in the Gingiva. Chronic periodontitis may exhibit many clinically visible signs, such as, changes in the contour of the tissue. View this figure on the CD and you will also see color changes. Compare this photograph with the one in Figure 11-2B.

Figure 11-2B. Minimal Visible Changes in Gingiva. In this example of chronic periodontitis, there are minimal visible tissue changes. Since periodontitis is a disease affecting the deeper tissues of the periodontium, the appearance of the surface tissue often is not a reliable indicator of disease severity. View this figure on the CD and compare it to Figure 11-2A.

Characteristics of Chronic Periodontitis:

- Most commonly seen in adults over 35 years of age but can occur in children and adolescents
- Initiated and continued by dental plaque but the host response plays an essential role in its pathogenesis
- Signs and symptoms include swelling, redness, gingival bleeding, periodontal pockets, bone loss, tooth mobility, suppuration (pus), dental calculus
- Bone loss may be evident on radiographs
- Disease progresses at a slow to moderate rate
- Attachment loss may occur in one area of a tooth's attachment, on several teeth, or the entire dentition
- It can be modified by other factors, especially cigarette smoking

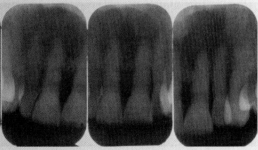

Figure 11-2C. Radiographic Evidence of Chronic Periodontitis. Dental radiographs of patients with chronic periodontitis usually reveal horizontal patterns of alveolar bone loss.

5. **Features of Chronic Periodontitis**
   A. The onset of the disease may be at any age; it is most commonly detected in adults older than age 35, but can occur in children and adolescents.
      1. The prevalence and severity of chronic periodontitis increases with age.
      2. The disease progresses at a slow to moderate rate but may have bursts of rapid progression (destruction).
   B. Signs and Symptoms of Chronic Periodontitis
      1. Tissue enlargement
      2. Tissue redness
      3. Gingival bleeding upon probing
      4. Periodontal pockets
      5. Bone loss, which may be visible on radiographs
      6. Tooth mobility
      7. Suppuration (discharge of pus)
      8. Presence of subgingival calculus
   C. The Inflammation May Affect Any Number of Teeth
      1. Localized inflammation may involve one site on a single tooth, several sites on a tooth, or several teeth.
      2. Generalized inflammation may involve the entire dentition.
      3. A patient may simultaneously have areas of health and areas with chronic periodontitis with tissue destruction.
   D. Chronic periodontitis may be modified by and/or associated with systemic diseases such as diabetes mellitus. It can be modified by other factors, especially cigarette smoking.
   E. Peri-implantitis is the term for chronic periodontitis in the tissues surrounding a dental implant.

6. **Etiology of Chronic Periodontitis**
   A. Although pathogenic bacteria are necessary for periodontitis, bacteria alone are not sufficient for the progression to chronic periodontitis.
   B. The onset and severity of chronic periodontitis are determined by the interaction between the plaque biofilm and the host immune response.
      1. Some individuals exhibit gingivitis for many years without disease progression to periodontitis.
      2. If the subgingival plaque biofilm is not removed, chronic periodontitis may be the result of the interaction between the bacteria and the host, resulting in tissue destruction and bone loss.

SEVERITY, EXTENT, AND PROGRESSION OF CHRONIC PERIODONTITIS

1. **Overview of the Concepts of Extent and Severity**
   A. Extent is the degree or amount of periodontal destruction and can be characterized based on the number of sites that have experienced tissue destruction.
   B. The severity, or seriousness, of the disease is determined by the rate of disease progression over time and the response of the tissues to treatment.
      1. Slight to moderate tissue destruction is characterized by a loss of up to one-third of the supporting periodontal tissues; probing depths of 4 to 6 mm with clinical attachment loss of up to 4 mm; and class I or II furcation involvement.
      2. Advanced tissue destruction is characterized by loss of greater than one-third of the supporting periodontal tissues; probing depths of 7 mm or greater with clinical attachment loss of 5 mm or more; and class III furcation involvement.
   C. Disease progression refers to the change or advancement of periodontal destruction. For example, how does the amount of attachment loss and bone destruction seen today compare to that seen several months ago? Is it the same, somewhat worse, or much worse?

2. **Extent of Destruction in Chronic Periodontitis**
   A. *Localized chronic periodontitis* is chronic periodontitis in which 30% or less of the sites in the mouth have experienced attachment loss and bone loss.
   B. *Generalized chronic periodontitis* is chronic periodontitis in which more than 30% of the sites in the mouth have experienced attachment loss and bone loss.
3. **Rate of Disease Progression.** *The rate of disease progression in chronic periodontitis appears to be slow.*
   A. The current view is that the tissue destruction seen in chronic periodontitis may not be continuous but rather occurs in short bursts during which there is breakdown of the periodontal ligament and alveolar bone destruction.
   B. Episodes of disease progression in chronic periodontitis occur randomly over time and at random sites in the mouth.

TREATMENT CONSIDERATIONS FOR INITIAL THERAPY

1. **Initial Therapy for Chronic Periodontitis**
   A. Initial care includes:
      1. Consultation with the patient's physician may be indicated if systemic risk factors are present. These might include smoking, uncontrolled or poorly controlled diabetes, systemic diseases, stress, or certain systemic medications.
      2. Individualized instruction, reinforcement, and evaluation of the patient's plaque control skills.
      3. Smoking cessation counseling should be offered to patients who smoke.
      4. Debridement of tooth surfaces.
      5. Antimicrobial agents may be used as an adjunct to initial therapy.
      6. Removal or control of local factors contributing to inflammation.
   B. A periodontal examination and re-evaluation of the initial therapy's outcomes should be performed after allowing an appropriate time interval for resolution of inflammation and tissue repair.
2. **Treatment Goals.** The goals for treatment of patients with chronic periodontitis are to:
   A. Control bacterial plaque to a level that is compatible with periodontal health
   B. Alter or eliminate any contributing risk factors for periodontitis
   C. Arrest the disease progression (*stop the attachment and bone loss from worsening*)
   D. Prevent the recurrence of periodontitis.
3. **Outcomes Assessment**
   A. The desired outcome of periodontal therapy for chronic periodontitis should result in:
      1. Significant reduction in gingival inflammation.
      2. Reduction of dental plaque to a level compatible with gingival health.
      3. Reduction of probing depths.
      4. *Prevention of further attachment loss.*
   B. The long-term outcome of periodontal therapy depends on patient compliance with self-care and periodontal maintenance (recall appointments) at appropriate intervals.
   C. Not all patients or sites will respond equally to therapy. Disease sites that have not responded successfully to treatment are characterized by:
      1. Inflammation of the gingiva.
      2. Increasing clinical attachment loss.
      3. Plaque levels that are not compatible with gingival health.
      4. In patients in whom the periodontal condition does not resolve, additional therapy may be required. In some cases, only specific sites in the dentition may require additional therapy.

RECURRENT AND REFRACTORY FORMS OF CHRONIC PERIODONTITIS

1. **Recurrent periodontitis**—new signs and symptoms of destructive periodontitis that reappear after periodontal therapy because the disease was not adequately treated and/or the patient did not practice adequate self-care.
2. **Refractory disease**—destructive periodontitis in a patient who, when monitored over time, exhibits additional attachment loss at one or more sites, despite appropriate, repeated professional periodontal therapy and a patient who practices satisfactory self-care and follows the recommended program of periodontal maintenance visits (Box 11-3).
   A. Under the 1989 classification system, refractory periodontitis was a separate disease category. It is now believed that refractory periodontitis is not a single disease entity, but rather that a small percentage of all forms of periodontitis may not respond to treatment.
   B. *In the 1999 classification system, the designation refractory can be applied to all types of periodontal disease that do not respond to treatment.* Cases of chronic periodontitis that do not respond to periodontal therapy are designated as *refractory chronic periodontitis.*

Box 11-3

Refractory Chronic Periodontitis

- Additional attachment loss in a patient despite all of the following:
  - Appropriate periodontal therapy, and
  - A patient who practices satisfactory self-care, and
  - An appropriate program of periodontal maintenance visits.

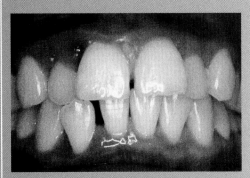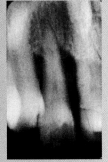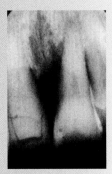

Figure 11-3A–3C. Refractory Chronic Periodontitis. Chronic periodontitis is considered refractory when the disease is not controlled by the conventional periodontal therapy normally recommended for patients with chronic periodontitis. In a refractory case, the patient experiences additional attachment loss despite appropriate periodontal therapy and satisfactory self-care. The dental radiographs of a patient with refractory periodontitis reveal *continuing evidence of bone loss over time despite appropriate therapy.*

SECTION 3: AGGRESSIVE PERIODONTITIS—HIGHLY DESTRUCTIVE FORM

CHARACTERISTICS OF AGGRESSIVE PERIODONTITIS

1. **Aggressive periodontitis** is a bacterial infection characterized by a rapid destruction of the periodontal ligament, rapid loss of supporting bone, high risk for tooth loss, and a poor response to periodontal therapy. Fortunately, aggressive periodontitis is less common than chronic periodontitis.
2. **Alternative Terminology.** Aggressive periodontitis was previously known as juvenile periodontitis.
3. **Characteristics**
   A. Aggressive periodontitis is characterized by:
      1. *Rapid destruction of the attachment and rapid loss of supporting bone*
      2. High risk for tooth loss
      3. A poor response to periodontal therapy
      4. No obvious signs or symptoms of systemic disease
      5. A lack of clinical signs of disease
         a. Affected tissue may have a normal clinical appearance
         b. Probing reveals deep periodontal pockets on affected teeth.
   B. Relatively small amounts of bacterial plaque are exhibited by the patient. The disease severity seems to be exaggerated given the light amount of plaque.
   C. Immune deficiencies and a genetic link have been shown to be possible modifying factors for this type of periodontal disease.

TREATMENT CONSIDERATIONS FOR AGGRESSIVE PERIODONTITIS

1. **Initial Therapy for Aggressive Periodontitis.** Treatment methods for aggressive periodontitis are similar to those used for chronic periodontitis.
   A. Consultation with a physician may be indicated for children and young adults who exhibit severe periodontitis. Due to the potential genetic link in aggressive periodontitis, evaluation and counseling of other family members is indicated.
   B. Care plan should include:
      1. Smoking cessation counseling should be offered to patients who smoke.
      2. Individualized instruction, reinforcement, and evaluation of the patient's plaque control skills.
      3. Debridement of tooth surfaces, combined with antimicrobial therapy.
      4. Removal or control of local factors contributing to inflammation.
      5. Surgical debridement of the soft tissue
   C. A periodontal examination and re-evaluation of the initial therapy's outcomes should be performed after allowing an appropriate time interval for resolution of inflammation and tissue repair.
2. **Treatment Goals.** Periodontitis is controlled if further attachment loss can be prevented—that is, no additional destruction of periodontal attachment and alveolar bone. Control of periodontitis may not be possible in aggressive periodontitis. *In such cases, a reasonable treatment goal is to slow the progression of the disease.*
   A. The desired outcome of periodontal therapy in patients with aggressive periodontitis is:
      1. Significant reduction in gingival inflammation.
      2. Reduction of dental plaque to a level compatible with periodontal health.
      3. *Prevention of further loss of attachment and supporting alveolar bone.*

    B. The best long-term outcome will be achieved when there is good patient compliance with self-care and periodontal maintenance (recall appointments) at appropriate intervals.

    C. Disease sites that *do not respond successfully to treatment* may occur and are characterized by:

      1. Inflammation of the gingiva.

      2. *Increasing attachment loss.*

      3. Plaque levels that are not compatible with gingival health.

      4. Increasing tooth mobility.

LOCALIZED AND GENERALIZED AGGRESSIVE PERIODONTITIS

The two forms of aggressive periodontitis are **localized aggressive periodontitis** and **generalized aggressive periodontitis**.

  1. Localized Aggressive Periodontitis

    A. **Features of Localized Aggressive Periodontitis (LAP) (Box 11-4)**

      1. Onset of disease around the time of puberty.

      2. Rapid tissue destruction around the permanent first molars and incisors.

      3. Frequently associated with the periodontal pathogen *Actinobacillus actinomycetemcomitans* (frequently abbreviated as Aa).

      4. Frequently associated with abnormal neutrophil function (immune dysfunction).

      5. Seems to affect more females than males.

    B. **Alternative Terminology.** LAP was previously known as localized juvenile periodontitis.

Box 11-4

Localized Aggressive Periodontitis

- Onset around the time of puberty
- Rapid tissue destruction
- Frequently associated with Aa
- Associated with abnormal neutrophil function
- More common in females than males
- Previously called localized juvenile periodontitis
- **Bone loss affects the first molars and incisors**

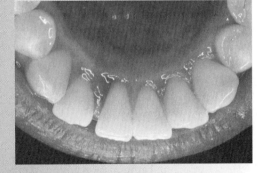

Figure 11-4A. Localized Aggressive Periodontitis. The photo shows a patient with LAP. Note that there are not any supragingival calculus deposits evident. Refer to the color version of this photo on the CD and you will notice some color and contour changes of the gingiva.

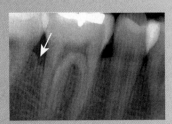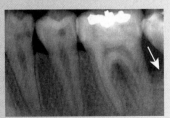

Figure 11-4B–4C. Radiographic Characteristics of Localized Aggressive Periodontitis. Patients with LAP have bone loss on the *first molar and incisor teeth*. The radiographs shown here reveal a pattern of bone loss on the first molars that is similar on both sides of the mandibular arch.

2. Generalized Aggressive Periodontitis
   A. **Features of Generalized Aggressive Periodontitis (GAP)** (Box 11-5)
      1. Onset usually occurs in persons younger than 30 years of age, but patients may be older
      2. Rapid tissue destruction around most teeth
      3. Frequently associated with the periodontal pathogens *A. actinomycetemcomitans* and *Porphyromonas gingivalis*
      4. Frequently associated with abnormal neutrophil function (immune dysfunction)
   B. **Alternative Terminology.** GAP was previously known as generalized juvenile periodontitis (GJP).

Box 11-5

Generalized Aggressive Periodontitis

- Disease onset usually occurs in persons under 30 years of age, but patients may be older
- Rapid tissue destruction around most teeth
- Associated with *Aa* and *P. gingivalis*
- Associated with abnormal polymorphonuclear leukocyte (PMN; neutrophil) function
- Previously known as generalized juvenile periodontitis
- Bone loss affects most teeth

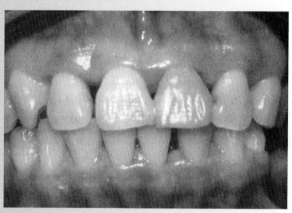

Figure 11-5A. Generalized Aggressive Periodontitis.
The rate of attachment loss and bone loss is rapid in GAP compared to chronic periodontitis.

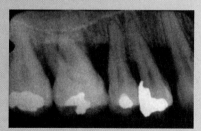 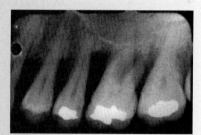

Figure 11-5B–5C. Radiographic Characteristics of Generalized Aggressive Periodontitis.
Radiographs of patients with GAP reveal severe alveolar bone loss *around most teeth*.

SECTION 4: LESS COMMON FORMS OF PERIODONTITIS

This group is composed of uncommon types of periodontitis including (i) periodontitis as a manifestation of systemic diseases, (ii) necrotizing periodontal diseases, (iii) abscesses of the periodontium, (iv) periodontitis associated with endodontic lesions, (v) developmental or acquired deformities and conditions, and (vi) occlusal trauma. Abscesses are discussed in Chapter 24.

PERIODONTITIS AS A MANIFESTATION OF SYSTEMIC DISEASES

1. **Periodontitis Associated with Systemic Disease**
   A. A number of systemic diseases and conditions are a contributing factor in the development of periodontitis.
   B. Systemic diseases and conditions that are capable of affecting the periodontium include undiagnosed or poorly controlled diabetes, Down syndrome, and acquired immunodeficiency syndrome. Refer to Chapter 8 for a detailed discussion of systemic disease as a contributing factor to periodontitis.
2. **Periodontitis Associated with Immune Dysfunction**
   A. Periodontitis associated with immune dysfunction is associated with systemic conditions that interfere with the body's resistance to bacterial infection (**Box 11-6**)
      1. Can occur in patients of any age.
      2. Is characterized by severe bone loss and tooth loss.
   B. In rare cases, periodontitis may be seen in young children beginning with the eruption of the primary teeth.
      1. Periodontitis around primary teeth is associated with systemic conditions that interfere with the body's resistance to bacterial infections.
      2. Rare systemic conditions that are associated with periodontitis in very young children include leukocyte adherence deficiency, congenital primary immunodeficiency, hypophosphatasia, chronic neutrophil defects, and cyclic neutropenia.
   C. Alternative Terminology. Periodontitis associated with immune dysfunction was previously known as generalized prepubertal periodontitis.

Box 11-6

Periodontitis Associated with Immune Dysfunction

- Occurs in patients of any age
- Seen in young children beginning with the eruption of primary teeth
- Characterized with severe bone loss and tooth loss
- Associated with systemic conditions that interfere with the body's resistance to bacterial infection
- Previously known as generalized prepubertal periodontitis

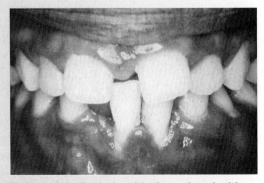

Figure 11-6. Periodontitis Associated with Immune Dysfunction. This photo shows the dentition of a young patient with PMN deficiency. Note the primary dentition is being lost and the permanent dentition is being exfoliated as soon as the permanent teeth erupt.

NECROTIZING PERIODONTAL DISEASES

1. **Necrotizing periodontal diseases** are destructive infections of periodontal tissues that involve **tissue necrosis** (localized tissue death).
   A. Types
      1. **Necrotizing ulcerative gingivitis (NUG)**—tissue necrosis that is limited to the gingival tissues.
         a. NUG is a painful infection, primarily of the interdental and marginal gingiva.
         b. It is characterized by partial loss of the interdental papillae (punched-out papillae), gingival bleeding, and pain (**Box 11-7**).
      2. **Necrotizing ulcerative periodontitis (NUP)**— tissue necrosis of the gingival tissues combined with loss of attachment and alveolar bone loss.
         a. NUP is a painful infection characterized by necrosis of gingival tissues, periodontal ligament, and alveolar bone.
         b. NUP is an extremely rapid and destructive form of periodontitis that can produce loss of periodontal attachment within days (**Box 11-8**).

Box 11-7

Necrotizing Ulcerative Gingivitis

- Sudden onset
- Pain
- Fiery red gingiva with spontaneous bleeding
- Necrosis of interdental papillae (cratered, punched-out papillae)
- Gray pseudomembrane
- Excessive salivation
- Fetid breath odor
- Fever, swollen lymph nodes

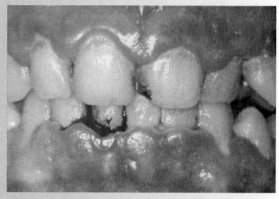

Figure 11-7. Necrotizing Ulcerative Gingivitis.

Box 11-8

Necrotizing Ulcerative Periodontitis

In addition to all of the signs and symptoms of NUG, patients with NUP may also experience:

- Rapid gingival recession
- Rapid, irregular bone loss
- Fever, swollen lymph nodes

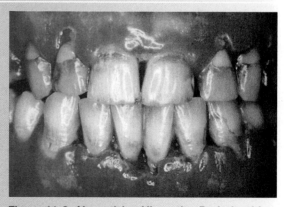

Figure 11-8. Necrotizing Ulcerative Periodontitis.

B. Both NUG and NUP are collectively referred to as necrotizing periodontal diseases because there is insufficient evidence that they are truly separate diseases. *It is suggested that NUG and NUP might possibly be stages of the same infection.*

C. Both NUG and NUP appear to be related to diminished systemic resistance to bacterial infection.

2. **Alternative Terminology.** These conditions previously have been known as trench mouth, Vincent's infection, and acute ulcerative necrotizing gingivitis (ANUG).

3. **Signs and Symptoms of Necrotizing Periodontal Diseases**

   A. Oral Signs and Symptoms

      1. **Gingival necrosis**—tissue death resulting in partial loss of interdental papillae, giving the appearance that the papillae have been punched-out or cratered.

      2. Fiery red gingiva with spontaneous gingival bleeding

      3. Intense oral pain that causes affected patients to seek dental treatment. This symptom is unusual since gingivitis and periodontitis normally are *not* painful.

      4. An unmistakable, fetid oral odor (bad breath).

         a. The pain associated with necrotizing periodontal diseases usually causes the individual to stop brushing.

         b. Materia alba, plaque, sloughed tissue, blood, and stagnant saliva collect in the oral cavity causing the oral odor.

      5. Excessive salivation

      6. Development of a **pseudomembrane**—a gray layer of tissue that covers the necrotic areas of the gingiva.

         a. The pseudomembrane may involve the gingiva of several teeth or it may cover the entire gingiva.

         b. It is easily wiped off with gauze, exposing an area of fiery red, shiny gingiva.

         c. The pseudomembrane is composed mainly of necrotic tissue cells, fibrin, leukocytes, and microorganisms.

      7. In the case of NUP, additional signs include rapid gingival recession, extremely rapid and irregular bone loss, delayed wound healing, and spread of infection to the adjacent oral mucosa.

   B. Systemic Signs and Symptoms

      1. Fever and malaise.

      2. Swollen lymph nodes.

4. **Etiology**

   A. Necrotizing periodontal diseases are associated with fusiform bacteria, *Provotella intermedia*, and spirochetes

   B. Predisposing Factors

      1. Cigarette smoking—most patients who experience NUG or NUP are smokers

      2. Increased levels of personal stress

      3. Poor nutrition

         a. In North America, NUG is associated with poor eating habits of young adults, such as college students.

         b. In developing countries, NUG occurs in very young children and appears to be related to poor nutritional status, especially a low protein intake.

      4. Fatigue

      5. Immune dysfunction or suppression. Immune dysfunction can exist in patients who are otherwise systemically healthy.

      6. Pre-existing gingivitis or tissue trauma

   C. Most Commonly Observed in:

      1. NUG: Persons between 15 and 25 years of age, particularly students and military recruits enduring times of increased stress.

      2. NUP: Individuals with systemic conditions including but not limited to human immunodeficiency virus (HIV) infection, severe malnutrition, and immunosuppression.

5. **Treatment of Necrotizing Periodontal Diseases**
   A. Care includes
      1. Irrigation
      2. Debridement of the necrotic tissues and tooth surfaces
      3. Patient self-care instruction
      4. Pain control
      5. Antibiotic therapy as appropriate for the management of systemic manifestations (fever, swollen lymph nodes).
   B. An excellent and very comprehensive description of dental hygiene care of the patient with necrotizing periodontal disease can be found in Wilkins. [1]
   C. Patient counseling should include instruction on proper nutrition, intake of fluids, and smoking cessation. A liquid dietary replacement, such as Ensure or Boost, can be recommended.

OCCLUSAL TRAUMA IN PATIENTS WITH PERIODONTITIS

1. **Secondary occlusal trauma** is injury as the result of occlusal forces applied to a tooth or teeth that have previously experienced attachment loss and/or bone loss.
2. *In this type of occlusal trauma, the periodontium was unhealthy before experiencing excessive occlusal forces* (**Box 11-9**).
3. Rapid bone loss and pocket formation result when excessive occlusal forces are applied to a tooth that has previously experienced attachment loss and/or bone loss.

Box 11-9

Secondary Occlusal Trauma

Clinical indicators of occlusal trauma may include one or more of the following:
* Tooth mobility (progressive)
* Fremitis (vibration felt when palpating a tooth, as the patient taps the teeth together)
* Tooth migration
* Fractured tooth
* Thermal sensitivity on chewing or percussion

Radiographic indicators may include one or more of the following:
* Widened periodontal ligament space
* Bone loss
* Root resorption

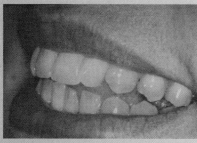
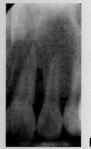

Figure 11-9. Secondary Occlusal Trauma. A: The woman pictured above puts repeated heavy pressure against her central incisor tooth. B: A dental radiograph of her central incisor shows severe bone loss around the central incisor that is subjected to the heavy pressure.

CHAPTER SUMMARY STATEMENT

Periodontitis is a bacterial infection of all parts of the periodontium that results in irreversible destruction of the periodontal ligament fibers and alveolar bone. The desired outcome of periodontal therapy is to stop the progression of the disease to prevent further attachment loss.

- Periodontitis may involve one area of a tooth's attachment, several teeth, or the entire dentition. A patient can simultaneously have areas of health and areas with periodontitis.
- Chronic periodontitis, the most common form of periodontitis, is characterized by pocket formation and/or gingival recession, slow to moderate rates of disease progression, and a favorable response to periodontal therapy.
- Aggressive periodontitis is characterized by a rapid destruction of the periodontal ligament, rapid loss of supporting bone, high risk for tooth loss, and a poor response to traditional periodontal therapy.

SECTION 5: FOCUS ON PATIENTS

CASE 1

A new patient has a diagnosis of severe generalized chronic periodontitis. The patient tells you that it is hard for him to believe he has serious periodontal problems since he has never had any discomfort and has never even noticed any dental problems. How could you respond to this patient's comments?

CASE 2

A patient who has recently moved to your city has an appointment with you regarding self-care instructions. The periodontal diagnosis is severe chronic periodontitis. In your discussion with the patient you learn that the patient is upset because she has been treated for periodontitis twice during the past decade in other dental offices. She is upset because now apparently she needs periodontal treatment again and she states she is confused about how this might be possible. How could you respond to this patient's concerns?

CASE 3

While reading a journal article you find a reference to a periodontal disease called localized juvenile periodontitis (LJP). Since this is not a disease category in the currently accepted disease classification system, how does this terminology relate to modern periodontal diagnoses?

Reference

1. Wilkins EM. Acute periodontal conditions. In *Clinical Practice of the Dental Hygienist*. 9th ed. Baltimore: Lippincott Williams & Wilkins; 2005.

SUGGESTED READING

1999 International Workshop for a Classification of Periodontal Diseases and Conditions. Papers. Oak Brook, Illinois, October 30-November 2, 1999. *Ann Periodontol.* 1999;4:1–112.

SECTION 6: CHAPTER REVIEW QUESTIONS

1. A bacterial infection of the periodontium characterized by a rapid destruction of the periodontal ligament, rapid loss of supporting bone, high risk for tooth loss, and a poor response to periodontal therapy is termed:
   A. Chronic periodontitis
   B. Aggressive periodontitis
   C. Necrotizing periodontal disease
   D. Recurrent periodontal disease

2. A bacterial infection of the periodontium characterized by a slow destruction of the periodontal ligament, slow loss of supporting bone and a good response to periodontal therapy is termed:
   A. Chronic periodontitis
   B. Aggressive periodontitis
   C. Necrotizing periodontal disease
   D. Recurrent periodontal disease

3. A destructive bacterial infection of the periodontium that involves tissue necrosis is termed:
   A. Chronic periodontitis
   B. Aggressive periodontitis
   C. Necrotizing periodontal disease
   D. Recurrent periodontal disease

4. New signs and symptoms of destructive periodontitis that reappear after periodontal therapy because the disease was not adequately treated and/or the patient did not maintain adequate self-care is termed:
   A. Refractory disease
   B. Recurrent disease

5. Chronic periodontitis in which 30% or LESS of the sites in the mouth have experienced attachment loss and bone loss is termed:
   A. Nonplaque-induced gingivitis
   B. Localized chronic periodontitis
   C. Generalized chronic periodontitis

6. Chronic periodontitis in which MORE than 30% of the sites in the mouth have experienced attachment loss and bone loss is termed:
   A. Nonplaque-induced gingivitis
   B. Localized chronic periodontitis
   C. Generalized chronic periodontitis

7. Chronic periodontitis in the tissues surrounding a dental implant is termed:
   A. Peri-implantitis
   B. Implant periodontitis
   C. Recurrent implantitis
   D. Refractory implantitis

8. Tissue destruction that is characterized by probing depths of 4 to 6 mm with clinical attachment loss of up to 4 mm is termed:
   A. Advanced tissue destruction
   B. Slight to moderate tissue destruction

Chapter

12 Clinical Periodontal Assessment

Refer to the CD packaged with this book for full color versions of the clinical photographs in this chapter.

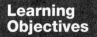
Learning Objectives

- Explain which members of the dental team are responsible for the clinical periodontal assessment.
- Compare and contrast a periodontal screening examination and a comprehensive periodontal assessment.
- Provide a brief overview of one type of periodontal screening examination.
- List the components of a comprehensive periodontal assessment.
- Describe how to assess each component of a comprehensive periodontal assessment.
- Explain how to calculate the width of attached gingiva.

- Explain how to calculate clinical attachment level given several different clinical scenarios.
- In a clinical setting, calculate and document the clinical attachment levels for a patient with periodontitis.

KEY TERMS

Clinical periodontal assessment
Legal responsibility
Treatment outcomes
Baseline data
Periodontal screening examination
Periodontal Screening and Recording
   System (PSR)
World Health Organization (WHO) probe
Color-coded reference mark

PSR Code
Comprehensive periodontal assessment
Exudate
Horizontal mobility
Vertical mobility
Fremitus
Gingival crevicular fluid
Attached gingiva
Clinical attachment level (CAL)

SECTION 1: INTRODUCTION TO PERIODONTAL ASSESSMENT

OVERVIEW OF THE ASSESSMENT PROCESS

1. The **clinical periodontal assessment** is essentially a fact-gathering process designed to provide a comprehensive picture of the patient's periodontal health status.
   A. This assessment is one of the most important functions performed by a clinician.
      1. The dental team must perform and document a clinical periodontal assessment for all patients.
      2. This procedure requires meticulous attention to detail since successful patient care is highly dependent on a thorough and accurate clinical periodontal assessment.
   B. The information gathered during the clinical periodontal assessment forms the basis of the individualized treatment plan for the patient.
2. **Objectives.** The objectives of the clinical periodontal assessment are to:
   A. Look for clinical signs of inflammation and damage to the periodontium
   B. Determine whether the patient's periodontium is healthy or diseased
   C. Document all clinical findings to serve as baseline data for the long-term monitoring of periodontal disease activity when evaluating the success of periodontal treatment.
3. **Two Types of Periodontal Assessment.** Two commonly used types of periodontal assessment are the periodontal screening examination and the comprehensive periodontal assessment.
   A. A periodontal screening examination is an efficient information-gathering process used to determine the periodontal health status of the patient (health or disease?).
   B. A comprehensive periodontal assessment is an intensive information-gathering process used to gather the detailed data needed to make a periodontal diagnosis (e.g., chronic periodontitis or aggressive periodontitis) and to document the periodontal health status to allow for long term monitoring of the patient.

RESPONSIBILITIES AND LEGAL CONSIDERATIONS

1. **Division of Responsibility within the Dental Team**
   A. **Responsibilities of the Dentist and Dental Hygienist.** Although the dental team in each dental office will function differently, it is helpful to look at the typical responsibilities of the dentist and dental hygienist in the assessment, diagnosis, and treatment planning steps.
      1. Typically, the dentist and dental hygienist share the responsibility for periodontal screening and comprehensive periodontal assessment.
      2. The dentist has the responsibility of assignment of a periodontal diagnosis, and the dentist with input from the dental hygienist plans the nonsurgical periodontal therapy.
   B. It is important for members of the dental team to understand that the dentist is **legally responsible** for all of the diagnosis and treatment planning that occurs in the office.
   C. Because of the extensive special training received by the dental hygienist, many dentists place part of the periodontal data collection in his or her capable hands.
2. **Legal Considerations**
   A. *Dentists and dental hygienists have a legal responsibility to complete an accurate and thorough periodontal assessment on every patient.*
      1. The failure to diagnose and properly treat periodontal disease may be one of the leading causes of dental malpractice.
      2. Dentists and hygienists must perform a clinical periodontal assessment in a manner that is consistent with the current standards of care set forth by the dental profession.

B. Without a thorough clinical periodontal assessment, periodontal diseases are not diagnosed or are misdiagnosed, leading to undertreatment or overtreatment of periodontal disease.

C. To be competent clinically, all dentists and dental hygienists must master the skills necessary to perform a thorough and accurate clinical periodontal assessment.

DOCUMENTATION

1. The clinical periodontal assessment is not complete until all of the information gathered during the assessment has been accurately recorded in the patient chart (Fig. 12-1). It is important to record and date all information accurately. Documentation is discussed in detail in Chapter 26.

2. Clinicians use the documented information to measure treatment outcomes and to monitor the patient's periodontal health status over time.

   A. Findings documented during the clinical periodontal assessment serve as baseline data against which to evaluate the success or failure of periodontal therapy. Baseline data refers to clinical information gathered prior to periodontal therapy that can be used for comparison to clinical information gathered at subsequent appointments.

   B. Documented findings also provide the baseline data used in the long-term monitoring of the patient's periodontal health status. An example of when patient monitoring may occur is at periodontal maintenance visits following successful treatment. Periodontal maintenance is discussed in Chapter 23.

1	2	3	4	5	6	7	8	9	10	11	12	13	14	15	16	**Maxilla**
			I			I	I	II	I		I					Mobility (I, II, III)
+	+		+			+	+	+		+	+	+		+	+	Bleeding/Purulence (+)
																Attachment Level (CEJ to BP)
635	634		338	535	537	626	625	537	625	536	725	524		435	535	Probing Depth (FGM to BP)

Facial / *Palatal* (tooth diagrams)

1	2	3	4	5	6	7	8	9	10	11	12	13	14	15	16	
+	+		+	+	+		+	+		+	+	+		+		Bleeding/Purulence (+)
																Attachment Level (CEJ to BP)
535	634		438	534	636	536	535	635	535	536	726	534		426	535	Probing Depth (FGM to BP)
																Plaque
	✓				✓	✓	✓	✓	✓	✓		✓		✓	✓	Supragingival Calculus
✓	✓		✓	✓	✓	✓	✓	✓	✓	✓	✓	✓		✓	✓	Subgingival Calculus
			4				4				4					PSR Code

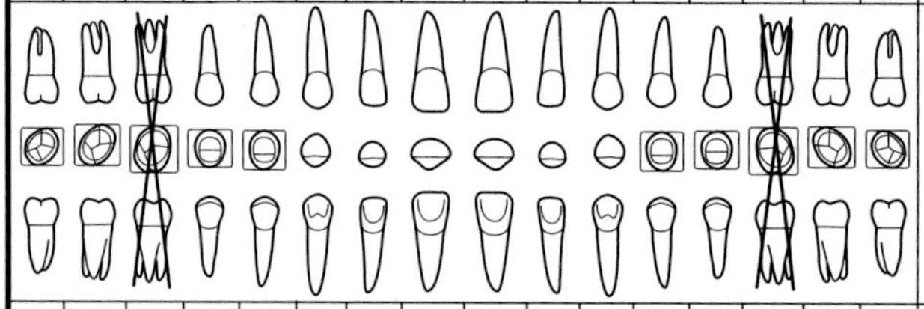

Right   *Left*

32	31	30	29	28	27	26	25	24	23	22	21	20	19	18	17	**Mandible**
		I				II	II	II	II							Mobility (I, II, III)
	+	+	+		+	+	+	+	+	+	+	+	+		+	Bleeding/Purulence (+)
																Attachment Level (CEJ to BP)
	535	536	545	524	535	635	545	536	637	635	524	535	635	636	635	Probing Depth (FGM to BP)

Lingual / *Facial* (tooth diagrams)

32	31	30	29	28	27	26	25	24	23	22	21	20	19	18	17	
	+	+		+	+	+	+	+	+	+	+		+	+	+	Bleeding/Purulence (+)
																Attachment Level (CEJ to BP)
	535	526	535	424	535	624	535	525	536	524	525	425	525	526	625	Probing Depth (FGM to BP)
																Plaque
					✓	✓	✓	✓	✓						✓	Supragingival Calculus
	✓	✓	✓	✓	✓	✓	✓	✓	✓	✓	✓	✓	✓	✓	✓	Subgingival Calculus
			4				4				4					PSR Code

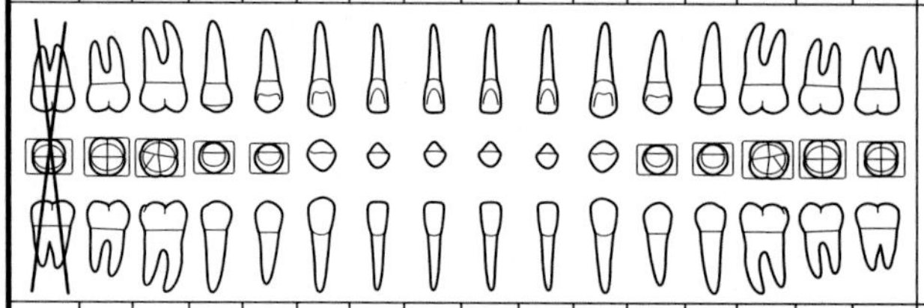

Figure 12-1. Documentation of Clinical Findings on a Periodontal Chart. This periodontal chart is an example of how clinical findings from the clinical periodontal assessment may be documented.

SECTION 2: THE PERIODONTAL SCREENING EXAMINATION

In some dental offices a periodontal screening examination is one of the first steps in evaluating the periodontal status of a patient. A **periodontal screening examination** is a periodontal assessment used to (i) determine the periodontal health status of the patient and (ii) identify patients needing a more comprehensive periodontal assessment. The **Periodontal Screening and Recording (PSR)** is an efficient, easy-to-use screening system for the detection of periodontal disease.

PERIODONTAL SCREENING AND RECORDING SYSTEM

1. **Characteristics of the PSR System**
   A. The PSR can help to identify those patients who need a comprehensive periodontal assessment.
   B. The results of this screening examination are used to separate patients into broad categories: (i) those that have periodontal health or gingivitis and (ii) those that have periodontitis.
   C. When the PSR screening examination indicates the presence of periodontal health or gingivitis, in many instances no further clinical periodontal assessment is needed beyond the PSR.
2. **Techniques for the PSR Screening Examination**
   A. Special Probe. A **World Health Organization (WHO) probe** is used for this examination. The WHO probe has a colored band (called the reference mark) located 3.5 to 5.5 mm from the probe tip. This **color-coded reference mark** is used when performing the PSR screening examination.
   B. One Code Per Sextant. Each sextant of the mouth is examined as a separate unit.
      1. The unique aspects of the PSR screening system are the manner in which the probe is read and the minimal amount of information that is recorded.
         a. Instead of reading and recording six readings per tooth, the clinician only needs to observe the position of the color-coded reference mark in relation to the gingival margin and a few other clinical features such as bleeding on probing, the presence of calculus, or the presence of an overhang on a restoration.
         b. Each of the sextants is examined as a separate unit during the PSR screening.
         c. *Only one score is recorded for each sextant in the mouth.* Each sextant is assigned a single PSR code; the highest code obtained for the sextant is recorded. An "X" is recorded if a sextant is edentulous.
   C. Probing Technique. The probe is walked circumferentially around each tooth in the sextant being examined. The color-coded reference mark is monitored continuously as the probe is walked around each tooth. At each site probed, the color-coded reference mark will be (a) completely visible, (b) partially visible, or (c) not visible at all.
   D. A **PSR code** is assigned to each sextant according to the criteria shown in Table 12-1. *The code assigned to a sextant should represent the most advanced periodontal finding on any tooth in that sextant.* The PSR codes may be recorded on a special PSR box chart (Fig. 12-2).
   E. The PSR codes are used to guide further clinical documentation.
      1. For some patients with low PSR codes in all sextants (codes 0, 1, or 2), the PSR screening is adequate documentation of the patient's periodontal health status (and a comprehensive periodontal assessment is not needed). Note, however, that occasionally the dentist may request a comprehensive periodontal assessment even when low PSR codes are found.

2. For patients with higher PSR codes in one or more sextants (codes 3 or 4), a comprehensive periodontal examination should be preformed as outlined in Section 3 of this chapter.

F. PSR codes can occasionally mislead a clinician.

1. As already pointed out, lower codes usually mean periodontal health or gingivitis, and higher codes usually mean periodontitis.

2. *When interpreting the results of the PSR, the clinician must be alert for teeth with gingival enlargement or with gingival recession. In the presence of either of these conditions the PSR can give misleading results.*

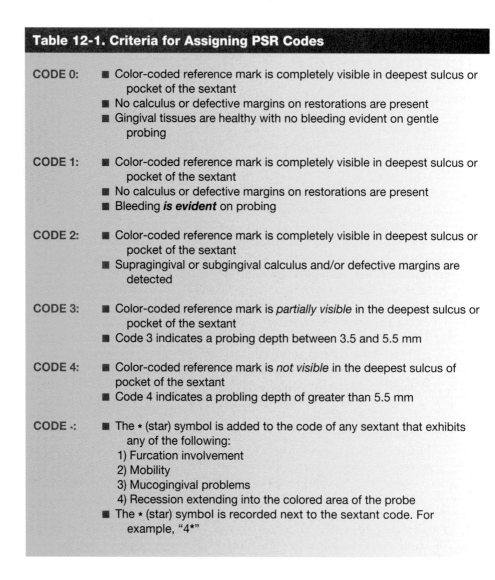

Table 12-1. Criteria for Assigning PSR Codes

CODE 0:
- Color-coded reference mark is completely visible in deepest sulcus or pocket of the sextant
- No calculus or defective margins on restorations are present
- Gingival tissues are healthy with no bleeding evident on gentle probing

CODE 1:
- Color-coded reference mark is completely visible in deepest sulcus or pocket of the sextant
- No calculus or defective margins on restorations are present
- Bleeding **is evident** on probing

CODE 2:
- Color-coded reference mark is completely visible in deepest sulcus or pocket of the sextant
- Supragingival or subgingival calculus and/or defective margins are detected

CODE 3:
- Color-coded reference mark is *partially visible* in the deepest sulcus or pocket of the sextant
- Code 3 indicates a probing depth between 3.5 and 5.5 mm

CODE 4:
- Color-coded reference mark is *not visible* in the deepest sulcus of pocket of the sextant
- Code 4 indicates a probling depth of greater than 5.5 mm

CODE ∗:
- The ∗ (star) symbol is added to the code of any sextant that exhibits any of the following:
  1) Furcation involvement
  2) Mobility
  3) Mucogingival problems
  4) Recession extending into the colored area of the probe
- The ∗ (star) symbol is recorded next to the sextant code. For example, "4∗"

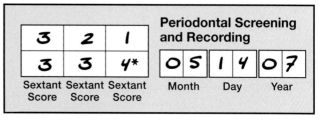

Figure 12-2. Periodontal Screening and Recording Box Chart. The PSR code is recorded in a box chart.

SECTION 3: THE COMPREHENSIVE PERIODONTAL ASSESSMENT

A **comprehensive periodontal assessment** is an intensive clinical periodontal assessment used to gather information about the periodontium. This section of the chapter outlines the clinical features that should be noted and documented during a comprehensive periodontal assessment. It is important to note that special precautions are necessary when examining dental implants. These examination techniques are not discussed in this chapter because they are presented in detail in Chapter 24.

The comprehensive periodontal assessment should always include probing depth measurements, bleeding on probing, presence of exudate, level of the free gingival margin and the mucogingival junction, tooth mobility, furcation involvement, presence of calculus and bacterial plaque, gingival inflammation, radiographic evidence of alveolar bone loss, and presence of local environmental risk factors.

COMPONENTS OF THE COMPREHENSIVE PERIODONTAL ASSESSMENT

1. **Probing Depth Measurements.** Probing depth measurements are made from the free gingival margin to the base of the pocket.
    A. Probing depths are recorded to the nearest full millimeter. Round up measurements to the next higher whole number (e.g., a reading of 3.5 mm is recorded as 4 mm, and a 5.5 mm reading is recorded as 6 mm).
    B. Probing depth measurements are recorded for six specific sites on each tooth: (i) distofacial, (ii) facial, (iii) mesiofacial, (iv) distolingual, (v) lingual, and (vi) mesiolingual.
2. **Bleeding on Probing**
    A. Bleeding on gentle probing represents bleeding from the soft tissue wall of a periodontal pocket where the wall of the pocket is ulcerated (i.e., where portions of the epithelium have been destroyed) (**Fig. 12-3**).

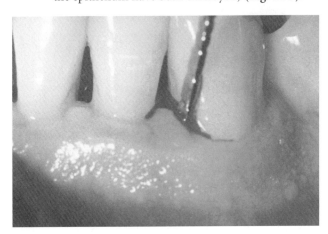

Figure 12-3. A Bleeding Site. Bleeding from the soft tissue wall is a sign of disease. This bleeding was evident upon gentle probing.

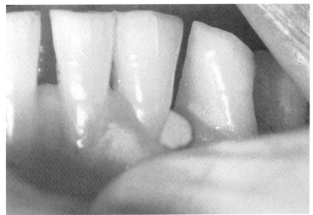

Figure 12-4. Exudate. Pressure with the clinician's finger on the gingiva reveals exudate from the gingival tissue adjacent to the lateral incisor. (Courtesy of Dr. Don Rolfs, Periodontal Foundations, Wenatchee, WA.)

    B. Bleeding can occur immediately when the site is probed or can be slightly delayed in occurrence, so an alert clinician will observe each site for a few seconds before moving on to the next site.
    C. Penetrating the soft tissue with excessive probing force also could cause bleeding. Probing pressure should be between 10 to 20 grams of pressure. Sensitive scales, available from scientific supply companies, can be used to calibrate probing pressure.

3. **Presence of Exudate**
   A. **Exudate**, sometimes referred to as suppuration, is pus. Pus represents dead white blood cells and can occur in any infection, including periodontal disease.
   B. Exudate can be recognized as a pale yellow material oozing from the orifice of a pocket. It is usually easiest to detect when the gingiva is manipulated in some manner. For example, light finger pressure on the gingiva can usually reveal exudate when present (**Fig. 12-4**).

4. **Level of the Free Gingival Margin**
   A. The level of the free gingival margin in relationship to the cementoenamel junction (CEJ) should be recorded on the dental chart. This level can simply be drawn on the facial and lingual surfaces of the dental chart.
   B. Several possible relationships exist between the free gingival margin and the CEJ:
      1. Free gingival margin is slightly coronal to (above) the CEJ—this is the natural level of the gingival margin.
      2. Free gingival margin is significantly coronal to the CEJ—this relationship is seen in some patients when the gingival tissue is edematous or enlarged.
      3. Free gingival margin is apical to the CEJ—this relationship, known as recession, leads to exposure of a portion of the root surface.

5. **Level of Mucogingival Junction**
   A. The level of the mucogingival junction represents the junction between the keratinized gingiva and the nonkeratinized mucosa. The level of the mucogingival junction is used in determining the width of the attached gingiva as will be described in Section 4.
   B. The mucogingival junction is usually readily visible since the keratinized gingiva is usually pale pink and opaque while the surface of the mucosa is thin, translucent tissue (**Fig. 12-5**).
   C. Occasionally, the mucogingival junction can be difficult to detect visually. In this case, the tissue can be manipulated by pulling on the patient's lip or pushing on the tissue with a blunt instrument to distinguish the moveable mucosa from the firmly attached gingiva.

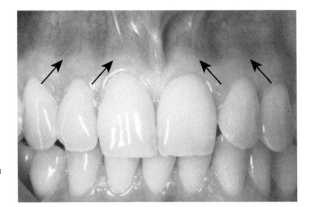

Figure 12-5. Mucogingival Junction. The mucogingival junction represents the junction between the keratinized gingiva with the nonkeratinized mucosa.

6. **Tooth Mobility and Fremitus**
   A. **Horizontal tooth mobility**, movement of the tooth in a facial to lingual direction, is assessed by trapping the tooth between two dental instrument handles.
      1. Alternating moderate pressure is applied in the facial-lingual direction against the tooth first with one, then the other instrument handle.
      2. Mobility can be observed by using an adjacent tooth as a point of reference during attempts to move the tooth being examined.
   B. **Vertical tooth mobility**, the ability to depress the tooth in its socket, is assessed using the end of an instrument handle to exert pressure against the occlusal or incisal surface of the tooth (**Fig. 12-6**).

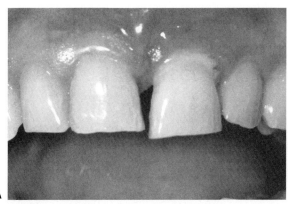
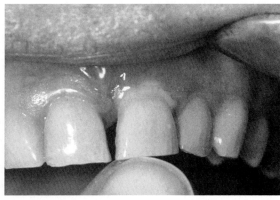

A   B

Figure 12-6. Vertical Tooth Mobility. A: The patient came to the dental office complaining of a loose tooth. Note the position of the maxillary left central incisor. B: The patient then demonstrated how he could push this tooth upward by applying pressure with his index finger against the incisal edge. This central incisor has vertical mobility. (Photographs courtesy of Dr. Don Rolfs, Periodontal Foundations, Wenatchee, WA.)

    C. Even though the periodontal ligament allows some slight movement of the tooth in its socket, the amount of this natural tooth movement is so slight that usually it cannot be seen with the naked eye. Thus, when visually assessing mobility, the clinician should expect to find no visible movement in a periodontally healthy tooth.
    D. There are many rating scales for recording clinically visible tooth mobility. One useful scale is indicated in **Table 12-2**.
    E. In some dental offices, the dentist may also wish to assess fremitus.
        1. **Fremitus** is a palpable or visible movement of a tooth when in function.
        2. Fremitus can be assessed by gently placing a gloved index finger against the facial aspect of the tooth as the patient either taps the teeth together or simulates chewing movements.

Table 12-2. Scale for Rating Visible Tooth Mobility

Classification	Description
Class 1	Slight mobility, up to 1 mm of horizontal displacement in a facial-lingual direction
Class 2	Moderate mobility, greater than 1 mm but less than 2 mm of horizontal displacement in a facial-lingual direction
Class 3	Severe mobility, greater than 2 mm of displacement in a facial-lingual direction or vertical displacement (tooth depressible in the socket)

7. **Furcation Involvement**
    A. A furcation probe is used to assess furcation involvement on multi-rooted teeth. Most molar teeth are, of course, multi-rooted, but some maxillary premolar teeth also develop with two roots creating the potential for a furcation involvement on some of these premolars also.
    B. Furcation probes are curved, blunt-tipped instruments that allow easy access to the furcation areas.

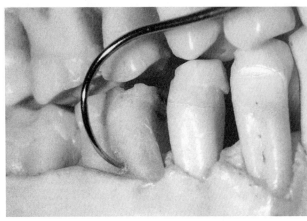
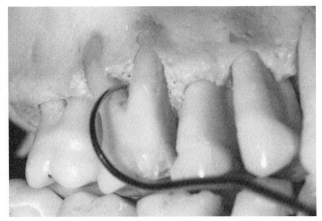

A   B

Figure 12-7. Use of Furcation Probes. **A:** Correct positioning of a furcation probe on a mandibular molar is demonstrated on a human skull. **B:** Correct positioning of a furcation probe on a maxillary molar is demonstrated on a human skull. (Courtesy of Dr. Don Rolfs.)

    C. Furcation involvement occurs on a multi-rooted tooth when periodontal infection invades the area between and around the roots, resulting in a loss of attachment and loss of alveolar bone between the roots of the tooth.

        1. Mandibular molars are usually bifurcated (mesial and distal roots), with potential furcation involvement on both the facial and lingual aspects of the tooth (**Fig. 12-7A**).

        2. Maxillary molar teeth are usually trifurcated (mesiobuccal, distobuccal, and palatal roots) with potential furcation involvement on the facial, mesial, and distal aspects of the tooth (**Fig. 12-7B**).

        3. Maxillary first premolars can have bifurcated roots (buccal and palatal roots) with the potential for furcation involvement on the mesial and distal aspects of the tooth.

    D. Furcation involvement frequently signals a need for periodontal surgery after completion of nonsurgical therapy, so detection and documentation of furcation involvement is a critical component of the comprehensive periodontal assessment.

    E. Furcation involvement should be recorded using a scale that quantifies the *severity (or extent) of the furcation invasion.* **Table 12-3** shows a commonly used scale for rating furcation invasions of multirooted teeth.

Table 12-3. Scale for Rating Furcation Involvement

Classification	Description
Class I	Curvature of the concavity can be felt with the probe tip; however the probe penetrates the furcation no more than 1 mm.
Class II	The probe penetrates into the furcation, but does not pass completely through the furcation.
Class III	Probe will pass completely through the furcation. In mandibular molars, the probe passes completely through the furcation between the mesial and distal roots. In maxillary molars, the probe passes between the mesiobuccal and distobuccal roots and will touch the palatal root.
Class IV	Same as class III furcation, except that the entrance to the furca is clinically visible because of the presence of gingival recession.

8. **Presence of Calculus Deposits on the Teeth**
   A. The presence of dental calculus on the teeth should be noted since these deposits must later be identified and removed as part of the nonsurgical therapy.
   B. Calculus is a local contributing factor in both gingivitis and periodontitis; thus, the identification and removal of these deposits is a critical component of successful patient treatment.
   C. Calculus deposits can be located through several techniques that include the following:
      1. Direct visual examination using a mouth mirror to locate *supra*gingival deposits.
      2. Visual examination while using compressed air to locate *supra*gingival deposits.
      3. Tactile examination using an explorer to locate subgingival calculus deposits.

9. **Presence of Plaque on the Teeth**
   A. The presence of bacterial plaque on the teeth should be noted during a comprehensive periodontal assessment since these deposits contain living periodontal pathogens that can lead to both gingivitis and periodontitis.
   B. Plaque deposits can be identified using disclosing dyes or by moving the tip of an explorer or a periodontal probe along the tooth surface adjacent to the gingival margin.
   C. There are many ways to record the presence of bacterial plaque, but most dental offices record the results of the plaque assessment in terms of the percentage of tooth surfaces with plaque evident at the gingival margin. A useful formula for recording plaque percentages is shown in Box 12-1.
      1. Note that in using the calculation shown in Box 12-1, a plaque score of 90% indicates that 90% of the total available tooth surfaces have plaque at the gingival margin.
      2. One goal of therapy would be for the patient to learn and perform plaque control measures that would bring the score as close to 0% as possible (or at least to bring the percentage of tooth surfaces with plaque as low as possible).

Box 12-1

Formula for Calculating Plaque Percentages

$$\frac{\text{Number of tooth surfaces with plaque}}{\text{Total number of tooth surfaces}} \times 100 = \text{percentage score}$$

   D. As discussed previously in this book, bacterial plaque is the primary etiologic factor for both gingivitis and periodontitis. Identification of the presence and distribution of bacterial plaque on the teeth is a critical piece of information needed when planning appropriate therapy and patient education.

10. **Gingival Inflammation**
   A. A thorough periodontal assessment includes recording the overt signs of inflammation. The overt signs of inflammation of the gingiva include erythema (redness) and edema (swelling) of the gingival margins resulting in readily identifiable changes in gingival color and contour.
   B. *It is always important to be aware that inflammation can be present in the deeper structures of the periodontium without necessarily involving any obvious clinical signs of inflammation of the gingival margin.*
      1. When assessing the presence of inflammation, it is important to remember that bleeding on probing also can be a sign of inflammation.
      2. Thus, when a clinician is identifying gingival inflammation, the visible signs such as color, contour, and consistency changes in the gingiva must be combined with the other signs such as bleeding on probing or the presence of exudate.

11. **Radiographic Evidence of Alveolar Bone Loss.** Radiographic interpretation is discussed in Chapter 13, so it will not be discussed in this chapter.
    A. It is important for the clinician to remember, however, that radiographs play an important role in arriving at the periodontal diagnosis and in developing an appropriate plan for nonsurgical periodontal therapy.
    B. *Radiographic evidence of alveolar bone loss is always an important part of a clinical periodontal assessment.*

12. **Presence of Local Contributing Factors**
    A. A thorough periodontal assessment will always include identification of local contributing factors.
    B. These factors are discussed in Chapter 7. The plan for treatment for any periodontal patient will always include measures to eliminate or to minimize the impact of these local factors.

SUPPLEMENTAL DIAGNOSTIC TESTS

Clinical periodontal assessment using the parameters discussed in Section 3 will result in an accurate periodontal diagnosis and can serve as a sound basis for designing an appropriate plan for therapy for the patient with gingival or periodontal disease. There are, however, a number of supplemental diagnostic tests that can be used for certain patients. *Clinicians might consider using some of these supplemental tests for patients that have periodontitis that is failing to respond to conventional periodontal therapy or periodontitis that shows other unusual signs of disease progression.*

There are a number of supplemental tests that have been suggested for use, and much research is continuing related to these types of tests. Most of these tests fall into three general types: (i) tests related to bacteria, (ii) tests that analyze gingival crevicular fluid content, and (iii) tests for genetic susceptibility to periodontal disease. *It is critical for the clinician to realize that based upon current research, none of these supplemental diagnostic tests should be ordered routinely on all patients with periodontal disease.*

1. **Tests Related to Bacteria.** Table 12-4 presents an overview of the tests related to bacteria. It is important to keep in mind that conventional periodontal therapy usually brings periodontal pathogens to low enough levels that disease progression can be halted without the need for identifying specific periodontal pathogens in most patients.

Table 12-4. Tests Related to Bacteria

TEST NAME	Purpose of Test	Special Considerations
Phase contrast microscopy study of plaque	Used for patient education and motivation	Test cannot identify specific bacterial species
Culture and sensitivity	Used to determine the sensitivity of bacteria to specific antibiotics	Sampling techniques for this test and the transport of bacterial samples to the laboratory are difficult
DNA (deoxyribonucleic acid) probe analysis	Used to identify specific periodontal pathogens in a person's mouth	Only a few bacterial species can be identified by this test

2. **Tests that Analyze Gingival Crevicular Fluid Content**
   A. Gingival Crevicular Fluid
      1. **Gingival crevicular fluid** is a fluid that flows into the sulcus from the gingival connective tissue; the flow is slight in health and increases in disease.
      2. Gingival crevicular fluid originates in connective tissue and flows into periodontal pockets. It has long been believed that this gingival crevicular fluid can contain markers for periodontal disease progression, and quite a bit of research time has been devoted to the study of this fluid.
   B. Gingival Crevicular Contents Being Studied
      1. Collagenase (an enzyme that breaks down collagen) is an example of one of the gingival crevicular fluid contents that has been studied, though no test for this is currently in use.
      2. Prostaglandin E2 (associated with arachidonic acid that is involved with inflammatory reactions such as those seen in periodontal disease) is another such gingival crevicular fluid ingredient that has been studied.
   C. The Future. It would be extremely helpful if clinicians had access to a diagnostic test that could indicate which patients are undergoing or are likely to undergo attachment loss. It is safe to assume that as more research is completed related to gingival crevicular fluid content, that some useful clinical tests will be developed in this area.

3. **Tests for Genetic Susceptibility for Periodontal Disease**
   A. Genetic Susceptibility
      1. It is obvious that a patient's genetic makeup affects susceptibility to many diseases including periodontal disease.
      2. This genetic makeup is inherited and cannot normally be altered.
   B. Tests for interleukin-1
      1. One test for genetic susceptibility to periodontal disease has been studied extensively and has resulted in a test that has been marketed to clinicians. (The PST Genetic Susceptibility Test from Interleukin Genetics Incorporated, Waltham, MA)
      2. This test identifies patients with genetic programming to produce high levels of interleukin-1 (an inflammatory mediator produced in response to the presence of periodontal pathogens).
         a. Higher levels of interleukin-1 in patients predispose the patients to more inflammation in the periodontium.
         b. It has been reported that 30% of the people in the United States have the genetic makeup to produce high levels of interleukin-1 in response to periodontal pathogens.

SECTION 4: CLINICAL FEATURES THAT REQUIRE CALCULATIONS

Some judgments that are made as part of the clinical periodontal assessment will require some calculations. The most common are the width of the attached gingiva and attachment level.

DETERMINING THE WIDTH OF ATTACHED GINGIVA

A. The **attached gingiva** is the part of the gingiva that is firm, dense, and tightly connected to the cementum on the cervical-third of the root or to the periosteum (connective tissue cover) of the alveolar bone. The attached gingiva lies between the free gingiva and the alveolar mucosa, extending from the base of the sulcus (or pocket) to the mucogingival junction.

    1. The function of the attached gingiva is to keep the free gingiva from being pulled away from the tooth.

    2. The width of the attached gingiva is not measured on the palate since it is not possible to determine where the attached gingiva ends and the palatal mucosa begins.

    3. *The attached gingiva **does not include** any portion of the gingiva that is separated from the tooth by a crevice, sulcus, or periodontal pocket.*

B. The width of the attached gingiva on a tooth surface is an important clinical feature for the dentist to keep in mind when planning many types of restorative procedures. If there is no attached gingiva on a tooth surface, the dentist is limited in the types of restorations that can be placed. Therefore, it is important to use the information collected during the comprehensive periodontal assessment to calculate this clinical feature.

C. The method for calculation of the width of attached gingiva is shown in Box 12-2. Note that the information needed to calculate the width of the attached gingiva already would have been recorded during the periodontal assessment.

Box 12-2

Width of the Attached Gingiva

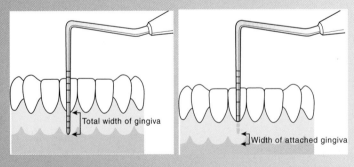

Formula: Calculate the width of the attached gingiva by subtracting the probing depth from the total width of the gingiva.

Step 1: Measure the total width of the gingiva from the gingival margin to the mucogingival junction.

Step 2: Measure the probing depth (from the gingival margin to the base of the pocket).

Step 3: Calculate the width of the attached gingiva by subtracting the probing depth from the total width of the gingiva.

(From Nield-Gehrig JS. *Fundamentals of Periodontal Instrumentation and Advanced Instrumentation,* 5th ed. Philadelphia: Lippincott Williams & Wilkins; 2004:454.)

CALCULATING THE ATTACHMENT LEVEL

1. **Definition.** The **clinical attachment level** (CAL) is an estimate of the periodontal support around the tooth as measured with a periodontal probe. This measurement is only an estimation of the actual histologic level of attachment still present. It is a means of estimating the level of the junctional epithelium.

2. Significance of Clinical Attachment Levels
   A. An attachment level measurement is a more accurate indicator of the periodontal support around a tooth than is a probing depth measurement.
      1. Probing depths are measured from the free gingival margin to the base of the sulcus or pocket. *The position of the gingival margin may change with tissue swelling, overgrowth of tissue, or recession of tissue. Since the position of the gingival margin can change (move), probing depths do not provide an accurate means to monitor changes in periodontal support over time in a patient.*
      2. CALs provide an accurate means to monitor changes in periodontal support over time. *CALs are calculated from measurements made from a **fixed point** on the tooth that does not change—the CEJ.*
   B. The presence of loss of attachment is a critical factor in distinguishing between gingivitis and periodontitis.
      1. Inflammation with *no attachment loss* is characteristic of gingivitis.
      2. Inflammation *with attachment loss* is characteristic of periodontitis.
      3. When attachment loss is 5 mm or greater, the patient should be referred to a periodontist.

3. **Calculating the Clinical Attachment Level**
   A. Recording the Gingival Margin on a Periodontal Chart.
      1. Technique to Determine the Gingival Margin Level. When tissue swelling or recession is present a periodontal probe is used to measure the distance the gingival margin is apical or coronal to the cementoenamel junction (**Figs 12-10 to 12-12**).
         a. **For gingival recession.** If gingival recession is present, the distance between the CEJ and the gingival margin is measured using a calibrated periodontal probe. This distance is recorded as the gingival margin level.
         b. **When the gingival margin is significantly coronal to the CEJ.** If the gingival margin significantly covers the cementoenamel junction, the distance between the margin and the CEJ is estimated using the following technique:
            1. Position the tip of the probe at a 45-degree angle to the tooth.
            2. Slowly move the probe beneath the gingival margin until the junction between the enamel and cementum is detected.
            3. Measure the distance between the gingival margin and the cementoenamel junction. This distance is recorded as the gingival margin level.
   B. Customarily, the notations 0, −, or + are used to indicate the position of the gingival margin on a periodontal chart (Box 12-3).

Box 12-3

Notations that Indicate the Position of the Free Gingival Margin

- A zero (0) indicates the free gingival margin is slightly coronal to the CEJ
- A negative number (−) indicates the free gingival margin significantly covers the CEJ
- A positive number (+) indicates the free gingival margin is apical to the CEJ (recession)

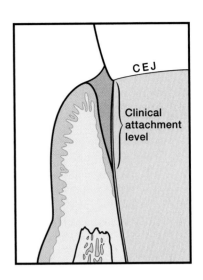

Figure 12-10. Calculating Clinical Attachment Level when the Gingival Margin is slightly coronal to the Cementoenamel Junction. When the gingival margin is slightly coronal to the CEJ, no calculations are needed since the probing depth and the clinical attachment level are equal.

For example:
Probing depth measurement: 6 mm
Gingival margin level: 0 mm
Clinical attachment loss: 6 mm

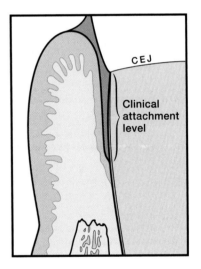

Figure 12-11. Calculating Clinical Attachment Level when the Gingival Margin is significantly coronal to the Cementoenamel Junction. When the gingival margin is significantly coronal to the CEJ, the CAL is calculated by **SUBTRACTING** the gingival margin level from the probing depth.

For example:
Probing depth measurement: 9 mm
Gingival margin level: − 3 mm
Clinical attachment loss: 6 mm

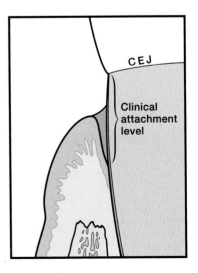

Figure 12-12. Calculating Clinical Attachment Level in the Presence of Gingival Recession. When recession is present, the CAL is calculated by **ADDING** the probing depth to the gingival margin level.

For example:
Probing depth measurement: 4 mm
Gingival margin level: + 2 mm
Clinical attachment loss: 6 mm

CHAPTER SUMMARY STATEMENT

The information gathered by the dental hygienist during the clinical periodontal assessment forms the basis for an individualized treatment plan for the patient. This chapter discusses two types of clinical periodontal assessment: a periodontal screening examination and the comprehensive periodontal assessment. The Periodontal Screening and Recording (PSR) is an efficient periodontal screening system for the detection of periodontal disease.

The comprehensive periodontal assessment is a complete clinical periodontal assessment used to gather information about the periodontium. The information collected in a comprehensive periodontal assessment includes probing depth measurements, bleeding on probing, presence of exudate, level of the free gingival margin and the mucogingival junction, tooth mobility, furcation involvement, presence of calculus and bacterial plaque, gingival inflammation, radiographic evidence of alveolar bone loss, and presence of local contributing factors. Supplemental diagnostic tests are indicated for certain patients. Some judgments made during a clincial periodontal assessment require calculation. These include the width of attached gingiva and clinical attachment levels. *Detection of clinical attachment level is important in determining whether gingivitis or periodontitis is present at a site of inflammation.*

The integration of the medical and personal patient histories with the clinical periodontal assessment is an important step in planning comprehensive patient care. In addition to risk factors identified during the clinical periodontal assessment (such as inflammation, bleeding, calculus, and attachment loss), other risk factors such as systemic disease (e.g., diabetes) and personal behaviors (e.g., smoking) are identified through the medical and personal histories. To develop a comprehensive treatment plan, the clinician must identify all risk factors associated with periodontal disease.

SECTION 5: FOCUS ON PATIENTS

CASE 1
While visiting a dental office, you observe a member of the dental team performing a periodontal assessment. You note that while searching for furcation invasion, the clinician is using a straight calibrated periodontal probe. What critical information might be lost because of instrument selection for this step in a periodontal assessment?

CASE 2
During a periodontal assessment you note severe inflammation of the gingiva over the facial surface of a lower right molar tooth. On the dental chart you are using there is no obvious mechanism to record this important piece of periodontal information. How should you proceed?

CASE 3
During a periodontal assessment of a periodontitis patient, you are trying to determine the clinical attachment level on the facial surface of a canine tooth. On the facial surface of the canine tooth you have measured 3 mm of gingival recession and a probing depth of 6 mm. How much attachment has been lost on the facial surface of this canine tooth?

SECTION 6: CHAPTER REVIEW QUESTIONS

1. Which member(s) of the dental team is/are responsible for the comprehensive periodontal assessment?
   A. The dental hygienist
   B. The dentist
   C. Both the dentist and the dental hygienist
   D. Either the dentist or the dental hygienist

2. The PSR (Periodontal Screening and Recording) requires that the clinician probe which of the following tooth surfaces?
   A. Only the facial surfaces of the teeth
   B. Only the lingual surfaces of the teeth
   C. Only the mesial and distal surfaces of the teeth
   D. All surfaces of the teeth

3. Probing depth measurements are recorded on how many surfaces of each tooth?
   A. 1 surface
   B. 2 surfaces
   C. 4 surfaces
   D. 6 surfaces

4. Which of the following is a synonym for exudate?
   A. Pus
   B. Blood
   C. Calculus
   D. Fremitus

5. Gingival recession means that the free gingival margin is
   A. Coronal to the CEJ
   B. At the same level as the CEJ
   C. Apical to the CEJ
   D. Even with the free gingival margin of the adjacent teeth

6. When measuring tooth mobility, the clinician should trap each tooth between
   A. Two fingers
   B. One finger and an instrument handle
   C. Two instrument handles
   D. The working ends of two probes

7. Furcation involvement is measured with what type of instrument?
   A. An explorer
   B. A curved periodontal probe
   C. A straight periodontal probe
   D. A Gracey curet

8. Attached gingiva is the part of the gingiva that is tightly connected to the cementum or periosteum.
   A. True
   B. False

9. Which of the following is the most accurate measurement of tooth support?
   A. Probing depths
   B. Clinical attachment levels

Chapter

13 Radiographic Analysis of the Periodontium

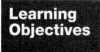
Learning Objectives

- Recognize the radiographic characteristics of normal and abnormal alveolar bone.
- Recognize and describe early radiographic evidence of periodontal disease.
- Distinguish between vertical and horizontal alveolar bone loss.
- Recognize potential etiologic agents for periodontal disease radiographically.
- Gain practical experience in radiographic assessment by applying information from this chapter in the clinical setting.

KEY TERMS

Radiolucent
Radiopaque

Cortical bone
Lamina dura

Crestal irregularities
Triangulation

SECTION 1: RADIOGRAPHIC APPEARANCE OF THE PERIODONTIUM

Dental radiographs are an important adjunct to the clinical assessment of the periodontium. To recognize disease, the dental hygienist must be able to recognize the normal radiographic appearance of the periodontium. Periodontal anatomy visible on radiographs includes the alveolar bone, periodontal ligament space, and cementum. The gingiva is a noncalcified soft tissue that cannot be seen on a radiograph.

1. **Radiolucent and Radiopaque Structures and Materials**
   A. **Radiolucent** materials and structures are easily penetrated by x-rays.
      1. Most of the x-rays will be able to pass through these objects and structures to expose the radiograph. Radiolucent areas appear as dark gray to black on the radiograph.
      2. Examples of radiolucent structures are the tooth pulp, periodontal ligament space, a periapical abscess, marrow spaces in the bone, and bone loss defects.
   B. **Radiopaque** materials and structures absorb or resist the passage of x-rays.
      1. Radiopaque areas appear light gray to white on the radiograph. These structures absorb most of the x-rays so that very few x-rays reach the radiograph.
      2. Examples of radiopaque structures and materials are metallic silver (amalgam restorations) and newer composite restorations, enamel, dentin, pulp stones, and compact or cortical bone.
2. **Identification of the Periodontium on Radiographs.** The components of the periodontium that can be identified on radiographs include the alveolar bone, periodontal ligament space, and cementum (**Fig. 13-1**).

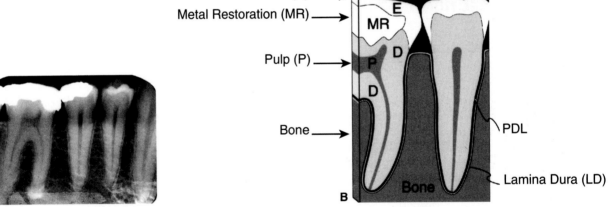

Figure 13-1. Radiographic Structures of the Periodontium.

   A. **Cortical Bone**
      1. **Cortical bone** is the outer surface of the bone and is composed of layers of bone closely packed together.
         a. On the maxilla, the cortical bone is a thin shell.
         b. On the mandible, the cortical bone is a dense layer.
      2. Radiographic Appearance of Cortical Bone
         a. Inferior border of the mandible appears on the radiograph as a thick white border.
         b. Interdental alveolar crests between the teeth of both jaws appear on the radiograph as a thin white line on the outside of crestal bone.
         c. The latticelike pattern of the cancellous bone that fills the interior portion of the alveolar process appears on the radiograph as a pattern of delicate white tracings within the bone.

B. Alveolar Crest. *The normal level of the alveolar bone is located approximately 2 mm apical to (below) the cementoenamel junction (CEJ).*

    1. If the coronal bone level is within 3 mm of the CEJ, the bone level is considered normal.

    2. It is unlikely that bone loss less than 3 mm can be detected on a radiograph.

C. Crestal Contour of the Interdental Bone

    1. The contour of the crest of the interproximal bone is a good indicator of periodontal health. *The contour of the interpoximal crest is parallel to an imaginary line drawn between the CEJs of adjacent teeth.*

    2. In posterior sextants, the contour of the interproximal crest is parallel to an imaginary line drawn between the CEJs of the adjacent teeth.

        a. Horizontal crest contour. The crest of the interproximal bone will have a horizontal contour when the CEJs of the adjacent teeth are at the same level (Fig. 13-2).

        b. Angular crest contour. The crest of the interproximal bone will have a vertical contour when one of the adjacent teeth is tilted or erupted to different height (Fig. 13-3).

D. Alveolar Crestal Bone

    1. Alveolar bone is the part of the jawbone that supports the teeth.

    2. The surfaces of the bony crests are smooth and covered with a thin layer of cortical (dense, hard) bone that may be seen as a thin, white line on a radiograph.

    3. *The most important radiographic feature of the alveolar crest is that it forms a smooth intact surface between adjacent teeth with only the width of the periodontal ligament space separating it from the adjacent root surface.*

        a. The crest of the interdental septa between incisors is thin and pointed.

        b. The crest of the interdental septa between the posterior teeth is rounded or flat (Fig. 13-4).

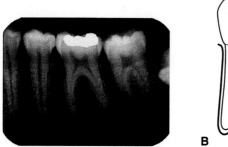 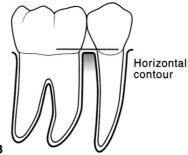

A   **B**

Figure 13-2. A: Normal Alveolar Bone Height. This radiograph shows a normal alveolar bone height that is 1.5 to 2 mm below and parallel to the cementoenamel junction. In this example, alveolar crest is a dense radiopaque line similar in density to the lamina dura surrounding the root of the tooth. **B: Horizontal Crest Contour.** The crest of the interproximal bone will have a horizontal contour when the CEJs of the adjacent teeth are at the same level.

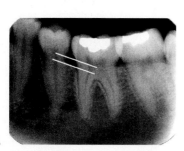 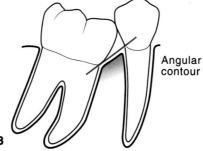

A   **B**

Figure 13-3. Angular Crest Contour. The crest of the interproximal bone will have a vertical contour when one of the adjacent teeth is tilted or erupted to different height.

E. **Lamina Dura**

1. The alveolar bone proper is the thin layer of dense bone that lines a normal tooth socket. In radiographs, the alveolar bone proper is identified as the **lamina dura**. On a radiograph, the lamina dura appears as a continuous white (radiopaque) line around the tooth root (**Fig. 13-5**).

2. On a radiograph, the lamina dura is continuous with the cortical bone layer of the crest of the interdental septa.

F. **Periodontal Ligament Space**

1. The space between the tooth root and the lamina dura of the socket is filled with the periodontal ligament tissue. The periodontal ligament tissue functions as the attachment of the tooth to the lamina dura of the socket.

2. Periodontal ligament tissue does not resist penetration of x-rays and, therefore, appears on the radiograph as a thin radiolucent black line surrounding the tooth root (**Fig. 13-5**).

3. In most cases, a widening of the periodontal ligament space (PDLS) on the radiograph indicates tooth mobility (**Fig. 13-6**).

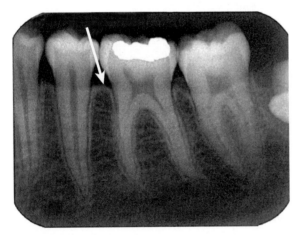

Figure 13-4. Alveolar Crest. The alveolar crest (indicated by an arrow) forms a smooth intact surface between adjacent teeth.

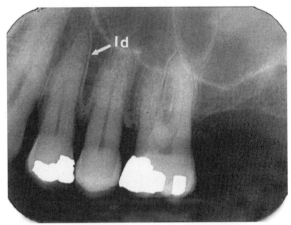

Figure 13-5. Lamina Dura and Periodontal Ligament Space. The lamina dura (ld) appears as a continuous white line around the tooth root. The dark space between the lamina dura and the root is the periodontal ligament space.

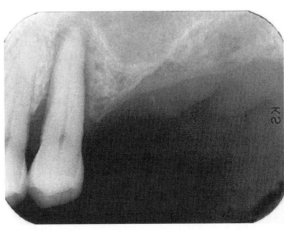

Figure 13-6. Widening of the PDL Space. This maxillary second premolar has a uniformly widened periodontal ligament space (PDL) that is characteristic of tooth mobility.

SECTION 2: USE OF RADIOGRAPHS FOR PERIODONTAL EVALUATION

TECHNIQUES FOR GOOD RADIOGRAPHIC QUALITY

1. **Long-Cone Paralleling Technique.** The long-cone paralleling technique provides a radiograph that is more anatomically accurate when compared with other intraoral techniques such as bisecting angle.
2. **Long-Gray scale-Low Contrast Images.** Long-scale contrast radiographic images have many visible shades of gray that make it easier to see subtle changes such as bone loss in periodontal disease. These images can be obtained using high kVp exposures (70 to 100 kVp) or using digital imaging software adjustments to maximize the gray scale of normally exposed images.

LIMITATIONS OF RADIOGRAPHS FOR PERIODONTAL EVALUATION

There are limitations in the use of the radiograph in the diagnosis of periodontal disease.

■ *A radiograph provides a two-dimensional image of a complex three-dimensional structure. The fact that the radiograph is a two-dimensional image can be misleading to the viewer.* For example, the buccal alveolar bone can hide bone loss on the lingual aspect of a tooth, and the palatal root makes it difficult to detect furcation involvement of a maxillary molar.

■ In addition, radiographs do not provide any information about the noncalcified components of the periodontium.

■ Radiographs *do not reveal* the following: the presence or absence of periodontal pockets, early bone loss, exact morphology of bone destruction, tooth mobility, early furcation involvement, condition of the alveolar bone on the buccal and lingual surfaces, or the level of the epithelial attachment.

1. **Periodontal Pockets**
   A. *The only reliable method of locating a periodontal pocket and evaluating its extent is by careful periodontal probing.*
   B. The periodontal pocket is composed of soft tissue so it will not be visible on the radiograph.
2. **Early Bone Loss**
   A. *The very earliest signs of periodontitis must be detected clinically, not radiographically.* By the time periodontal bone loss becomes detectable on the radiograph, it usually has progressed beyond the earliest stages of the disease.
      1. Interseptal bony defects smaller than 3 mm usually cannot be seen on radiographs.
      2. Bone height on the facial and lingual aspects is difficult to evaluate radiographically because the teeth are superimposed over the bone.
   B. *A radiograph cannot accurately display the shape of bone deformities because it is not three-dimensional.*
3. **Early Furcation Involvement**
   A. Radiographs usually *show more interradicular bone*—bone between the roots of the teeth—than is actually present. The facial and lingual aspects of the alveolar bone will often be superimposed over the furcation and hide bone loss from view.
   B. *Variations in alignment of the x-ray beam may conceal the presence or extent of furcation involvement.*
   C. Furcation involvement (bone loss between the roots) is detected by clinical examination with a furcation probe. The furcation area of a tooth should be examined with a furcation probe even if the radiograph shows a very small radiolucency or an area of diminished radiodensity at the furcation (**Fig. 13-7**).

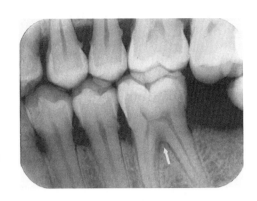

Figure 13-7. Furcation Involvement. The radiolucency on the mandibular first molar should be evaluated using a furcation probe.

4. **Extensive bone loss**
    A. *Crestal bone loss of 5 mm or greater may cause the coronal bone to be poorly visualized or not seen at all on normal bitewing radiographs*
    B. Vertically oriented bitewings may be used in these situations
    C. An adaptor is available for most film holders to accomplish this
    D. The long axis of the film is rotated 90 degrees to be perpendicular to the occlusal plane instead of the short axis (**Fig. 13-8**).
    E. Vertical bitewing radiographs show more of the coronal bone than regular bitewings especially when the teeth are widely separated by the film holder (**Fig. 13-9**).
5. **Disease Activity**
    A. Just as clinical attachment levels only indicate past disease destruction, *radiographs do not show **disease activity**, but only the **effects of the disease**.*
    B. *Because of these limitations, the radiographic examination is never a satisfactory substitute for a clinical periodontal assessment.*

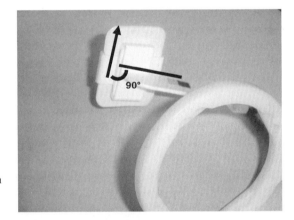

Figure 13-8. Film Placement for Vertical Bitewing. A #2 periapical film positioned for taking a vertical bitewing radiograph. Note how the film is rotated 90 degrees from the usual orientation.

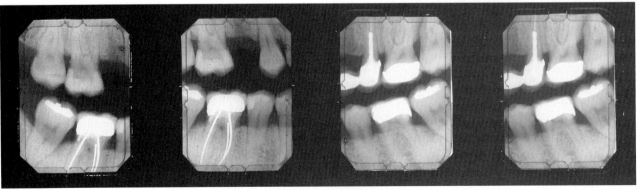

Figure 13-9. Four-Film Vertical Bitewing Series. Note how much coronal bone is visible on these vertical bitewings despite the separation of the teeth by the positioning device.

BENEFITS OF RADIOGRAPHS FOR PERIODONTAL EVALUATION

Despite the radiograph's limitations, the periodontal examination is incomplete without accurate radiographs. Radiographs will demonstrate the following: most of the bony changes associated with periodontitis, the tooth root morphology, relationship of the maxillary sinus to the periodontal deformity, widening of periodontal ligament space, advanced furcation involvement, periodontal abscesses, and local factors such as overhanging restorations, marginal ridge height discrepancies, open contacts, and calculus (Table 13-1).

Table 13-1. Benefits of Radiographs in the Detection of Periodontal Disease	
Condition	**Radiographic Sign(s)**
Early bony changes	Break or fuzziness at the crest of the interdental alveolar bone Widening of the periodontal ligament space at crestal margin Presence of fingerlike radiolucent projections into the interdental alveolar bone
Horizontal bone loss	Can be measured from a plane that is parallel to a tooth-to-tooth line drawn from the CEJs of adjacent teeth
Vertical bone loss	Seen as more bone loss on the interproximal aspect of one tooth than on the adjacent tooth; bone level is at an angle to a line joining the CEJs
Bone defects	Are radiolucent due to bone loss and therefore visible on radiographs, although three-dimensional structure may be hard to determine
Furcation involvement	Loss of bone in furcation area may be detectable as triangular radiolucency especially on mandibular molars

1. **Assessment of Bony Changes.** Early radiographic signs of periodontitis are (i) fuzziness at the crest of the alveolar bone, (ii) a widened periodontal ligament space (PDLS), and (iii) radiolucent areas in the interseptal bone (Fig. 13-10).
   A. Crestal Irregularities. Crestal irregularities are the appearance of breaks or fuzziness instead of a nice clean line at the crest of the interdental alveolar bone.

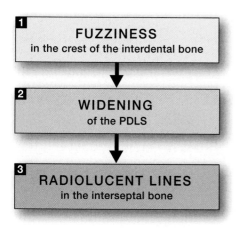

Figure 13-10. Early Radiographic Signs. Sequence of radiographic changes that occur in periodontitis.

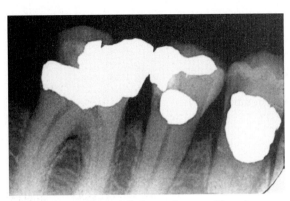

Figure 13-11. Triangulation. The crestal bone between these mandibular teeth demonstrates triangulation, a pointed, triangular appearance.

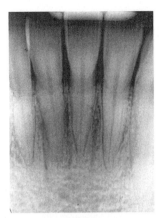

Figure 13-12. Fingerlike Radiolucent Projections. The nutrient canals within the bone are seen as fingerlike projections extending between and beyond the roots of the mandibular incisors on this radiograph.

    B. Triangulation (Funneling). **Triangulation** is the widening of the PDLS caused by the resorption of bone along either the mesial or distal aspect of the interdental (interseptal) crestal bone (**Fig. 13-11**).

    C. Interseptal Bone Changes

        1. Another radiographic sign of periodontitis is the existence of fingerlike radiolucent projections extending from the crestal bone into the interdental alveolar bone (**Fig. 13-12**).

        2. These fingerlike radiolucent lines represent a reduction of mineralized tissue (bone) adjacent to blood vessel channels within the alveolar bone.

        3. If chronic periodontitis goes untreated and much of the alveolar bone around the tooth is destroyed, the tooth will seem to float in space on the radiograph. This represents the terminal stage of the disease process.

2. Extent or Direction of Bone Loss. The extent or direction of bone loss is determined using the CEJ of adjacent teeth as the points of reference.

    A. Horizontal Bone Loss

    Horizontal bone loss is bone destruction that is parallel to an imaginary line drawn between the CEJs of adjacent teeth (**Fig. 13-13**).

    B. Vertical Bone Loss

    Vertical (or angular) bone loss occurs when there is greater bone destruction on the interproximal aspect of one tooth than on the adjacent tooth (**Fig. 13-14**).

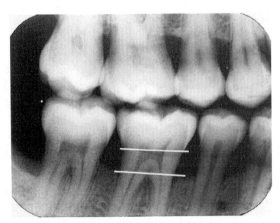

Figure 13-13. Horizontal Bone Loss. Horizontal bone loss is bone destruction that is parallel to an imaginary line drawn between the CEJs of adjacent teeth.

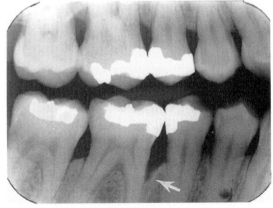

Figure 13-14. Vertical Bone Loss. The arrow points to vertical bone loss on the mesial surface of the mandibular first molar.

3. **Assessment of Bone Loss**
    A. The radiograph is an indirect method of detecting bone loss. *Periodontitis is a disease process with active and inactive periods, so the radiograph is only a snapshot of an instant in time in the disease process.*
    B. The radiograph reveals the bone *remaining* rather than the amount of bone actually lost.
    C. Bone loss occurs on all surfaces; however, the tooth root tends to mask (or hide) bone loss on the facial and lingual surfaces of the tooth.
    D. Mesial or distal bone loss is evaluated primarily by examining the interproximal septal bone on the radiograph. The amount of bone loss is *estimated* as the difference between the level of the remaining bone and the normal bone height.
4. **Assessment of Furcation Involvement**
    A. Furcation involvement will not be seen on the radiograph until the bone resorption extends past the furcation area.
        1. Furcation involvement of mandibular molars is easier to detect on a radiograph than is furcation involvement of maxillary molars. This is because mandibular molars have only two roots, a mesial root and a distal root (**Fig. 13-15**).
        2. Furcation involvement on maxillary molars is more difficult to detect on a radiograph. Maxillary molars have three roots, a mesiobuccal, distobuccal, and palatal root. The palatal root is often superimposed over the furcation of the tooth on the radiograph and masks (hides) any radiolucency there.

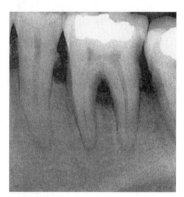

Figure 13-15. Furcation Involvement. The furcation involvement is easily visible on the mandibular first molar in this radiograph.

    B. It is a general rule that furcation involvement is often *greater* than what the radiograph reveals.
    C. If using the radiograph to aid in the detection of furcation involvement, the following rules should be kept in mind:
        1. If there is a slight thickening of the periodontal ligament space in the furcation area, the area should be examined clinically with a furcation probe.
        2. If severe bone loss is evident on the mesial or distal surface of a multirooted tooth (especially maxillary molars), furcation involvement should be suspected.
5. **Recognition of Local Contributing Risk Factors.** Several local contributing risk factors that may be revealed by the radiograph are calculus deposits, faulty restorations, and food packing areas.
    A. Calculus Deposits
        1. *The only accurate way to detect calculus deposits is with an explorer*, however, large calculus deposits *may be visible* on a radiograph.
            a. The radiograph may show large, heavy interproximal calculus deposits.
            b. Calculus deposits may be visible on the facial and lingual surfaces of teeth when there is severe bone loss on these surfaces.
        2. The ability to visualize calculus radiographically depends on the degree of mineralization within the calculus and the angulation factors of the x-ray beam.

B. Faulty Restorations. Inadequate dental restorations and prostheses are common causes of gingival inflammation, periodontitis, and alveolar bone resorption. In many cases, faulty restorations can be detected on a radiograph (**Fig. 13-16**).

C. Trauma from Occlusion
   1. The radiograph is used only as a supplemental aid in recognizing trauma from occlusion.
   2. Radiographic signs of trauma from occlusion include the following:
      a. Increased width of the periodontal ligament spaces on the mesial and distal sides of the tooth due to resorption of the lamina dura.
      b. Vertical or angular bone destruction.

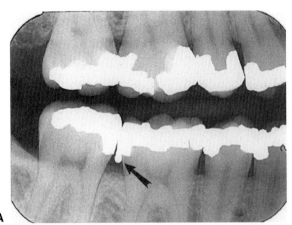
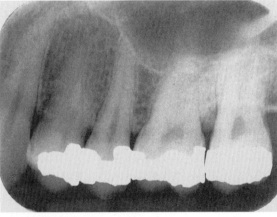

A   **B**

Figure 13-16. Faulty Restorations. A: The distal surface of the mandibular first molar, indicated by the arrow, has a faulty restoration that creates a food trap and harbors plaque biofilm. B: The distal proximal tooth surface of the maxillary first molar and the mesial tooth surface of the second molar have not been restored to their original shape and contour. These faulty contours create an open contact that can allow food impaction.

CHAPTER SUMMARY STATEMENT

When the limitations of radiographs are recognized, they can be an important diagnostic aid in the examination and diagnosis of patients with periodontitis. Radiographs are extremely useful tools in the detection of bony changes due to periodontitis such as crestal irregularities, triangulation, interseptal bone loss, assessment of bone defects, and furcation involvement.

SECTION 3: FOCUS ON PATIENTS

CASE 1

Mr. Jones is a new patient in your dental office. He brings with him some recent full-mouth radiographs that reveal no evidence of alveolar bone loss. While studying a copy of the patient's dental chart, you note that there is a diagnosis of chronic periodontitis. How might you explain the apparent discrepancy between the lack of radiographic evidence of bone loss and the diagnosis of periodontitis?

CASE 2

During a periodontal assessment for a new patient, you detect clinical attachment loss. When you suggest that the patient needs dental radiographs, the patient objects because she does not want to be exposed to "unnecessary x-rays." How should you respond?

CASE 3

While reviewing a new set of dental radiographs for a patient, you note numerous sites of obvious bone loss. The bone loss appears to be vertical (or angular), where there is much more bone loss on one tooth surface compared with the immediately adjacent tooth surface. How might the dental team use this vertical pattern of bone loss when developing the periodontal diagnosis?

SECTION 4: CHAPTER REVIEW QUESTIONS

1. All of the following are **radiolucent** materials and structures, EXCEPT:
   A. Tooth pulp
   B. Enamel
   C. Periodontal ligament space
   D. Marrow spaces in the bone

2. The normal level of the alveolar bone is approximately _____ apical to the cementoenamel junction.
   A. 0.5 mm
   B. Less than 1 mm
   C. 2 mm
   D. 3 mm

3. When one of two adjacent teeth is tilted or erupted to a different height than its neighboring tooth, the crest of the interproximal bone will have a _____ crest contour.
   A. Angular
   B. Horizontal
   C. Parallel
   D. Vertical

4. The alveolar bone proper is the thin layer of dense bone that lines a normal tooth socket. On a radiograph, the alveolar bone proper is identified as the:
   A. Alveolar bone proper
   B. Periodontal ligament space
   C. Cortical bone
   D. Lamina dura

5. On a radiograph, widening of the periodontal ligament space is an indication of:
   A. Tooth mobility
   B. A partially erupted tooth
   C. Triangulation
   D. Subgingival calculus

6. On a radiograph, when the crestal bone between two adjacent teeth has a pointed, triangular appearance, this is termed:
   A. Tooth mobility
   B. A partially erupted tooth
   C. Triangulation
   D. Subgingival calculus

7. Radiographs may useful in visualizing all of the following signs of periodontitis, EXCEPT:
   A. Periodontal pockets
   B. Horizontal bone loss
   C. Vertical bone loss
   D. Recognition of local contributing risk factors

8. The best method for detection of subgingival calculus deposits is:
   A. Dental radiograph
   B. Periodontal explorer

14 Periodontal Care Modifications for Systemic Conditions

Learning Objectives

- Discuss and provide several examples of how systemic conditions can increase an individual's susceptibility to periodontal disease.
- Give several examples of medications that can produce changes in the periodontium.
- Discuss and provide several examples of how periodontal pathogens can have an adverse effect on an individual's systemic health.

KEY TERMS

Bacteremia	Calcium channel blockers	Cyclosporin
Bacterial endocarditis	Antiarrhythmic drugs	Azathioprine
Well controlled diabetes	Aspirin therapy	Corticosteroid
"Ask. Advise. Refer."	Phenytoin	Osteoradionecrosis (ORN)
Quitlines	Hemodialysis	

SECTION 1: RELATIONSHIP BETWEEN SYSTEMIC AND PERIODONTAL DISEASE

There can be a very strong two-way relationship between systemic disease and periodontal problems that can affect the outcome of periodontal treatment. One half of this relationship is the concept that systemic conditions can increase the likelihood that an individual will develop periodontitis. The other half of this relationship is the concept that periodontal disease can have an adverse effect on an individual's systemic health.

SYSTEMIC CONDITIONS CAN IMPACT THE PERIODONTIUM

1. As discussed in Chapter 8, systemic conditions can increase an individual's susceptibility to periodontal disease. Proven systemic risk factors that increase susceptibility include tobacco use, diabetes mellitus, osteoporosis, hormone alteration, psychological stress, and genetic influences.
2. The medications that are used to treat systemic diseases also can produce changes in the periodontium. An example is the overgrowth of the gingival tissue seen in individuals taking phenytoin (Dilantin) to control convulsions or seizures in the treatment of epilepsy.

PERIODONTAL DISEASE CAN ADVERSELY AFFECT SYSTEMIC HEALTH

1. Periodontal disease is a bacterial infection.
2. Periodontal pathogens may have an adverse effect on an individual's systemic health.
   A. Periodontal disease may affect an individual's general health when pathogenic oral bacteria enter the bloodstream and spread to cause infections in other parts of the body.
   B. Periodontal infection may contribute to the development of heart disease, premature, underweight babies, poorly controlled diabetes, and respiratory diseases.
   C. Dental hygienists need to be knowledgeable about the effect of periodontitis on systemic conditions and take responsibility for assisting patients in maintaining overall health.
3. **Bacteremia**
   A. Bacteremia is the presence of bacteria in the bloodstream. Bacteria and byproducts from the oral cavity are commonly introduced into the bloodstream during routine tooth brushing, flossing, subgingival irrigation, and most invasive dental procedures, including hand and ultrasonic instrumentation and periodontal therapy.
   B. The extent to which oral bacteria enter the bloodstream appears to be directly related to severity of gingival inflammation. Oral bacteria can enter the bloodstream through inflamed or ulcerated tissue or by direct invasion of the gingival connective tissue. The best means to prevent bacteremia of oral origin is through the maintenance of periodontal health.
   C. Individuals at increased risk for systemic complications from oral infections include immunosuppressed individuals; hospitalized patients unable to perform adequate plaque control, those with artificial joint or heart valve replacements, and those taking antibiotics that alter the oral flora.
   D. *In planning periodontal care, it is important to assure that the planned treatment will not be harmful to an individual's systemic health.*

4. **Infective Endocarditis**
   A. **Bacterial endocarditis** is a bacterial infection caused by bacteria that adhere to the lining of the heart chambers and the heart valves. Infective endocarditis affecting the left side of the heart may have a rapid onset and a fatal outcome.
   B. Oral organisms are common etiologic agents of infective endocarditis. Oral bacteria that have been associated with infective endocarditis include *Streptococcus sanguis*, *Haemophilus aphrophilus*, as well as gram-negative oral bacteria including *Actinobacillus actinomycetemcomitans*, *Eikenella corrodens*, *Capnocytophaga*, and *Fusobacterium nucleatum*.
   C. Maintenance of good periodontal health is the best way to reduce the risk of oral bacteremia in patients who are susceptible to infective endocarditis.

SECTION 2: CARE MODIFICATIONS BY SYSTEMIC CONDITIONS

This section concentrates on systemic conditions that are most likely to require modification in the care plan for the provision of periodontal therapy, including periodontal instrumentation of tooth surfaces. The fictitious patient case described in Box 14-1 demonstrates how the two-way relationship between systemic disease and periodontal disease is an important consideration in periodontal care.

Box 14-1

Maria: An Example of the Two-Way Relationship

Maria is a cheerful 52-year-old who has never been to your office before. You discover she is very proud of her two grandchildren, so the conversation goes along about kids and the interesting things they do. Upon further questioning, you discover Maria has had diabetes for about 3 years and takes an oral hypoglycemic medication. Also, her maternal grandmother and an older sister have diabetes. Maria smokes about one pack of cigarettes every 2 days.

Clinically, Maria exhibits periodontitis. No other oral problems are detected by the oral or radiographic examinations.

When the dentist and hygienist plan periodontal care for this patient, they will first want to determine how well her diabetes is controlled. Many offices can perform a blood sugar test with a drop of blood from a simple finger prick. The blood sugar (glucose) value obtained will immediately indicate if the patient's diabetes is controlled or if she needs to see her physician before treatment can begin. Knowledge of the blood sugar levels is important because the dental healthcare provider cannot expect a good response to periodontal therapy in an uncontrolled diabetic.

Maria is the perfect example of an individual in whom there is a two-way relationship between her systemic disease and her periodontal disease. Education opportunities to address with Maria include (i) how diabetes affects the periodontium and (ii) how periodontal disease could make it more difficult to control her blood sugar levels and increase her risk for complications from the diabetes.

Maria should also be advised about the adverse effects of smoking on diabetes and the periodontium and about smoking cessation resources.

DIABETES MELLITUS

1. **Diabetes.** Diabetes is a disease in which the body does not produce or properly use insulin, a hormone that is needed to convert sugar, starches, and other food into fuel for use by the body. It is important to record the type of diabetes, duration of diabetes, history of diabetic complications, medications, and method of metabolic monitoring used by the patient.

2. **Control of Blood Glucose Levels.** It important for the diabetic to monitor blood glucose levels carefully. Blood sugar tests measure how well an individual's body is processing glucose. There are two tests commonly used to measure blood glucose levels (**Table 14-1**).

   A. Hemoglobin A_{1c} (pronounced hemoglobin A-one-C)

      1. A hemoglobin A_{1c} test is a simple laboratory test used to monitor if blood glucose is under control. The hemoglobin A_{1c} test measures the amount of sugar that is attached to the hemoglobin in red blood cells, with the results given as a percentage. The percentage that occurs in people without diabetes is usually about 6%.

      2. The hemoglobin A_{1c} goal for most people with diabetes is less than 7%. Patients with diabetes who can lower their hemoglobin A_{1c} values below 7% decrease their chances of complications from diabetes such as blindness, nerve damage, and kidney damage. If scores are above 8%, the diabetic is much more susceptible to infection and a slower healing time.

   B. A Finger-Stick Test

      1. The finger-stick test is a simple test that can be done in the periodontal office using a blood glucose meter.

      2. Ideal goals for most diabetics when using a blood glucose meter are 80 to 120 mg/dL (mg/dL = milligrams per deciliter)

   C. Patient Education Regarding Glucose Levels. Dental hygienists should advise individuals with diabetes of the importance of stable glucose levels for the health of the periodontium. Explain that glucose levels over the target range increase the likelihood of developing periodontitis.

Table 14-1.	**Blood Glucose Levels in Diabetes**
Test	**Glucose Levels**
Hemoglobin A_{1c}	Goal for most individuals with diabetes is a glucose level less than 7% High susceptibility to infection occurs when the glucose level is above 8%
Finger-Stick Test	Glucose level at appointment time: Target range = 80 to 120 mg/dL Increased risk of infection = 180 to 300 mg/dL Unacceptable range = greater than 300 mg/dL

3. **Periodontal Treatment Considerations**
   A. Establish Communication with the Patient's Physician
      1. The physician should be contacted before treatment to determine if antibiotic premedication is needed. The results of the patient's most recent hemoglobin A_{1c} test should be obtained and recorded in the patient's dental chart.
      2. Periodontal therapy, including periodontal debridement of tooth surfaces, should be postponed until the diabetes is well controlled. Diabetes is **well controlled** if the blood glucose levels are stabilized within the recommended range.
         a. The patient with poorly controlled diabetes should not receive elective periodontal care.
         b. The patient with poorly controlled diabetes will be more susceptible to bacterial and fungal infections, such as gingivitis, periodontitis, and candidiasis. Patients with poorly controlled diabetes do not heal as well following periodontal surgery.
   B. Day of the Appointment
      1. Ask the patient to bring his or her blood glucose meter to the appointment to test glucose blood levels before beginning the dental procedure.
      2. Instruct the patient to eat a normal breakfast and take medication as prescribed.
   C. Postappointment Considerations. The patient may be unable to eat following periodontal therapy, predisposing him or her to hypoglycemia. The patient's physician should be consulted prior to therapy for recommendations about alterations in the patient's medication regimen.
4. **Oral Cavity as a Source of Infection in Individuals with Diabetes**
   A. The presence of any infection, including periodontitis, may make it difficult for the individual to control his or her glucose blood level.
      1. It is important to inform the physician of the degree of periodontal disease.
      2. The importance of periodontal treatment to eliminate the periodontal infection should be explained to the patient.
   B. Untreated periodontal disease may make it more difficult for individuals with diabetes to control their glucose levels, thus increasing their chances of complications from diabetes.[1]

TOBACCO USE

1. **Effect of Tobacco Use on Response to Periodontal Therapy.** As discussed in Chapter 6, smoking appears to be one of the most important risk factors in the development and progression of periodontal disease.
2. **Effect of Quitting on the Periodontium**
   A. The past effects of smoking on the periodontium, such as bone loss, cannot be reversed; however, smoking cessation is beneficial to the periodontium.
      1. Several years after quitting, former smokers are no more likely to have periodontal disease than persons who have never smoked. This indicates that quitting seems to gradually erase the harmful effects of tobacco use on periodontal health.
      2. Evidence that periodontal health does improve with smoking cessation has led the American Academy of Periodontology to recommend tobacco cessation counseling as an important component of periodontal therapy.
   B. Quitting restores the body's inflammatory response. (Smokers have a reduced inflammatory response that masks the normal signs of inflammation, such as redness and bleeding.)
      1. Ten to 12 weeks after cessation of smoking, the patient may note gingival inflammation and bleeding that may last for several months.
      2. Hygienists should explain that cessation of smoking will lead to a revitalized immune response and possible inflammation and bleeding. This change is a

> sign that the immune response is returning to normal; inflammation should subside in time with conscientious self-care and regular professional care.

3. About 1 year after smoking cessation, the gingiva becomes less fibrotic and assumes a more normal anatomy.

3. **Patient Education.** Dental hygienists should advise patients of tobacco's negative effects on the periodontium and the benefits of quitting tobacco use. ("As your clinician, I need you to know that quitting smoking is the most important thing you can do to protect your current and future dental health.")

   A. *Smoking may well be the major preventable risk factor for periodontal disease.*

   B. Periodontal conditions will most likely continue to worsen as long as smokers continue to use tobacco.

   C. Smokers who plan to continue smoking should be informed that meticulous self-care and frequent professional visits are critical.

4. **Periodontal Treatment Considerations**

   A. Dental healthcare providers should ask about and record the tobacco-use status of every patient.

   B. Every person who smokes should be offered smoking cessation treatment at every office visit.

      1. In a nonjudgmental manner, the dental hygienist should inquire if the individual is thinking about quitting. For those who are contemplating quitting, this may allow them to express and clarify their intentions. At this point, an action plan for smoking cessation can be developed.

      2. Smoking cessation guidelines in English and Spanish are available through the U.S. Department of Health and Human Services on the Internet (http://www.ahcpr.gov/guide/) or by telephone (1-800-358-9295).

      3. **"Ask. Advise. Refer."** is the American Dental Hygienists' Association's (ADHA's) smoking cessation initiative designed to encourage dental hygienists to educate patients about smoking cessation resources.

      4. **Quitlines** are toll-free telephone centers staffed by trained smoking cessation experts. A list of quitlines is provided in Chapter 28 of this book.

         a. Smokers are more likely to quit if advised to do so by health professionals. Virtually no expertise is needed to refer patients to a telephone quitline or website.

         b. It takes as little as 30 seconds to refer a patient to a quitline or website.

CARDIOVASCULAR DISORDERS

1. **General Recommendations for Patients with Cardiovascular Disorders.** The primary concern for the management of a patient with a cardiovascular disorder during periodontal therapy is to maintain the patient's optimum blood pressure, heart rate, and heart rhythm. A stress-reduction protocol (Box 14-2) should be used for individuals with cardiovascular problems.
2. **Effects of Medical Therapies on the Periodontium**
   A. Medications
      1. Calcium channel blockers, medications used to control high blood pressure, are associated with gingival overgrowth in some patients.
      2. Antiarrhythmic drugs used to treat individuals with irregular heartbeats have side effects such as gingival overgrowth or xerostomia that may impact the periodontium.
      3. Anticoagulant drugs are substances that prevent or delay coagulation of the blood.
         a. Anticoagulant therapy is frequently used for patients with a history of prosthetic heart valves, valvular disorders, myocardial infarction (heart attack), cerebrovascular accident (stroke), or thromboembolism (blood vessel blocked by a clot).
         b. No modification of anticoagulant therapy is usually required for patients however, consultation with the patient's physician is recommended prior to treatment.
      4. Aspirin therapy is commonly recommended for individuals with a history of myocardial infarction (heart attack) or for the prevention of clot formation as an adjunct to anticoagulant drugs. In this case, bleeding during periodontal therapy—including periodontal instrumentation—could be a problem; consult with the patient's physician to determine if the aspirin dosage should be adjusted prior to periodontal therapy.
   B. Medical Devices
      1. A pacemaker is a device surgically placed in the chest of a patient to regulate an irregular heartbeat.
      2. In a recent position paper, the American Academy of Periodontology recommends that dental health care workers avoid exposing patients with cardiac pacemakers to magnetostrictive ultrasonic devices.[2]

Box 14-2

Strategies for Stress Reduction

- **Good Communication.** Use empathy and effective communication to establish trust and determine the cause(s) of the patient's anxiety.
- **Reduce Anxiety.** Premedicate as needed with an antianxiety medication for use (i) the night before the appointment to aid the patient in getting a good night's sleep and (ii) the day of the appointment.
- **Scheduling.** Schedule appointments early in the day (so that patient will be well rested and not have all day to worry about the upcoming treatment).
- **Suggestions for Patient.** Suggest that the patient eat a normal meal before the appointment and allow ample travel time to get to the dental office or clinic.
- **Length of Treatment.** Keep appointments short.
- **Pain Control.** Ensure good pain control before, during, and after the appointment, as appropriate, including the use of pain medications, local anesthesia, and/or nitrous oxide.

3. **Oral Cavity as a Source of Infection in Individuals with Heart Disease and Stroke**
   A. Individuals with periodontitis may be more at risk for heart disease and have nearly twice the risk of having a fatal heart attack than persons without periodontal disease.[3]
   B. Dental hygienists should inform their patients that periodontal disease might be a risk factor for heart disease. Preventive care is important not only to save teeth, but also might reduce the risk of heart disease and stroke.

CHRONIC OBSTRUCTIVE PULMONARY DISEASE

1. Periodontal Treatment Considerations
   A. Chronic obstructive pulmonary disease (COPD) is a chronic disorder of the lungs in which the airways become blocked and narrowed, making it more difficult to move air through them. Chronic bronchitis and emphysema are two common examples of COPD.
   B. A stress reduction protocol should be used for individuals with COPD.
   C. The use of ultrasonic or sonic instruments is contraindicated for individuals with COPD. An individual with COPD would have a high infection risk if he or she were to aspirate septic material or microorganisms from dental plaque into the lungs.
   D. Nonemergency periodontal treatment should be postponed if the patient has an upper respiratory infection.
2. **Oral Cavity as a Source of Infection in Individuals with Respiratory Disease**
   A. Pneumonia can be caused by the aspiration of oral bacteria into the lower respiratory tract.
   B. Good plaque control is important in reducing the incidence of lung infection.
      1. Persons in hospital intensive care units, persons in nursing homes, and other bedridden individuals are often not able to perform plaque control procedures, resulting in more bacterial plaque.
      2. Caregivers should be instructed in appropriate plaque control techniques. Plaque removal every 48 hours may be an effective way of preventing respiratory infection for hospitalized or nursing home patients.

CEREBROVASCULAR ACCIDENT (STROKE)

1. **Cerebrovascular Accident (Stroke).** A cerebrovascular accident (CVA) is the sudden death of brain cells due to a problem with the blood supply. When blood flow to the brain is impaired, oxygen and important nutrients cannot be delivered. The result is abnormal brain function. A cerebrovascular accident results in a sudden loss of neurologic function (speech, movement, or sensation) for a period of 24 hours or longer.

2. **Periodontal Treatment Considerations**
   A. A medical consultation should always be obtained for a patient with a history of stroke. Patients who have suffered a stroke are frequently given anticoagulants, such as coumadin, and may need alteration of their medication regimen before periodontal therapy.
   B. Stroke patients may experience difficulty in swallowing, chewing, facial weakness, and weakness in the hands and arms.
      1. These problems may result in changes in diet and oral self-care. Modified oral health aids, such as brushes with large handles, electric toothbrushes, and floss holders, may be helpful.
      2. Daily antimicrobial rinses may be helpful in controlling supragingival plaque.
   C. Patients with a history of stroke are particularly susceptible to the harmful effects of stress. Therefore, stress reduction techniques should be incorporated such as the scheduling of short, early morning appointments.
   D. To avoid a medical emergency, monitor blood pressure at every appointment. No periodontal treatment should be done if the blood pressure reading is 160/100 or greater.

3. **Oral Cavity as a Source of Infection in Individuals with Heart Disease and Stroke**
   A. Any infection, including periodontitis, should be treated because bacterial infections may trigger clot formation and trigger another stroke.
   B. Based on an analysis of the first National Health and Nutrition Examination Survey (NHANES III), researchers found periodontal disease to be a significant risk factor for cerebrovascular disease (stroke), in particular nonhemorrhagic stroke.[4]
   C. Dental hygienists should inform their patients that periodontal disease might be a risk factor for stroke. Preventive care is important not only to save teeth, but also might reduce the risk of heart disease and stroke.

EPILEPSY

1. **Epilepsy.** Epilepsy is a brain disorder that occurs when the electrical signals in the brain are disrupted. This change in the brain leads to a seizure. Seizures can cause brief changes in a person's body movements, awareness of his or her surroundings, emotions, and/or senses (such as taste, smell, vision, or hearing).

2. **Periodontal Treatment Considerations**
   A. **Phenytoin** (FEN-i-toyn) is an anticonvulsant medication used to control convulsions or seizures in the treatment of epilepsy.
   B. Gingival hyperplasia—overgrowth of the gingiva—is one of the most common side effects of phenytoin (**Fig. 14-1**). It has been estimated that 40% to 50% of the millions of individuals who take phenytoin will develop gingival overgrowth to some extent. Overgrowths appear to be more common in children and young adults.
   C. The best treatment of medication-associated gingival enlargement is to discontinue the associated drug.
      1. Sometimes the patient's physician may prescribe an alternative medication that is less likely to be associated with gingival enlargement.
      2. Discontinuing or changing the medication, however, is often not practical with most patients because of the medication's important role in medical treatment.
      3. Therefore, plaque control and surgical treatment of gingival enlargement are the most practical choices.
      4. Surgical elimination of the tissue overgrowth is often required.
         a. Unfortunately, the gingival overgrowth is likely to recur within 1 to 2 years even in the presence of good plaque control, especially if the patient is younger than 25.
         b. If plaque control is inadequate, the re-growth will occur rapidly.
         c. The patient should be advised of the likelihood of the recurrence of the gingival overgrowth following surgery.
   D. Educating patients about the oral side effects of medications is critical to reducing the medication-related risks of periodontal disease.
      1. Plaque control is critical in the treatment and prevention of medication-associated tissue overgrowth. Meticulous self-care combined with frequent professional care including periodontal debridement of tooth surfaces is vital.
      2. Antimicrobial mouth rinses may be valuable adjuncts to mechanical plaque control.

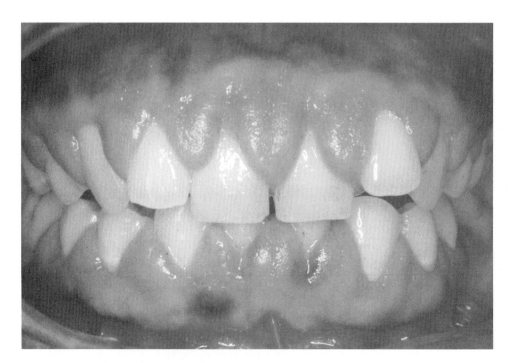

Figure 14-1. Gingival Hyperplasia. Gingival overgrowth is a common side effect of phenytoin.

LIVER DISEASE

1. **Liver Disease.** The liver acts as the body's refinery, regulating life processes including converting food for use by the body's cells, processing drugs into forms that are easier for the body to use, and detoxifying and excreting of poisonous substances from the body. There are many forms of liver disease including viral hepatitis, cirrhosis, liver disorders in children, gallstones, alcohol-related liver disorders, and cancer of the liver.
2. **Periodontal Treatment Considerations**
   A. Bleeding.
      1. The patient's physician should be consulted prior to any periodontal therapy. The liver produces most of the clotting factors for the blood. In patients with liver disease, excessive bleeding may occur with invasive dental procedures.
      2. The liver plays a principal role in digestion of proteins. Swallowing of blood during periodontal therapy should be minimized, since the ability to metabolize blood proteins is diminished in patients with liver disease.
   B. Since the liver's ability to metabolize drugs is limited in patients with liver disease, the physician should be consulted prior to the use of any drugs including pain medications, antibiotics, and local anesthetics. Acetaminophen (Tylenol) is hepatotoxic (potentially destructive of liver cells) and should be avoided in patients with severe liver disease.
   C. Patients with liver disease are at increased risk of infection. Patients should be educated about the importance of meticulous plaque control.

PREGNANCY

1. **Periodontal Treatments Considerations**
   A. Inflammation of the gingiva increases in pregnant women in the presence of small amounts of bacterial plaque.
      1. In most cases, increased gingival inflammation only occurs in patients who had evidence of gingivitis before becoming pregnant.
      2. If the patient has healthy gingiva prior to pregnancy and maintains good plaque control throughout pregnancy, she should remain free of gingival inflammation.
   B. Periodontal debridement of tooth surfaces and patient education should be an important part of prenatal care. In a recent survey, 99% of obstetricians felt that pregnant patients should continue to receive routine dental care.[5]
      1. The dental hygienist should stress the importance of thorough plaque control and its role in the prevention of plaque-induced gingivitis during pregnancy.
      2. A common misconception is that calcium is taken from the teeth for the baby; the dental hygienist should explain that minerals within the teeth are not metabolically available.
2. **Oral Cavity as a Source of Infection in Pregnant Individuals**
   A. Periodontal disease is an infection, and all infections pose a risk to the health of the baby. Products produced by periodontal bacteria in the mother's oral cavity may enter the bloodstream, cross the placenta, and harm the fetus.
   B. Pregnant women who have periodontal disease may be seven times more likely to have a baby that is born too early and too small.[6]
   C. One possible mechanism for the association between periodontitis and adverse pregnancy outcomes involves the role of prostaglandin E_2 (PGE_2) in initiating normal labor.
      1. During normal pregnancy, PGE_2 plays an important role in regulating the onset of labor, uterine contractions, and delivery. Fluid levels of PGE_2 rise steadily throughout pregnancy and once a critical threshold is reached, induce labor, cervical dilation, and delivery.
      2. As discussed in Chapter 6, PGE_2 plays an important role in periodontal inflammation and bone loss. It is possible that periodontal disease may affect pregnancy by serving as a reservoir of PGE_2.

3. One study found that mothers who delivered low-birthweight babies had twice the levels of PGE_2 in their gingival crevicular fluid than mothers who delivered normal-birthweight infants.[7]
4. Dental hygienists should inform female patients that healthy gums might lead to a healthier body and a healthier baby. Women considering pregnancy should have a periodontal screening and establish good plaque control habits before becoming pregnant. Prenatal care should include meticulous self-care and frequent professional care.

KIDNEY DISEASE AND HEMODIALYSIS

1. **Kidney Disease and Hemodialysis**
   A. Kidney disease is a disorder in which the kidney is unable to excrete waste products and to maintain the correct balance of water and salts in the body.
   B. **Hemodialysis** is a method of filtering unwanted waste products from the blood using a machine that acts as an artificial kidney.
2. **Periodontal Treatment Considerations**
   A. Patients with renal inflammation may have a reduced ability to withstand the stress of dental treatment; therefore, stress reduction techniques should be used.
   B. Prophylactic antibiotic coverage is recommended prior to periodontal treatment for hemodialysis patients.
      1. Dialysis patients have an increased incidence of bacterial endocarditis.
      2. Bacteria introduced into the bloodstream during dental procedures can produce inflammation of the arteries at the site of the hemodialysis shunt or fistula.
   C. Dialysis patients may form dental calculus more rapidly than healthy individuals, so frequent periodontal maintenance intervals are recommended.
   D. Periodontal treatment—including periodontal instrumentation of tooth surfaces—should be scheduled in consultation with the patient's urologist.

BLEEDING DISORDERS

1. **Bleeding Disorders.** Common inherited bleeding disorders are hemophilia A, hemophilia B, and von Willebrand disease. Not all coagulation disorders are inherited. Patients with severe liver disease may have prolonged bleeding times.
2. **Oral Manifestations of Bleeding Disorders**
   A. Petechiae—small red or purplish discolorations of the mucous membrane
   B. Ecchymoses—bruising of the mucous membrane
   C. Spontaneous gingival bleeding
   D. Prolonged massive bleeding during periodontal procedures
3. **Periodontal Treatment Considerations**
   A. Special measures need to be taken to prevent excessive bleeding during and after periodontal treatment. Bleeding can be a problem with such procedures as periodontal instrumentation of root surfaces, local anesthetic injection, or periodontal surgery. Bleeding usually will not be a problem with probing.
      1. Consultation with the physician is recommended prior to treatment.
      2. Laboratory assessment of blood coagulation times and platelets may be indicated.
   B. One of the most important considerations is that patient education needs to be provided at an early age. Meticulous plaque control is vital in preventing inflammation and disease initiation.

LEUKEMIA

1. **Leukemia.** Leukemia is cancer of blood-forming tissue such as bone marrow. Types of leukemia are grouped by the type of cell affected and by the rate of cell growth. Leukemia is either acute or chronic.
2. **Periodontal Considerations**
   A. Oral manifestations include oral ulcerations, palatal petechiae, and spontaneous gingival bleeding.
   B. The gingival tissues may have a boggy, fiery red appearance or may be light pink to white in color.
   C. Individuals with leukemia have increased susceptibility to infection.

ORGAN TRANSPLANTATION

1. **Organ Transplantation.** Organ transplantation is the surgical transfer of an organ (heart, kidney, liver) from one person to another. Unfortunately, the body has a tendency to treat the transplanted organ as a foreign substance and to destroy (reject) it.
2. **Periodontal Treatment Consideration**
   A. **Effects of Medications**
      1. Transplant patients take antirejection drugs called **immunosuppressants** and may be more prone to infection including periodontal disease. The most commonly used immunosuppressive drugs include cyclosporin, azathioprine, and corticosteroids.
         a. **Cyclosporin** may cause gingival overgrowth as well as severe liver damage, predisposing the patient to anemia and bleeding disorders.
         b. **Azathioprine** may cause anemia, placing the patient at risk for infection and bleeding.
         c. **Corticosteroid** use is associated with an increased potential for infection and an inability to adjust to stress, including the stress of dental procedures.
      2. Stress reduction techniques should be employed.
   B. Bacterial infections of a periodontal origin present a systemic health risk to organ transplant recipients.
      1. Patients should be counseled about the importance of meticulous self-care and frequent periodontal maintenance visits.
      2. Ideally, optimal oral health should be established prior to transplantation surgery.

CANCER

1. Patients undergoing radiation therapy or chemotherapy may experience a variety of oral problems that impact the periodontium including:
   A. Mucositis—inflammation of the mucous membrane. The most important factor in reducing mucositis is periodontal debridement of tooth surfaces and meticulous self-care prior to the start of radiation therapy or chemotherapy.
   B. Xerostomia—oral dryness. Xerostomia makes mastication and speech more difficult, increases the incidence of oral candidiasis, increased plaque accumulation, and dentinal sensitivity.
   C. Reduced healing capacity. Radiation therapy results in reduced blood flow to the irradiated tissues with a reduction in wound healing capacity. Radiation of the jaws can result in a complication known as **osteoradionecrosis** (ORN) that renders the oral bone less capable of resolving trauma or infection and can result in severe destruction of bone. The mandible is especially prone to ORN. The risk of ORN continues for the remainder of the patient's life. Tooth extraction or periodontal surgical procedures after radiation treatment involves a high risk of developing ORN.

   D. Bacterial, fungal, and viral infections of the oral cavity. Candidiasis is the most common fungal infection in cancer patients. Chlorhexidine rinses are helpful in controlling candidiasis.

2. Bacterial infections of a periodontal origin present a systemic health risk to patients with cancer. Patients should be counseled about the importance of meticulous self-care and frequent periodontal maintenance visits.

3. Dental health care providers will need to coordinate planned periodontal therapy with the patient's physician. Appropriate periodontal care can play a key role in improving the patient's quality of life after cancer therapy.

4. Management of these patients should include frequent periodontal maintenance visits, dietary counseling, and the use of 0.4% stannous fluoride or 1% sodium fluoride in custom trays. It is important that any periodontal therapy or tooth extractions be completed before the start of radiation therapy or chemotherapy.

CHAPTER SUMMARY STATEMENT

There is strong two-way relationship between systemic disease and periodontal problems.

- On one hand, systemic conditions can increase an individual's susceptibility to periodontal disease. The medications that are used to treat systemic diseases also can produce changes in the periodontium. Systemic conditions may require modification in periodontal therapy—including periodontal instrumentation of tooth surfaces—to ensure that periodontal therapy will not be harmful to the patient's systemic health.
- On the other hand, periodontal pathogens may have an adverse effect on an individual's systemic health. Dental health care providers should educate patients about the health implications of periodontal disease. Currently, the major goal of periodontal therapy is to prevent disease progression and preserve the teeth. In the future, a major goal of periodontal therapy may be to enhance general systemic health.

SECTION 3: FOCUS ON PATIENTS

CASE 1
Edward is a 53-year-old who is being seen for a diagnostic workup. The patient informs you that he has a new medical diagnosis of angina (chest pain). He explains that his chest pain occurs only when he is under stress. How should you proceed?

CASE 2
Louise is a new patient in the periodontal practice. At her first appointment, she is upset because she says that her physician insisted that she consult with a periodontist. She goes on to say that she is afraid of dental care and would just like to go home. She does not understand why her physician "made her come" to the periodontal office. How might you respond to Louise?

CASE 3
You receive a telephone call from a patient who requests information about an upcoming appointment. The patient informs you that he has just begun hemodialysis and wants to know if this will have any effect on his appointment. Your review of the patient's dental chart reveals that his periodontal diagnosis is moderate plaque-induced gingivitis and that the patient has an appointment with you for periodontal instrumentation. How might you respond to the patient?

References

1. Flier JS. An overview of insulin resistance. In: Moller DE, ed. *Insulin resistance.* New York: Wiley; 1993:1–8.
2. Drisko CL, Cochran DL, Blieden T, et al. Position paper: Sonic and ultrasonic scalers in periodontics. Research Science and Therapy Committee of the American Academy of Periodontology. *J Periodontol.* 2000;71:1792–1801.
3. Genco R, Chadda S. Periodontal disease as a predictor of cardiovascular disease in a Native American population [abstract 3158]. *J Dent Res.* 1997;76(Spec No):514–519.
4. Wu TJ, et al. Periodontal disease and risk of cerebrovascular disease: A prospective study of representative sample of U.S. adults. *Am J Epidermiol.* 1999;149(11 (Suppl S).
5. Shrout MK, Comer RW, Powell BJ, et al. Treating the pregnant dental patient: Four basic rules addressed. *J Am Dent Assoc.* 1992;123:75–80.
6. Dasanayake AP. Poor periodontal health of the pregnant woman as a risk factor for low birth weight. *Ann Periodontol.* 1998;3:206–212.
7. Offenbacher S, Jared HL, O'Reilly GP, et al. Potential pathogenic mechanisms of periodontitis associated pregnancy complications. *Ann Periodontol.* 1998;3:233–250.

SECTION 4: CHAPTER REVIEW QUESTIONS

1. The presence of bacteria in the bloodstream is:
   A. Bacteremia
   B. Bacterial endocarditis

2. All of the following are true about smoking, EXCEPT:
   A. Smokers do not respond as well to periodontal instrumentation as nonsmokers.
   B. Smokers are twice as likely to lose teeth as nonsmokers.
   C. After quitting, smokers are still more likely to have periodontal disease than non-smokers.
   D. Smokers tend to harbor higher levels of *Bacteroides forsythus* than nonsmokers.

3. Using a finger-stick test, the ideal glucose blood level is:
   A. Less than 60 mg/dL
   B. 80 to 120 mg/dL
   C. 180 to 300 mg/dL
   D. Greater than 300 mg/dL

4. Untreated periodontal disease may make it more difficult for individuals with diabetes to control their blood glucose levels.
   A. True
   B. False

5. All of the following medications can cause gingival hyperplasia, EXCEPT:
   A. Calcium channel blockers
   B. Phenytoin
   C. Cyclosporin
   D. Insulin

6. All of the following medications can cause excessive bleeding during periodontal treatment, EXCEPT:
   A. Aspirin
   B. Coumadin
   C. Blood thinners
   D. Phenytoin

7. Bacterial infections of a periodontal origin present a systemic health risk to individuals with which of the following systemic conditions?
   A. Cancer
   B. Diabetes
   C. Pregnant women
   D. All of the above

8. Systemic diseases can increase an individual's risk of periodontitis. Periodontitis, however, cannot have an adverse effect on an individual's overall health.
   A. Both these statements are true.
   B. Both these statements are false.
   C. The first sentence is true; the second sentence is false.
   D. The first sentence is false; the second sentence is true.

15 Evidence-Based Periodontal Care

**Learning
Objectives**

- Identify the three components of evidence-based decision making.
- Summarize the five elements in the framework of the evidence-based decision making process.
- Formulate questions using the PICO process.
- Compare and contrast the different levels of evidence.
- Appraise clinical evidence and determine its usefulness in clinical practice.
- Describe mechanisms for applying evidence into practice.
- Evaluate your ability to make an evidence-based decision about periodontal care.
- Discuss ethical issues related to evidence-based decision making.
- Define skills needed to implement evidence-based decision making.

KEY TERMS

Evidence-based dental care
Evidence-based decision making
Clinical expertise
PICO process
MEDLINE
Cochrane Collaboration

PubMed
Clinical practice guidelines
Peer-reviewed
Systematic review
Randomized controlled trials
Experimental group

Control group
Cohort study
Case-controlled study
Case series or report
Animal study
In vitro studies
Clinically relevant

SECTION 1: WHAT IS EVIDENCE-BASED PERIODONTAL CARE?

1. Evidence-based dental care (EBDC) is an approach to periodontal care in which dental professionals and patients make decisions about periodontal care based on the best available information. Providing evidence-based dental care requires that dental hygienists question and think about what they are doing and be open to learning new techniques.

Box 15-1

Concepts of Evidence-Based Care

- The primary aim of the evidence-based approach to periodontal care is to encourage dental health care providers (i) to look for and make sense of scientific evidence about best treatment practices, clinical techniques, equipment, and products and (ii) to apply the evidence to provide the best possible periodontal care.[1]
- In evidence-based dental care, evidence is not just used to help the clinician make good decisions about patient care. Equally important is providing scientific evidence about treatments, drugs, and devices to patients so that they can make more informed decisions about which periodontal care is best for them.

2. **Why Do We Need Evidence-Based Dental Care?** Two forces are changing dental health care. First, information about new techniques, tests, procedures, and products for periodontal care is emerging at an astonishing rate. Second, patients are taking an active role in decision making about periodontal treatment.
   A. Direct Access to Rapidly Emerging Clinical Research Information
      1. **Explosion of Information.** Every year, in each dental specialty, over 500 reports on clinical trials are published in more than 50 separate dental journals. This amounts to nearly 10 journal articles per week for 52 weeks per year and those numbers are increasing by 10% to 20% per year.[2]
      2. **Direct Access to Information**
         a. In the past, dental health care providers relied on what they learned in school and the advice of recognized experts to determine how to provide care. Patients had little or no input into this process. Knowledge of new or cutting edge research was limited to a few practitioners with access to an educational or health care institution.
         b. Today, with the advent of the Internet, clinicians have access to the results of federally funded clinical trials on treatment methods, equipment, and materials. PubMed, a gateway to more than 10 million research citations, can be accessed by anyone for free.
         c. *Practicing dental hygienists are expected to remain current with new techniques, devices, and materials that will result in improvements in periodontal care.* Dental hygienists in private practice cannot continue to use the same treatments and techniques learned in dental hygiene school year after year. The best practice 2 years ago may not represent the highest standard of care today.
   B. Active Patient Role in Decision-Making
      1. Today's patient expects to be a partner in the decision making process about his or her own periodontal care. Patients arrive at the dental office with information downloaded from the Internet.
      2. Before the widespread use of information technology, patients depended on the expertise of a health care provider for advice, and in most cases accepted that advice without question.

PATIENT-CENTERED CARE

1. It is the dental hygienist's responsibility to understand the evidence and its implications for periodontal treatment. Ultimately, however, it will be the patient who chooses which therapy he or she prefers.
2. In helping a patient decide which treatment is right for him or her, there are several elements that should be discussed, including:
    A. The evidence about a particular treatment option
    B. The treatment of choice based on the evidence
    C. All possible treatment alternatives
    D. The risks of no treatment at all
3. In selecting the treatment option that is right for them, patients frequently have concerns such as:
    A. Cost. Patients usually are concerned about what a treatment will cost. In addition, patients decide if the treatment has benefits that they perceive as being worth the cost.
    B. Pain. Assurances about pain control and management help lessen these concerns.
    C. Time lost from work. Different jobs and work environments have varying levels of flexibility in allowing employees time off for health-related matters.
    D. Impact on family. Caregivers of young children or elderly family members may feel that they do not have the time to devote to periodontal treatment. Individuals with chronic health problems may believe that periodontal care is no longer a priority.

EVIDENCE-BASED DECISION MAKING

Dental hygienists need to access and appraise the research and then communicate the findings to their patients so they can partner in the decision making process. To help provide a framework for sorting through this process, a tool called evidence-based decision making has been developed.

1. The recognized definition of **evidence-based decision-making** is, "the integration of best research evidence with clinical experience and patient values."[2] The goals of evidence-based decision making are outlined in Box 15-2.
2. Evidence-based dental care involves the combination of three elements: (i) the best research evidence, (ii) clinical experience of the dental professional, and (iii) patient values and preferences regarding treatment.
    A. Failing to include all three of these elements would be like making a periodontal diagnosis based only on bleeding without considering attachment loss or having current radiographs. The value of each is limited without putting all three into context.
    B. According to the father of evidence-based medicine, David Sackett, MD, "When these three elements are integrated, clinicians and patients form a diagnostic and therapeutic alliance which optimizes clinical outcomes and quality of life."[2]

THREE ELEMENTS OF EVIDENCE-BASED DECISION MAKING

1. Evidence
    A. The cornerstone of evidence-based decision making is patient-centered clinical research.[2]
    B. The types of periodontal care options evaluated in patient centered clinical research are generally related to:
        1. The accuracy or precision of diagnostic tests.[2] An example of this in periodontal care is the decision whether to pursue supplemental diagnostic tests, such as the DNA probe analysis discussed in Chapter 12.

   2. The ability of diagnostic techniques to predict future disease.[2] An example of this is whether the presence of bleeding on probing or additional attachment loss can be used to predict the future disease.

   3. The effectiveness and safety of therapeutic or preventive regimens.[2] An example of this is daily use of an oral irrigation device. Is this device effective and safe when used at home by the patient on a daily basis?

2. **Clinical Expertise.** Clinical expertise is the ability of a clinician to grow in skill and knowledge through experience.

   A. Ideally, a clinician uses his or her clinical experiences in making better treatment decisions.

   B. The limitation is that not all individuals are able to learn and grow from experience. To acquire practical wisdom the clinician needs to learn how to be reflective and analyze his or her own performance.

3. **Patient Values**

   A. The glue that holds the evidence-based decision together is the incorporation of patient values.

   B. If due consideration is not given to the individual preferences and concerns that the patient expresses, the likelihood of the patient fully accepting the clinician's recommendation is diminished.

   C. Acknowledging patient values helps build trust, enhance dialogue, and improve compliance and satisfaction.

   D. Incorporating patient values into the decision making process requires good listening skills and empathy. Aspects to consider include:

   1. Visualizing the experience through the patient's eyes (putting yourself in the patient's position). This includes eliciting a patient's past experiences, feelings, fears, and expectations.[3]

   2. Understanding the patient as a person. This means understanding the patient's attitude toward treatment and the influence of family, employment, socioeconomic factors, and culture on his values and expectations.[3]

Box 15-2

Goals of Evidence-Based Decision Making for Periodontal Care

1. Less emphasis on clinical experience for periodontal care planning.
2. More emphasis on valid scientific findings for periodontal care planning.
3. Improved treatment decisions based on evidence.
4. Minimized potential harm to the patient.
5. Improved periodontal treatment outcomes.

SECTION 2: THE PROCESS OF EVIDENCE-BASED DECISION MAKING

Using an evidenced-based approach to periodontal care involves a process. The framework for this process involves five basic steps.[4–6] These five steps are summarized in Box 15-3.

Box 15-3

Five Basic Steps in Evidence-Based Dental Care

1. Ask a clear and focused question
2. Search for the best evidence
3. Appraise the evidence
4. Act on the evidence
5. Evaluate your performance

Box 15-4

The PICO Process

P = Patient or Problem
I = Intervention
C = Comparison
O = Outcome

STEP 1: ASK A CLEAR AND FOCUSED QUESTION

In order to find the best information to help patients, it is fundamental to learn how to ask the right questions. This is more challenging than it seems. It involves converting problems into answerable questions.

1. **Use Four Components to Structure the Question.** The structure for asking a clear and focused question entails four critical components, known as the PICO process.[4,5] Box 15-4 highlights the elements of the PICO process. Utilization of the PICO process involves the combination of four separate components to form an answerable question.
    A. P stands for the patient or problem
       1. An example of the P component might be: *A periodontal maintenance patient with bleeding and gingivitis.*
       2. The patient's problem is narrowed by influencing characteristics such as disease or health status, age, race, gender, previous conditions, past, and current medications.

    B. I stands for the intervention
- **1.** An intervention is a specific diagnostic test, treatment, adjunctive therapy, medication, product, or clinical procedure.
- **2.** An example of an intervention being questioned is: *brushing and daily home irrigation.*

    C. C stands for the comparison
- **1.** Identifies the specific alternative therapy or device that you wish to compare to the main intervention.
- **2.** An example of the C segment of the question is: *compared to brushing and flossing.*

    D. O stands for outcome
- **1.** Identifies the measurable outcome you plan to accomplish, improve, or influence.
- **2.** An example of the O segment of the question is: *reduce gingivitis and bleeding within four weeks.*

2. Formulate the Question. Once each of the PICO components has been determined, the clinician combines them into an answerable question. Using the above examples, the question would read: *For a periodontal maintenance patient with bleeding and gingivitis, will brushing and daily home irrigation OR brushing and flossing provide a better reduction in bleeding and gingivitis within four weeks?*

STEP 2: FIND GOOD EVIDENCE

A critical component of evidence-based care is an understanding of what constitutes quality research. It is of primary importance to be able to locate the best sources of evidence.

1. Sources of Evidence. There are hundreds of articles related to dental hygiene care published every month. Although it is impossible to review everything, it is important to know how to locate the articles with the most relevance for periodontal care. There are several sources of evidence available, each with different merit.

    A. Computerized Biomedical Databases. Computerized databases have made it easy to distribute and access information.
- **1.** MEDLINE is the English-language database for biomedical information. MEDLINE can be accessed free of charge through several gateways. One example is **PubMed**, a gateway hosted by the National Library of Medicine (NLM) at **http://www.nlm.nih.gov**
- **2.** The **Cochrane Collaboration** (**http://www.cochrane.org**) prepares, maintains, and disseminates comprehensive and systematic reviews of the effects of health care, including medical and dental care.

    B. Clinical Practice Guidelines. In recent years, professional organizations have begun developing documents called Clinical Practice Guidelines to assist practitioners with evidence-based decision making.
- **1. Clinical Practice Guidelines** are user-friendly statements that bring together the best scientific evidence and other knowledge necessary to assist clinicians and patients in arriving at decisions on appropriate periodontal care.[2]
  - **a.** Well-written clinical practice guidelines do not tell the clinician which decision to make, instead the statement (i) identifies the range of potential care options for a specific health problem, (ii) provides evidence that the clinician can combine with his or her own clinical judgment and experience, and (iii) assists the clinician in educating the patient about treatment options.
  - **b.** The three elements of evidence, clinical judgment, and patient preferences help the clinician and patient to make an informed recommendation regarding periodontal care.

2. Clinical practice guidelines can assist clinicians in various areas.
   a. Assist clinicians in learning about the newest research findings
   b. Combine the results of many studies into a convenient, usable format
   c. Identify therapies with the strongest evidence and most predictable outcome
   d. Decrease variations in treatment recommendations among practitioners
3. Professional associations are a good resource for locating the most relevant practice guidelines. It is the responsibility of the individual practitioner to keep current with practice guidelines.
C. Scientific journals
   1. Published by professional associations but sometimes sponsored by commercial underwriting.
   2. Peer-reviewed (also called refereed) by a panel of experts with no financial ties to the journal. **Peer-reviewed** journals use a panel of experts to review research articles for study design, statistics, and conclusions.
   3. Viewed as high quality; good sources for randomized clinical trials or systematic reviews.
   4. Access to journals may require travel to dental libraries.

2. **Levels of Evidence.** The importance or merit of a research study usually is evaluated through its design. Systematic reviews and randomized controlled trials represent the best levels of evidence. Case reports and expert opinion are the lowest levels of evidence. Figure 15-1 illustrates the levels of evidence.

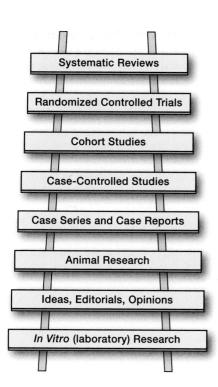

Figure 15-1. Levels of Evidence. The levels of evidence are represented as a ladder of evidence in this drawing. Each level of evidence can be thought of as rungs on a ladder. The higher the rung, the better the level of evidence.

A. A systematic review—the highest level of evidence—provides a summary of individual research studies that have investigated the same phenomenon or question in order to obtain a reliable overview of a problem. Findings from systematic reviews may be used for decision making about the provision of care.

   1. This type of review serves as a mechanism for combining the results of smaller studies that may have produced unclear or conflicting results into useful information.

   2. A systematic review provides better insight into effectiveness of the intervention—such as a specific diagnostic test, treatment, adjunctive therapy, medication, product, or procedure—and its merit for use in clinical practice.[9]

   3. A systematic review is *not* the same as a literature or narrative review. Literature or narrative reviews generally do not follow a rigorous methodology, lack the ability to be reproduced, and the conclusion reached cannot be verified.

B. Randomized controlled trials (RCT) are studies in which subjects are randomly assigned to either an experimental or control group.

   1. The experimental group receives the new intervention, such as a new diagnostic test or treatment. The control group receives the standard intervention. The two groups are followed for a period of time to determine if there are differences between the results.

   2. The design of the RCT helps minimize bias and determine cause and effect relationships.

C. A cohort study involves identifying two groups (cohorts) of subjects.

   1. The individuals in one group have a certain condition or received a particular treatment or both. The individuals in the other group do not have the condition and/or did not receive a particular treatment. The two groups are followed over a period of time to determine if there are differences in the outcomes.

   2. Cohort studies are limited because randomization is not possible. Groups may differ in the variables not under study, such as socioeconomic status, and that may affect the outcome. There may be loss of subjects over time.

D. A case-controlled study looks back in time (retrospective) at people who already have a certain condition and investigates potential risk factors associated with the disease. This type of study is a method of study for very rare disorders or those with long lag times between exposure and outcome.[8,9]

   1. Case-controlled studies can be less reliable in outcome because a statistical relationship shown between the disease condition and a risk factor does not mean that risk factor is the cause of the disease condition.

   2. Another problem with this type of study is that it relies on the memories of subjects or the documentation in a medical history.

   3. Case-controlled studies can be done quickly and inexpensively via medical history review.

E. Case series and case reports consist of collections of reports on the treatment of individual patients or reports on a single patient.[8,9]

   1. These studies are observational and may describe a rare disease, new intervention, or adverse effects. There is no control group in this type of study for comparison of outcomes.

   2. The data collected in this type of study is gathered in an uncontrolled manner. Therefore, there is no statistical validity and the results cannot be generalized to the larger population.

F. **Animal studies** are research studies conducted on animals.
   1. This type of study usually is conducted in the early phases of the development of an intervention to determine safety.
   2. Results from animal studies cannot be generalized to the human population.
G. **Ideas, editorials**, or **opinions** are *not* scientific studies.
   1. Many interventions that are used in dentistry have not been tested.
   2. Good ideas and opinions can open new avenues for clinical care. However, these ideas and opinions have not been validated in the literature and remain simply opinion.
H. **In-vitro studies** are conducted in the laboratory setting. Humans are not used.
   1. For example, this type of study might be used to determine the plaque removal efficacy of a toothbrush via a mechanical brushing machine.
   2. The results from laboratory studies cannot be generalized to the human population.

STEP 3: REVIEW AND CRITICALLY APPRAISE THE EVIDENCE

1. Good science depends on controls. A research study only provides useful information to periodontal care, if that study is designed and executed correctly.
   A. Very few studies, particularly when dealing with human subjects, can control all the variables in the study 100%. Hence most scientific studies have some flaws.
   B. Good investigators disclose the limitations of their studies and inherent biases or flaws, generally in the discussion section of the study. The process of critical appraisal helps the clinician sort out the relevant or valid papers from those of poor quality.
2. When evaluating a study, three key questions need to be asked about how the study was performed and its application to a clinical situation.[6]
   A. *Are the results of the study valid or believable?* Appraisal at this stage involves reviewing the study design and methodology.
   B. *What are the results?* The results section of a study is the portion of an article where the hard (numerical) data are reported. The types of statistical tests used to determine the data should be clearly explained.
   C. *Will the results help me in caring for my patients?* The discussion section of a study should provide a precise and clearly stated conclusion and a synopsis of how the results apply to clinical practice. A satisfactory explanation of how the results match the final conclusions should be described in-depth. An analysis of the conclusion should include a discussion about the following.
      1. Generalization of the results to the general population. Not all results can be generalized to the general population as a whole, and the authors should provide an explanation of this phenomenon.
      2. Consistency of results. Discrepancies with previously published studies should be explained, including the factors contributing to the different results and what the difference might mean.
      3. Applicability to clinical practice. Dental hygienists need to evaluate whether the result is **clinically relevant** to periodontal care. That is, if the finding is important enough to affect a treatment decision (to cause the clinician to incorporate it in the patient's treatment). Consideration might be given to whether the results are new or groundbreaking or whether they provide building blocks to enhance practice. From the patient perspective, consideration might be given to whether the intervention improves the welfare or compliance of the patient or reduce treatment or treatment costs.

STEP 4: APPLY THE EVIDENCE

1. It is important to realize that even good evidence rarely provides absolutes about a given therapy.
2. Once the evidence has been carefully evaluated, it is up to the dental hygienist, using experience and clinical judgment, to decide if the evidence is appropriate for each individual patient situation. Many research studies exclude individuals with complex medical problems or those taking some regular medications.

STEP 5: EVALUATE YOUR PERFORMANCE

The final step in evidence-based decision making is self-evaluation. The dental hygienist should ask these key questions about how he or she provides care.

1. *Is what I am doing right?*
   A. How sure am I that what I do is right?
      1. Do I know where to access systematic reviews?
      2. Do I attend continuing education courses?
      3. Do I keep up with journal reading?
      4. Am I active in my professional association?
   B. How well developed is my clinical judgment? Am I able to combine evidence and clinical experience to make a good decision?
   C. Do I listen to my patients?
      1. Do I provide them with enough information and direction to make a good decision?
      2. Do I respect their autonomy and choices?
2. *What do I need to stop doing?*
   A. Am I holding on to what I do because "that's what I learned in school" even though it was several years ago?
   B. Is what I am doing making the best use of office and patient resources, both financial and human?
3. *What do I need to keep doing but change how I do it?*
   A. Are there better, more efficient or cost-effective tools available such as specific diagnostic tests, treatments, adjunctive therapies, medications, products, or procedures than what I am currently using?
   B. Do I have the appropriate amount of time scheduled or equipment provided for the highest level of patient care?

CHAPTER SUMMARY STATEMENT

Evidence-based dental care is an approach to periodontal care in which dental professionals and patients make decisions about care based on the best available information. The evidence-based decision-making process requires the integration of best clinical research, practitioner expertise, and patient values. Providing evidence-based dental care requires that dental hygienists question and think about what they are doing and be open to learning new techniques. Hygienists must spend the time to search and assess the research literature. Acquiring the skills to find high levels of evidence and being willing to listen to patients and incorporate their values is essential to this process. By using an evidence-based approach to periodontal care, hygienists can meet the challenges of continuing to provide quality care in a rapidly changing field of dental health care.

SECTION 3: FOCUS ON PATIENTS

CASE 1

You have just started working in a new office and find that the other dental hygienist in the practice, Debbie, "doesn't believe" in using the ultrasonic equipment. Debbie states she has been practicing for 20 years, that is what she learned in school, and she knows what she sees: good results with hand scaling. It is a little intimidating since you have less experience (only 5 years) but have routinely used ultrasonic instruments and mention to her "that is what you learned in school." For a while you pass it off as no big deal, a difference of opinions, but because Debbie didn't use the ultrasonic equipment, the equipment in the office is old and does not function at the level it should. You speak to your employer about getting a new machine, but he said, "Debbie doesn't use it, why do you?"

1. How would you answer your employer?
2. What types of evidence would you try to locate to justify your position?
3. Where would you search?
4. What types of key words would you use?
5. How would you manage your conflict with Debbie?

CASE 2

Mr. Fred Jones is a long-standing patient in your practice. He had periodontal surgery 7 years ago and is sporadic about his maintenance visits. His last visit was over 2 years ago. The initial examination shows calculus and stain, minimal bleeding, and generalized 5- to 6-mm probing depth including some furcation areas. You explain to Mr. Jones that he will need to return for additional treatment (periodontal debridement). He tells you that, "he knew you were going to say that" and then brings out an article from a consumer health magazine that his wife showed to him. The article describes a new product that you have never heard of and states that this technique is supposed to be a substitute for scaling and root planing. "Can I have that treatment?" he asks.

1. What steps would you take to learn about the product in Mr. Jones' article?
2. What type of merit does the magazine have?
3. What type of information would you look for in the article?
4. What would you say to Mr. Jones regarding this article?

CASE 3

Your patient, Ms. Karen Jones, is a healthy, nonsmoking 30-year-old. Her only medication is birth control pills of 5 years' duration, and a daily multivitamin. She has been coming in for regular maintenance every 6 months. She brushes two times per day and flosses when she remembers, perhaps once per week and she states she finds the procedure difficult. The examination shows some 4-mm probing depths and significant bleeding. As you have done several times in the past, you show the patient how to use the manual brush and floss and really "lay it on the line" about improving oral health and warn her she will need to come in more frequently if her habits do not improve. The patient states that "she tries" and is visibly upset when she leaves office. While you hate to see her upset, you hope she finally got the message.

About a month after her visit, you get a message that Karen Jones would like you call her. When you reach Karen, she tells you she has been "researching" her gum problem, and she has found out she has several alternatives to a manual toothbrush and floss. Karen reports she has looked on the Internet, and talked to a relative who is also a dental hygienist. She has learned about automatic toothbrushes, automatic flossing devices, and oral irrigators, and how they could help her. In fact, she has purchased one of everything, and feels her mouth is improving. Not only that, the power-flossing device makes the task so much easier. "Why didn't you tell me about this?" she demands. "I am unhappy, and going to have my records transferred elsewhere!"

1. What are some of the reasons the dental hygienist may have for not telling Karen about these products?
2. Ethically, is not telling a patient about all self-care products that have evidence to support their use the same as not telling a patient about all available professional treatment options? Why or why not?
3. What steps could the dental hygienist take to improve her knowledge on self-care products?

CASE 4

You have just joined a new, large group dental practice with 10 office settings. Because of your experience and previous work with a periodontal practice, you have been assigned to serve on the practice's product review committee. Every quarter, the committee meets with different sales representatives who want the dental practice to either utilize or dispense their products. When you see the agenda for the upcoming meeting, you see that all the representatives that day will be from toothbrush companies. You find out you will be choosing the brush that all 10 offices will recommend for the next year. Before you know it, your co-workers are lobbying you to pick the brush that they like—and you have not even heard the sales presentations yet.

1. What steps can you take prior to the meeting to help you make a good decision for the practice?
2. What types of questions should you ask the sales consultants?
3. What types of questions, if any, should you ask your colleagues?
4. What benefit might you get from asking patients about their preferences?
5. What type of evidence would you like to see for each product?
6. How will you support your decision to your colleagues?

References

1. Richards D, Lawrence A. Evidence based dentistry. *Br Dent J.* 1995;179:270–273.
2. Sackett D, Strauss S, Richardson W, et al. *Evidence-Based Medicine: How to Practice and Teach EBM.* New York: Churchill Livingstone; 2000.
3. Stevenson AC. Compassion and patient-centered care. *Aust Fam Physician* 2002;31:1103–1106.
4. Practicing EBD. Center for Evidence-Based Dentistry. Available at: www.cebd.org Last accessed May 10, 2005.
5. Forrest JL, Miller SA. Evidence-based decision making in action. Part 1: Finding the best clinical evidence. *J Contemp Dent Pract.* 2002;3:10–26.
6. Forrest JL, Miller SA. Evidence-based decision making in action. Part 2: Evaluating and applying the clinical evidence. *J Contemp Dent Pract.* 2003;1:42–52.
7. Davies HTO, Crombie IK. What is a systematic review. May 2003. Available at: www.evidence-based-medicine.co.uk Last accessed May 10, 2005.
8. Sutherland SE. Evidence-based dentistry: Part IV: Research design and levels of evidence. *J Can Dent Assoc* 2001;67:375–378.
9. Glossary of evidence-based terms. *J Evid Base Dent Pract.* 2004;4:331–335.

SECTION 4: CHAPTER REVIEW QUESTIONS

1. Identify the three key components of the evidence-based decision making process and give a brief explanation and example of each.

2. Name the five processes involved in arriving at an evidence-based decision and give an example of what you would do for each component.

3. Develop an answerable question relevant to patient care using the PICO process.

4. Which type of evidence has the most clinical relevance? Why?

5. What sources would you use to find the best evidence?

6. What elements of a study would you review in determining the validity of study results?

7. What are Clinical Practice Guidelines and where would you look for them?

8. What are some of the reasons practitioners fail to apply evidence?

9. What questions would you ask to evaluate your performance in evidence-based decision making?

10. Is there a Code of Ethics for dental hygienists? Where would you find it?

16 Decision Making During Treatment Planning

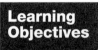

Learning Objectives

- List the three fundamental diagnostic questions used in assigning a periodontal diagnosis.
- Explain how to arrive at appropriate answers to each of the fundamental diagnostic questions.
- List the phases of treatment.
- Define the term periodontal disease site.
- Define the term informed consent.
- Describe the scope of information that should be provided to the patient.

KEY TERMS

Clinical decision-making process
Overt signs of inflammation
Hidden signs of inflammation
Signs of periodontal disease
Symptoms of periodontal disease
Silent disease

Natural level of gingival attachment
Attachment loss
Localized periodontal disease
Generalized periodontal disease
Disease sites
Master treatment plan

Assessment and preliminary therapy phase
Nonsurgical periodontal therapy phase
Surgical therapy phase
Restorative phase
Periodontal maintenance phase
Informed consent

SECTION 1: DECISIONS RELATED TO ASSIGNING A PERIODONTAL DIAGNOSIS

OVERVIEW OF THE DECISION-MAKING PROCESS FOR PERIODONTAL CARE

1. **Clinical decision making** and treatment planning is the process whereby the dentist and dental hygienist use the information gathered during the clinical periodontal assessment to identify treatment strategies that meet the individual needs of the patient.
    A. It is the dentist's legal responsibility to arrive at a periodontal diagnosis; however, it is both the dentist's and the dental hygienist's responsibilities to plan the nonsurgical therapy.
    B. In an efficient dental practice, the entire team must be familiar with the diagnostic decision making process and the fundamental principles for planning nonsurgical periodontal therapy.
2. **Patient's Role in Decision Making**
    A. An equally important component of the treatment planning process is the patient's involvement in the decision making process.
    B. Dental health care providers have an obligation to encourage patients to participate fully in treatment decisions and goals.
3. **Decision Making Is an Ongoing Process**
    A. Clinical decision making and treatment planning is an ongoing process because patients are followed for years or decades in most dental practices.
    B. The periodontium consists of dynamic tissues and an individual's periodontal care needs may change over time.
    C. The dental team must be aware that a perfectly sensible periodontal diagnosis and plan for therapy at one point in time may require modification at a later date.
4. **Assigning a Periodontal Diagnosis**
    A. The first step in treatment planning is assigning a correct periodontal diagnosis.
        1. *Determination of a periodontal diagnosis can be simplified by asking and answering three fundamental clinical questions in a systematic manner* (**Figure 16-1**)
        2. These three fundamental questions are used to guide the dental team through the diagnostic process. Many decisions including assigning a periodontal diagnosis and planning nonsurgical therapy revolve around the answers to these important questions.

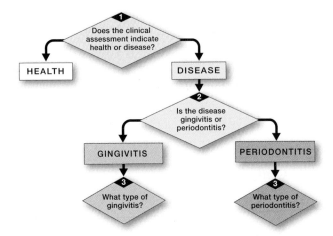

Figure 16-1. Decision Tree. A decision tree using three fundamental questions for determining an initial periodontal diagnosis.

ASSIGNING A PERIODONTAL DIAGNOSIS: FUNDAMENTAL DIAGNOSTIC QUESTIONS

1. **The First Basic Diagnostic Question:** *"Does the clinical assessment indicate health or disease in the periodontium?"*
    A. The answer to the first question should be based on the signs of inflammation that are noted and recorded during the clinical assessment.
        1. The dental team should be familiar with the difference between the signs of a disease and the symptoms of a disease.
            a. **Signs of periodontal disease** are the features of a disease that can be observed or are measurable by the clinician. Examples include gingival erythema (redness), edema, bleeding, loss of attachment, mobility, and loss of alveolar bone support.
            b. **Symptoms of periodontal disease** are features of a disease that are noted by the patient.
                1. Examples of symptoms include pain, itching gums, blood on the bed pillow, and a bad taste in the mouth.
                2. Because periodontitis does not cause symptoms in many patients, some clinicians refer to periodontitis as a **silent disease**.
                3. Calling periodontitis a silent disease underscores the fact that *periodontitis can exist in patients who are totally unaware of its presence.*
        2. Signs of inflammation include both **overt signs** of inflammation (readily visible) and **hidden signs** of inflammation (not readily visible) (Table 16-1).
            a. Examples of overt signs of inflammation are changes in the color, contour, and consistency of the gingival tissue.
            b. Examples of hidden signs of inflammation are alveolar bone loss, bleeding on probing, and purulence or exudate.

Table 16-1. Signs of Inflammation in the Periodontium

Overt (Readily Visible) Signs	Hidden Signs
Color change in the gingiva	Bone loss
Contour changes in the gingiva	Purulence (exudates)
Change in consistency in the gingiva	Bleeding on probing

    B. Health
        1. If the clinical periodontal assessment reveals no signs of inflammation in the periodontium, then the answer to Question #1 is health.
        2. This means that inflammatory disease is not present and that the patient is probably not in need of further diagnostic decisions.
    C. Disease
        1. If the clinical periodontal assessment reveals either overt or hidden signs of inflammation in the periodontium, then the answer to Question #1 is, of course, disease.
        2. This means that some type of inflammatory disease is present and that further diagnostic decisions will need to be made.
    D. Additional Diagnostic Measures. Even in the absence of inflammatory disease in the periodontium, some patients will require additional diagnostic measures. For example, a patient with no inflammation but with severe gingival recession accompanied by cervical abrasion of the teeth may need to be evaluated for possible use of traumatic toothbrushing techniques.

2. **The Second Basic Diagnostic Question:** *"If the clinical assessment indicates disease, is the disease gingivitis or is it periodontitis?"*

A. Attachment Loss. The answer to this question is based on clinical evidence of attachment loss as determined from the clinical findings recorded during the clinical assessment. The **natural level of the gingival attachment** to the tooth is slightly coronal to the cementoenamel junction (CEJ). **Attachment loss** refers to migration of the attachment apparatus apical to (below) the level of the CEJ (**Fig. 16-2**).

1. Gingivitis. If the clinical assessment reveals no attachment loss in the presence of inflammation, then the answer to Question #2 is gingivitis.

2. Periodontitis. If the clinical assessment revealed attachment loss in the presence of inflammation, then the answer to Question #2 is periodontitis.

B. It is important for the dental team to use dental radiographs during the clinical assessment.

1. In most patients with moderate to severe periodontitis, alveolar bone loss will be evident on the radiographs.

2. Even before radiographic changes occur, however, attachment loss will be detectable to the alert clinician. The members of the dental team must be able to detect periodontitis long before there is obvious radiographic evidence of alveolar bone loss.

3. **The Third Basic Diagnostic Question:** *"If the patient has gingivitis, what type of gingivitis?"* or *"If the patient has periodontitis, what type of periodontitis?"*

A. The classification of types of gingival disease and the types of periodontitis was discussed in Chapters 9 through 11.

B. The dentist will use these disease classifications to assign a specific periodontal diagnosis based on the clinical features outlined in those chapters.

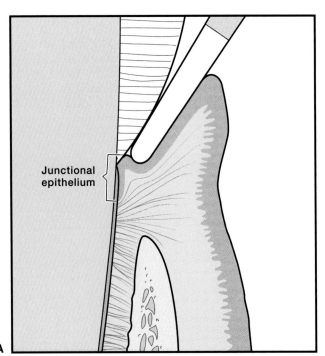
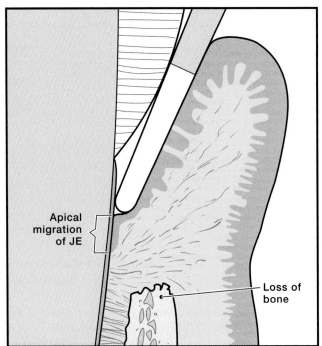

Figure 16-2. Level of Attachment. A: Natural Level of Attachment. The natural level of the junctional epithelium is *slightly coronal* to the cementoenamel junction (CEJ). Note that the probe tip does not reach the CEJ if the attachment is at its natural level. B: Attachment Loss. In attachment loss, the junctional epithelium is *apical* to the level of the CEJ. Note that the probe tip extends beyond the CEJ if the attachment apparatus has migrated apically.

DOCUMENTING THE PERIODONTAL DIAGNOSIS

1. Documenting the periodontal diagnosis is a critical skill for the dental team, and adhering to a standard format for such documentation is helpful. The following are some guidelines for documenting periodontal diagnoses.
   A. Use the correct diagnostic term as outlined in the classification scheme, such as chronic periodontitis or aggressive periodontitis.
   B. Include descriptive modifiers such as slight (mild), moderate, or severe to describe the *severity* of the disease. **Table 16-2** shows how the terms slight, moderate, and severe should be used as part of documentation of a periodontal diagnosis. The term *clinical attachment loss* (CAL) is used to underscore that these measurements are clinical measurements and may not coincide exactly with histologic measurements.
   C. Include descriptive modifiers such as **localized** or **generalized** to describe the *extent* of the disease.
      1. **Table 16-2** shows how the terms localized and generalized should be used as part of documentation of the extent of periodontal disease. **Disease sites** are the individual teeth or specific surfaces of a tooth that are experiencing periodontal destruction.
      2. Examples of appropriate periodontal diagnoses might be *generalized moderate chronic periodontitis* or *localized severe aggressive periodontitis.*

Table 16-2. Use of Modifiers in Documenting Disease Severity and Extent

	Descriptive Modifier	Definition
Disease Severity	Slight	1 to 2 mm clinical attachment loss
	Moderate	3 to 4 mm clinical attachment loss
	Severe	5 mm or more of clinical attachment loss
Disease Extent	Localized	30% or less of the sites in the mouth are involved
	Generalized	More than 30% of the sites in the mouth are involved

2. Using the Case Type System for Periodontal Patients
   A. Case Types. Although the case type system is somewhat limited in value, it has been standard practice in the United States to assign a periodontal case type to all periodontal patients. These case types are sometimes used in insurance reporting and in communication with third-party payers. Assigning a periodontal case type is included in the initial decision making process in most dental offices and is included here for additional information.
      1. Case Type I. Patients with gingivitis only.
      2. Case Type II. Patients with slight (mild) periodontitis.
      3. Case Type III. Patients with moderate periodontitis.
      4. Case Type IV. Patients with severe periodontitis.
   B. The value of the case type system is very limited because the case type alone does not specify the precise periodontal disease classification. For example, a Case Type III patient could be a patient with chronic periodontitis or a patient with aggressive periodontitis. A designation of Case Type III only signifies that the disease is of moderate severity.
   C. *It is important for all members of the dental team to use the written periodontal diagnosis (e.g., generalized moderate chronic periodontitis) when describing the periodontal status of a patient and to use the case type only as a supplemental description.*

SECTION 2: DECISIONS RELATED TO TREATMENT SEQUENCING

THE PERIODONTAL MASTER TREATMENT PLAN

1. The **master treatment plan** is a sequential outline of the measures to be carried out by the dentist, the dental hygienist, and the patient to eliminate disease and restore a healthy periodontal environment.
   A. The master treatment plan is used to coordinate and sequence all treatment and educational measures and to estimate the length of time required for comprehensive treatment.
   B. Although some of the treatment included in the master treatment plan does not involve the dental hygienist, it is important that the hygienist understand how all phases of treatment contribute to the goal of restoring a healthy periodontal environment.
2. **Patient Consent for Treatment.** The patient is a critical player in any plan involving periodontal therapy, and communications with the patient are vital as the treatment plan is developed.
3. **Phases of Periodontal Treatment.** The phases of treatment and treatment measures are summarized in **Table 16-3**.

Table 16-3. Five Phases of Periodontal Master Treatment Plan

Phase	Measures and Procedures
Assessment phase and preliminary therapy	Assessment data collection Treatment of emergency conditions Medical care of systemic conditions Extraction of hopeless teeth
Nonsurgical periodontal therapy (Phase I)	Self-care education Nutritional counseling Smoking cessation counseling Periodontal debridement (instrumentation) Antimicrobial therapy Correction of local risk factors Fluoride therapy Caries control and temporary restorations Occlusal therapy Minor orthodontic treatment Evaluation of Phase I therapy
Surgical therapy (Phase II)	Periodontal surgery Endodontic surgery Dental implant placement
Restorative therapy (Phase III)	Dental restorations Fixed and removable prostheses Re-evaluation of overall response to treatment
Phase IV: Periodontal maintenance (Phase IV)	Ongoing care at specified intervals

PHASES OF TREATMENT

1. **Assessment and Preliminary Therapy**
   A. The **assessment and preliminary therapy phase** includes assessment data collection and care for immediate treatment needs such as emergency care and extractions. Clinical periodontal assessment is discussed in Chapter 12.
   B. This stage of care also has been referred to as emergency therapy.
2. **Nonsurgical Periodontal Therapy**
   A. The **nonsurgical periodontal therapy phase** of treatment includes all the *nonsurgical* measures used to help control gingivitis and periodontitis. This phase includes dental hygiene care and educational measures.
   B. This stage of care also is called *Phase I therapy*, *bacterial control*, and *anti-infective therapy*. Nonsurgical periodontal therapy is covered in Chapters 17 and 18.
3. **Surgical Therapy**
   A. The **surgical therapy phase** of treatment includes periodontal surgery, placement of dental implants, and root canal therapy.
      1. The master treatment plan may include nonperiodontal procedures that will not be performed by the periodontist.
      2. Root canal therapy would be provided by a general dentist or an endodontist.
   B. This stage of care is also known as *Phase II* therapy. Periodontal surgical procedures are discussed in Chapter 21.
4. **Restorative Therapy**
   A. The **restorative phase** of treatment may include splinting of teeth, restorations, and replacement of missing teeth by fixed or removable prostheses.
      1. Portions of this stage of treatment might not be provided by the periodontist.
      2. The patient is referred to his or her general dentist or a prosthodontist for restorations and replacement of missing teeth.
   B. This stage of care also is called *Phase III* therapy.
5. **Phase IV: Periodontal Maintenance**
   A. The **periodontal maintenance phase** of treatment includes all measures used by the dental team and the patient to keep periodontitis under control (following thorough treatment) and therefore to maintain the teeth functioning throughout life. *The goal of this stage of treatment is to prevent the recurrence of periodontal diseases.*
   B. This stage of care also is known as *Phase IV* therapy. Periodontal maintenance is discussed in detail in Chapter 23.

DOCUMENTATION OF TREATMENT

Documentation of assessment data and all educational and treatment services performed should be entered in the patient record as they are performed. This documentation is referred to as the **progress notes** or **chart notes**. Documentation of periodontal care is presented in Chapter 26.

SECTION 3: INFORMED CONSENT FOR PERIODONTAL TREATMENT

The patient is a critical player in any plan involving periodontal therapy, and communications with the patient are vital as the treatment plan is developed. A breakdown in communication often leads to lawsuits. According to experts on malpractice litigation, keeping the lines of communication open with the patient is a vital component in avoiding lawsuits. Studies demonstrate that patients who believe that they have been well informed regarding their condition and who have had their questions answered, are more compliant with treatment recommendations, have a higher trust in their health care provider, and are more satisfied with their care. These factors lead to better treatment outcomes and reduced malpractice risk.

1. **Informed consent** is a patient's voluntary agreement to proposed treatment after achieving an understanding of the relevant facts, benefits, and risks involved.
   A. An individual's consent is informed only if the recommended treatment, alternate treatment options, and the benefits and risks of treatment have been thoroughly described to the person in language understood by the patient.
   B. Informed consent must be voluntary. Informed consent originates from (i) a person's legal right to direct what happens to his or her body and (ii) the ethical duty of the dental healthcare provider to involve the individual in his or her own dental care.
   C. **Scope of Information.** The most important goal of informed consent is to provide an individual an opportunity to be an informed participant in his or her health care decisions. It is generally accepted that complete informed consent includes a discussion of the following elements:
      1. The diagnosis and an explanation of the periodontal condition that warrants the proposed treatment.
      2. An explanation of the purpose of the proposed periodontal treatment.
      3. A description of the proposed treatment and the individual patient's role and responsibilities during and after periodontal treatment.
      4. A discussion of the known risks and benefits of the proposed periodontal treatment.
      5. An assessment of the likelihood that the proposed treatment will accomplish the desired objectives. When discussing treatment outcomes it is important not to appear to guarantee treatment outcomes to the patient. Remember that individual patients will respond differently to treatment.
      6. A presentation of alternative treatment options, if any, and the known risks and benefits of these options.
      7. A discussion of the prognosis if no treatment is provided.
      8. A discussion of the actual costs associated with the proposed treatment.
      9. Reinforcement of the individual's right to refuse consent to the proposed treatment. Patients often feel powerless. To encourage the patient's voluntary consent, the dental health care provider should make it clear to the patient that he or she is participating in a decision, not merely signing a consent form.
2. **Informed refusal** is a person's right to refuse all or a portion of the proposed treatment after the recommended treatment, alternate treatment options, and the likely consequences of declining treatment have been explained in language understood by the patient. A patient has a legal right to refuse proposed periodontal care.
3. **Ethics and Informed Consent.** The doctrine of informed consent reminds dental health care providers to respect patients by fully and accurately providing information relevant to their health care decisions. It is generally accepted that informed consent includes:
   A. Information that is provided in understandable language. It is the dental health care provider's responsibility to present all information necessary for informed consent to the individual in a way that is understood by him or her.
      1. Use simple, straightforward sentences.

   2. Use commonly recognizable terms. Avoid the use of jargon or technical terms, and explain terms that may not be easily understood.
   3. Use a translator if the patient does not speak English or speaks with little understanding.
   B. An opportunity for the patient to answer and ask questions. Foster an open exchange of information and encourage the patient to ask questions.
   C. Assessment of the patient's understanding of information provided. Use open-ended and nondirective questions.
      1. *"What more would you like to know?"*
      2. *"What are your concerns?"*
      3. *"What is your next question?"*
4. **Format for Consent Process.** Informed consent may be either verbal or written.
   A. Many dental healthcare providers prefer to have the patient sign and date a written consent form for documentation of the consent process. In addition, the written consent document should be signed and dated by the dentist and a witness (generally, another staff member).
   B. Once signed, a written consent document becomes part of the individual's permanent dental record.
   C. If a written consent document is not used, the patient's verbal consent should be documented in the patient chart. An example of documentation of verbal consent is, *"Discussed the diagnosis; purpose, description, benefits, and risks of the proposed treatment; alternative treatment options; the prognosis of no treatment; and costs. The patient asked questions and demonstrates that he understands all information presented during the discussion. Informed consent was obtained for the attached treatment plan.*

CHAPTER SUMMARY STATEMENT

When assigning a periodontal diagnosis, there are three fundamental diagnostic questions that should be asked and answered by the dental team. Those questions are:

(1)   *"Does the clinical assessment indicate health or disease in the periodontium?"*

(2)   *"If the clinical assessment indicates disease, is the disease gingivitis or is it periodontitis?"*

(3)   *"If the patient has gingivitis, what type of gingivitis?"* or *"If the patient has periodontitis, what type of periodontitis?"*

   It is important for the dental hygienist to understand how all phases of periodontal treatment contribute to the goal of restoring a healthy periodontal environment. The patient is a critical player in any plan involving periodontal therapy, and communications with the patient are vital as the treatment plan is developed. Informed consent is a patient's voluntary agreement to proposed treatment after achieving an understanding of the relevant facts, benefits, and risks involved.

SECTION 4: FOCUS ON PATIENTS

CASE 1
Periodontal assessment of a new patient reveals generalized plaque-induced gingivitis. There are moderate calculus deposits and heavy plaque deposits on most teeth. The patient has a history of smoking two packs of cigarettes each day. What plan for non-surgical therapy might your dental team develop for this patient?

CASE 2
Periodontal assessment of a new patient with poorly controlled diabetes mellitus reveals localized moderate chronic periodontitis. The patient's plaque control is poor, and there are light calculus deposits on supragingival and subgingival tooth surfaces. There is a large overhang on a restoration in a premolar tooth. What plan for nonsurgical therapy might your dental team develop for this patient?

CASE 3
Periodontal assessment of a new patient reveals localized signs of gingival inflammation but no attachment loss. The findings also include a site of gingival recession and toothbrush abrasion on the facial surface of a canine tooth. At this site of recession there is no sign of inflammation of the gingiva. How should this site of gingival recession due to traumatic brushing affect the basic diagnostic questions?

Suggested Readings

Parameters of Care. American Academy of Periodontology. *J Periodontol.* 2000;71(5 Suppl):i–ii, 847–883.

Marcus M, Spolsky V. Concepts of quality and the provision of periodontal care: A survey. *J Periodontol.* 1998;69:228–240.

Nevins M, Becker W, Kornman K. *Proceedings of the World Workshop in Clinical Periodontics, Princeton, New Jersey, July 23–27, 1989.* Chicago: The American Academy of Periodontology; 1989.

Newman MG. Improved clinical decision making using the evidence-based approach. *Ann Periodontol.* 1996;1:i–ix.

Palmer RM. Periodontal treatment: non-surgical or surgical? *Dent Update.* 1997;24:III–VII.

SECTION 5: CHAPTER REVIEW QUESTIONS

1. Overt signs of inflammation include color, contour, and _____.
   A. Purulence
   B. Alveolar bone loss
   C. Consistency

2. The key to answering the second basic diagnostic question is
   A. Gingival bleeding
   B. Attachment loss
   C. Tooth mobility

3. Migration of the attachment apparatus apical to the level of the CEJ is termed:
   A. The natural level of the gingival attachment
   B. Change in consistency
   C. Attachment loss

4. Signs of periodontal disease are features of the disease that can be observed by:
   A. The patient
   B. The clinician
   C. Both (a) and (b)

5. The natural level of the gingival attachment is located:
   A. At the CEJ
   B. Apical to the CEJ
   C. Slightly coronal to the CEJ

6. **Localized** periodontitis is defined as periodontal disease that affects:
   A. 30% or less of the sites in the mouth
   B. More than 30% of the sites in the mouth

7. Case Type II patients are defined as patients having:
   A. Gingivitis only
   B. Slight (mild) periodontitis
   C. Moderate periodontitis

8. Management of emergency care is provided during which phase of treatment?
   A. Assessment phase and preliminary therapy
   B. Nonsurgical periodontal therapy phase
   C. Restorative therapy phase

Chapter

17 Nonsurgical Periodontal Therapy

Learning Objectives

- Define the term nonsurgical periodontal therapy.
- State a fundamental philosophy for developing a plan for nonsurgical periodontal therapy.
- List indications for nonsurgical periodontal therapy.
- Describe a typical plan for nonsurgical periodontal therapy for a patient with plaque-induced gingivitis.
- Describe typical plans for nonsurgical periodontal therapy for patients with slight chronic periodontitis and with moderate chronic periodontitis.
- Explain the terms scaling, root planing, periodontal debridement, and deplaquing.
- Describe the type of healing to be expected following successful instrumentation of tooth surfaces.

- List two local risk factors that may occur in a patient needing nonsurgical periodontal therapy.
- Explain the term dental hypersensitivity and explain how this condition can appear as a result of periodontal debridement.
- Describe a strategy for managing dentinal hypersensitivity.
- Explain why re-evaluation of the patient's periodontal condition is important.
- List the steps in a re-evaluation appointment.
- Describe three decisions made during the re-evaluation appointment.
- List two types of patients that should be considered for referral to a specialist in periodontics.

KEY TERMS

Nonsurgical periodontal therapy
Treatment plan
Periodontal maintenance
Periodontal debridement
Deplaquing
Long junctional epithelium

Nonresponsive disease sites
Dentinal hypersensitivity
Dentinal tubules
Odontoblastic process
Smear layer
Re-evaluation

PRINCIPLES OF NONSURGICAL PERIODONTAL THERAPY

1. **Nonsurgical periodontal therapy** includes all nonsurgical treatment and educational measures used to help control gingivitis and periodontitis such as patient self-care, periodontal debridement, and chemical plaque control. As the name implies, periodontal surgery is not a part of nonsurgical therapy.
   A. *Nonsurgical periodontal therapy has the broad overall objective of eliminating disease and returning the periodontium to a healthy state that can then be maintained by a combination of professional and patient care.*
      1. Other terms used to describe nonsurgical periodontal therapy are initial periodontal therapy, initial therapy, hygienic phase, anti-infective phase, cause-related therapy, and soft tissue management.
      2. Nonsurgical periodontal therapy, however, is the preferred terminology for this phase of periodontal care.
   B. Philosophy for Developing a Plan for Nonsurgical Periodontal Therapy
      1. The fundamental philosophy for developing a sensible plan for nonsurgical periodontal therapy should be to plan treatment that will provide for the control, elimination, or minimization of each primary etiologic factor, each local risk factor, and each systemic risk factor identified in a patient at the time of the clinical assessment.
      2. Procedures included in a plan for nonsurgical periodontal therapy should be selected to meet the needs of the individual patient and should include those measures most likely to help bring the identified disease under control.
2. **Indications for Nonsurgical Periodontal Therapy**
   A. Nonsurgical periodontal therapy should be planned for all patients with plaque-associated gingivitis and for all patients with chronic periodontitis.
   B. For most patients with more advanced periodontal disease such as severe chronic periodontitis, control of the periodontitis will require thorough nonsurgical periodontal therapy followed by periodontal surgery.
      1. Although periodontal surgery is frequently indicated for patients with more advanced periodontitis, all patients with chronic periodontitis should undergo nonsurgical periodontal therapy prior to periodontal surgical intervention. Nonsurgical periodontal therapy is frequently successful in minimizing the extent of surgery needed.
      2. Other Types of Periodontitis. *Members of the dental team should be aware that nonsurgical periodontal therapy is not the treatment of choice for all patients with periodontitis.*
         a. Nonsurgical periodontal therapy is not necessarily the best therapy for patients with other types of periodontitis, such as aggressive periodontitis.
         b. Patients with types of periodontitis other than chronic periodontitis should be referred to a periodontist. Criteria for referral are discussed later in this chapter.
3. **Goals of Nonsurgical Periodontal Therapy.** The goals of nonsurgical periodontal therapy are summarized in Box 17-1.

Box 17-1

Goals of Nonsurgical Periodontal Therapy

Goal 1: To minimize the bacterial challenge to the patient
Goal 2: To eliminate or control local environmental risk factors for periodontal disease
Goal 3: To minimize the impact of systemic risk factors for periodontal disease
Goal 4: To stabilize the attachment level

A. Goal 1: To control the bacterial challenge to the patient
  1. Control of the bacterial challenge involves intensive training of the patient in appropriate techniques for self-care and professional removal of calculus deposits and bacterial products from tooth surfaces.
  2. Removal of calculus deposits and bacterial products contaminating the tooth surfaces is an important step in achieving control of the bacterial challenge. Calculus deposits are always covered with living bacterial biofilms that are associated with continuing inflammation if not removed.
B. Goal 2: To minimize the impact of systemic factors
  1. It is apparent that there are certain systemic diseases or conditions that can increase the risk of developing periodontitis or can increase the risk of developing severe periodontitis where periodontitis already exists. Two examples of systemic factors are uncontrolled diabetes mellitus and smoking.
  2. A thorough plan for nonsurgical therapy always includes measures to minimize the impact of systemic risk factors. For example, a periodontitis patient with a family history of diabetes mellitus should be evaluated to rule out undiagnosed diabetes as a contributing factor to the periodontitis. Also, a patient who smokes should receive smoking cessation counseling.
C. Goal 3: To eliminate or control local risk factors
  1. Local environmental risk factors can increase the risk of developing periodontitis in localized sites. For example, defective restorations can lead to plaque retention in the localized area of the defective restoration.
  2. Plaque retention in a site, over time, allows periodontal pathogens to live, multiply, and damage the periodontium.
  3. Local environmental risk factors should be eliminated as part of the plan for nonsurgical periodontal therapy.

   D. Goal 4: To stabilize the attachment level
   1. The ultimate goal of nonsurgical periodontal therapy is to stabilize the level of attachment.
   2. Stabilization of the attachment level involves control of all of the factors listed in the other goals of nonsurgical periodontal therapy.
4. **Components of Nonsurgical Periodontal Therapy**
   A. The Patient's Role in Nonsurgical Periodontal Therapy. The patient maintains responsibility for daily self-care, and the dental team assumes responsibility for regular professional care. The important topic of plaque control for the periodontal patient is presented in Chapter 18.
   B. Professional Therapy in Nonsurgical Periodontal Therapy
   1. Dental health care providers should keep in mind that the precise treatment plan for nonsurgical periodontal therapy must always be customized for the unique needs of each individual patient.
   2. Nonsurgical instrumentation is a major part of professional nonsurgical periodontal therapy and is discussed in the next section.
   C. Box 17-2 shows a list of some of the nonsurgical therapy procedures that the dental team can utilize for patients.

Box 17-2

Nonsurgical Therapy Procedures

   1. Customized self-care instructions
   2. Periodontal debridement (instrumentation) of tooth surfaces and pocket space
   3. Correction of systemic risk factors
   4. Correction of local environmental factors

TYPICAL TREATMENT PLANS FOR NONSURGICAL PERIODONTAL THERAPY

Although it is critical for a treatment plan for nonsurgical therapy to meet the needs of each individual patient, beginning clinicians often find it helpful to review examples of typical plans for nonsurgical therapy.

1. A **treatment plan** for nonsurgical periodontal therapy is a sequential outline of the services and procedures to be carried out by the dentist, the dental hygienist, and the patient. These services and procedures are designed to restore the periodontal health of the patient.

2. **Examples of Typical Treatment Plans**

   A. Typical Plan for a Patient with Plaque-Induced Gingivitis. The typical plan for nonsurgical therapy for a patient with plaque-induced gingivitis might include the following:

      1. Customized self-care instructions and patient education and motivation.
      2. Periodontal instrumentation.
      3. Elimination of plaque retentive factors such as overhanging restorations, caries, and ill-fitting dental prostheses.
      4. Correction of systemic risk factors.
      5. Re-evaluation of patient's periodontal status.
         a. The dental team is always obligated to re-evaluate the results of nonsurgical periodontal therapy to ensure that all appropriate measures have been included and to identify other measures that might be needed.
         b. It is wise for the dental team to include this re-evaluation step in the plan for nonsurgical therapy so that the patient has a clear idea from the outset the therapy to be accomplished and also how the results of the treatment will be assessed.

   B. Typical Plan for a Patient with Slight (Mild) Chronic Periodontitis. It is important to customize the nonsurgical therapy for the needs of each patient, but again it would be helpful to look at a typical plan for a patient with slight periodontitis. This typical plan would include the following:

      1. Customized self-care instructions and patient education and motivation.
      2. Periodontal instrumentation. This periodontal debridement usually includes root planing in areas of attachment loss.
      3. Control of local risk factors to include: removal of overhanging restorations, restoration of caries, treatment of trauma from occlusion, correction of systemic risk factors, and re-evaluation of patient's periodontal status.

   C. Typical Plan for a Patient with Moderate Chronic Periodontitis

      1. This typical plan includes the possibility of periodontal surgery following non-surgical periodontal therapy.
         a. As the severity of periodontitis increases, it becomes more likely that some periodontal surgery will be needed to bring the disease under control.
         b. Even patients who are headed toward surgery at some later date will require thorough nonsurgical therapy to minimize the inflammation as much as possible before the surgical intervention.
      2. The typical plan for a patient with moderate chronic periodontitis might include the following:
         a. Customized self-care instructions and patient education and motivation.
         b. Periodontal instrumentation. This periodontal debridement usually includes root planing in areas of attachment loss.
         c. Control of local risk factors.
         d. Possible periodontal surgery depending on the findings at the re-evaluation.

   D. Typical Plan for a Patient with Severe Chronic Periodontitis. For the patient with severe periodontitis, the nonsurgical periodontal therapy would be similar to that for moderate chronic periodontitis. The need for periodontal surgical therapy would be re-evaluated, however, after the completion of nonsurgical periodontal therapy. Surgical periodontal therapy is discussed in Chapter 21.

SECTION 2: NONSURGICAL INSTRUMENTATION

OBJECTIVE AND RATIONALE FOR PERIODONTAL INSTRUMENTATION

1. **Objective of Periodontal Instrumentation**
   A. The objective of the mechanical removal of calculus and bacterial plaque is the physical removal of microorganisms and their products to prevent and treat periodontal infections.
      1. *Because of the structure of biofilms, physical removal of bacterial plaque is the most effective mechanism of control.*
      2. Subgingival plaque within pockets cannot be reached by brushes, floss, or mouth rinses.
         a. For this reason, frequent periodontal debridement of subgingival root surfaces to remove or disrupt bacterial plaque *mechanically* is an essential component of the treatment of periodontitis.
         b. In fact, periodontal debridement is likely to remain the most important component of nonsurgical periodontal therapy for the foreseeable future.
   B. Removal of deposits from tooth surfaces is a critical step in any plan for nonsurgical periodontal therapy. Calculus deposits harbor living bacterial biofilms; thus, if the calculus remains, so do the pathogenic bacteria, making it impossible to re-establish periodontal health.
2. **Rationale for Periodontal Instrumentation.** The scientific basis for performing periodontal debridement includes all of the following.
   A. Arrest the progress of periodontal disease.
   B. Induce positive changes in the subgingival bacterial flora (count and content).
   C. Create an environment that permits the gingival tissue to heal, therefore eliminating inflammation.
      1. Convert the pocket from an area experiencing increased loss of attachment to one in which the clinical attachment level remains the same or even gains in attachment.
      2. Eliminate bleeding.
      3. Improve the integrity of tissue attachment.
   D. Increase effectiveness of patient self-care.
   E. Permit re-evaluation of periodontal health status to determine if surgery is needed.
   F. Prevent recurrence of disease through periodontal maintenance therapy. **Periodontal maintenance** includes all measures used by the dental team and the patient to keep periodontitis under control.

INSTRUMENTATION TERMINOLOGY

There has been some evolution in the terminology associated with calculus removal and plaque removal over the past few years. The careful reader will be wise to note that there are different sets of terminology that appear in the dental hygiene journals and textbooks compared to the dental journals and textbooks. The differences in this terminology revolve around the terms described below.

1. **Traditional Terminology**
   A. **Scaling**, as defined in the American Dental Association (ADA) Procedure Codes, is instrumentation of the crown and root surfaces of the teeth to remove plaque, calculus, and stains.
   B. **Root planing**, as defined in the ADA Procedure Codes, is a treatment procedure designed to remove cementum or surface dentin that is rough, impregnated with calculus, or contaminated with toxins or microorganisms.
      1. As traditionally defined, root planing involved the routine, intentional removal of cementum and the instrumenting of all root surfaces to a glassy smooth texture.
      2. Until recently it was thought that bacterial products were firmly held in cemental surfaces exposed by periodontitis. It was believed that vigorous root planing with intentional removal of cementum was always needed to ensure the removal of all calculus as well as all bacterial products from the root surfaces.
      3. *It is now clear that vigorous root planing is not universally needed to re-establish periodontal health in a site of periodontitis.* Rather than vigorous root planing and removal of most or all of the cementum, it is now known that the bacterial products can be removed from the root surfaces by using modern techniques with ultrasonic instruments combined with a minimal amount of actual root planing.
2. **Emerging Terminology.** Periodontal debridement is a newer term that has been used in the dental hygiene literature since 1993 to replace the term scaling and root planing.
   A. **Periodontal debridement** is defined as the removal or disruption of bacterial plaque, its byproducts, and plaque retentive calculus deposits from coronal surfaces, root surfaces, and within pocket space and tissue wall to the extent needed to re-establish periodontal health and restore a balance between the bacterial flora and the host's immune responses.
      1. Periodontal debridement includes instrumentation of every square millimeter of root surface for removal of plaque and calculus, but does not include the deliberate, aggressive removal of cementum.
      2. Conservation of cementum is a goal of periodontal debridement.
         a. Some clinicians believe that conservation of cementum enhances periodontal healing, repair, or regeneration.[1]
         b. In health, an important function of cementum is to attach the periodontal ligament fibers to the root surface. During the healing process after disease, cementum is thought to contribute to repair of the periodontium.[2]
         c. Research studies indicate that the complete removal of cementum from the root surface, exposing the ends of dentinal tubules, may allow bacteria to travel from the pulp into the periodontal pocket. This infusion of bacteria from the pulp may exacerbate alveolar bone loss.[3–5]

      3. During periodontal debridement, the extent of instrumentation should be limited to that needed to obtain a favorable tissue response. Root surfaces should be instrumented only to a level that results in resolution of tissue inflammation.

  B. Deplaquing is the disruption or removal of subgingival microbial plaque and its byproducts from cemental surfaces and the pocket space.

3. Considerations Regarding Emerging Terminology

  A. Insurance Coding Systems. Insurance codes are entered on insurance forms. Dental treatment is listed under the appropriate procedure number. Insurance codes are discussed in detail in Chapter 27.

    1. Although the term periodontal debridement as defined in the dental hygiene literature describes modern periodontal therapy better than the older terms, it has not yet replaced these older terms as recognized by the ADA. Periodontal debridement is not a currently recognized ADA procedure name.

    2. Because of these problems with the ADA codes, most dentists and periodontists have been reluctant to embrace the new terminology. Some authors and clinicians have redefined the term root planing so that its meaning is similar to that of periodontal debridement. This approach of redefining the term root planing can be confusing, however, because it is difficult to determine which definition any one person is using.

  B. Reference for Insurance Codes. In the United States, insurance codes are published in the book *American Dental Association Current Dental Terminology 2005*. These codes are very specific and should be reviewed carefully before specific dental treatment is coded.

TISSUE HEALING: END POINT OF INSTRUMENTATION

1. Tissue Health as End Point. The goal of instrumentation is to render the root surface and pocket space acceptable to the tissue so that healing occurs. *There is widespread agreement that the end point for this instrumentation is simply a return to soft tissue health.*

2. Healing After Instrumentation

  A. After periodontal debridement some healing of the periodontal tissues will occur.

    1. The primary pattern of healing after periodontal debridement is through the formation of a **long junctional epithelium** (Fig. 17-1).

    2. *There is no formation of new bone, cementum, or periodontal ligament during the healing process that occurs after periodontal debridement.*

  B. Nonsurgical periodontal therapy can result in reduced probing depths due to the formation of a long junctional epithelium combined with the gingival recession that often occurs following nonsurgical periodontal therapy.

3. **Assessing Tissue Healing.** Tissue healing does not occur overnight, and in most cases it is not possible to assess tissue response for at least 1 month after the completion of instrumentation.

   A. An appointment for re-evaluation should be scheduled for 4 to 6 weeks after completion of instrumentation. The re-evaluation appointment is discussed in Section 3 of this chapter.

   B. **Nonresponsive sites** are sites that show continued loss of attachment and may exhibit clinical signs of inflammation and/or bleeding upon probing following thorough nonsurgical periodontal therapy.

      1. Nonresponsive sites should be carefully re-evaluated with an explorer for the presence of residual calculus deposits or roughness.

      2. If the root surface is rough, more vigorous root planing of the site may be indicated.

      3. Nonresponsive sites should be thoroughly deplaqued with an ultrasonic instrument (unless ultrasonic instrumentation is contraindicated for this patient).

      4. If the site is still nonresponsive a few weeks after reinstrumentation, the dental hygienist should try to determine what other factors might be contributing to the disease process, such as host factors. Periodontal surgical treatment is frequently indicated in these sites.

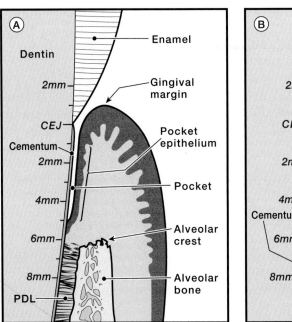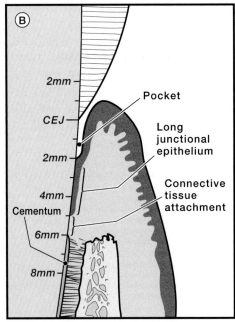

Figure 17-1. Healing After Nonsurgical Periodontal Debridement. A: Before therapy, the periodontal pocket has a probing depth of 6 mm. B: After periodontal therapy the tissue healing is through the formation of a long junctional epithelium. This results in a probing depth of 2 mm. Note that there is no formation of new bone, cementum, or periodontal ligament during the healing process that occurs after periodontal debridement.

DENTINAL HYPERSENSITIVITY

1. **Description of Dentinal Hypersensitivity**
    A. **Dentinal hypersensitivity** is a short, sharp painful reaction that occurs when some areas of exposed dentin are subjected to mechanical (touch of toothbrush bristles), thermal (ice cream), or chemical (acidic grapefruit) stimuli. For example, an individual may experience pain when brushing a certain tooth or when eating sweet, sour, or acidic foods. Breathing in cold air while walking outside on a cold day might produce a similar painful reaction.
    B. Hypersensitivity is associated with exposed dentin; however, not all exposed dentin is hypersensitive.
        1. Exposed dentin is dentin that is exposed to the oral cavity due to an absence of the enamel (crown) or cementum (root) that normally covers it.
        2. Dentin may be exposed on a tiny or extensive area of the tooth.
    C. The pain of hypersensitivity is sporadic. A patient may experience sensitivity for a time and then, other periods when sensitivity is not a problem.
2. **Precipitating Factors for Sensitivity**
    A. Gingival Recession
        1. *Patients frequently encounter dentinal hypersensitivity when periodontal therapy results in tissue healing that exposes small areas of the tooth root.*
        2. This type of sensitivity results most often following periodontal surgical therapy, but can also be associated with nonsurgical periodontal therapy.
    B. During and Following Nonsurgical Debridement
        1. *Instrumentation of root surfaces also can result in dentinal hypersensitivity.* The possibility of creating dentinal hypersensitivity underscores that conservation of cementum should be a goal of nonsurgical instrumentation. During instrumentation, local anesthesia can be used to control the discomfort if needed to complete thorough instrumentation.
        2. Most commonly, however, instrumentation of root surfaces does not result in dentinal hypersensitivity.
            a. Sensitivity may not occur in most instances because instrumentation of root surfaces may result in a smear layer of dentin over the root surfaces.
            b. This so-called **smear layer** refers to crystalline debris from the tooth surface that covers the dentinal tubules and inhibits fluid flow, thus preventing the sensitivity.
3. **Origin of Hypersensitivity**
    A. Evidence suggests that the origin of dentinal hypersensitivity is explained by the hydrodynamic theory of dentin sensitivity.
        1. The **dentinal tubules** penetrate the dentin like long, miniature tunnels extending through the dentin.
        2. The dentinal tubules are partially filled with an **odontoblastic process**—the thin tail of cytoplasm from a cell in the tooth pulp—that extends from the pulp to the dentoenamel or dentocementum junction (**Fig. 17-2**).

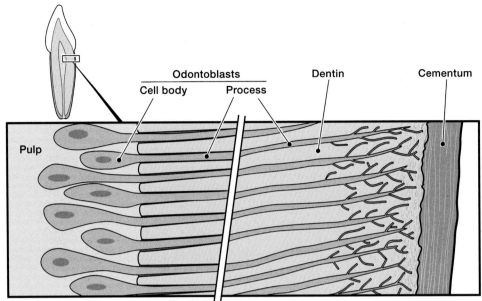

Figure 17-2. Odontoblastic Process. The odontoblastic cell process in the dentinal tubule extends from the pulp to the junction of the dentin with the enamel or cementum.

    B. Changes in temperature create hydrodynamic forces within the fluid-filled dentinal tubules that stimulate nerve endings within the pulp associated with the odontoblastic processes, thus resulting in pain.

  4. Strategies for Treatment of Dentinal Hypersensitivity

    A. When dentinal tubules are exposed, most tooth surfaces go through a natural process of crystallization and occlusion (blocking) of the open dentinal tubules.

      1. This natural process takes several weeks, and many remedies are designed to occlude the dentinal tubules temporarily and give the natural process time to take place.

      2. Fortunately, most dentinal hypersensitivity is mild and resolves within a few weeks if the exposed root surfaces are kept plaque free. In its more severe forms, however, dentinal hypersensitivity can result in a patient's inability to perform thorough self-care.

B. Chemicals can be used to help seal the dentinal tubules and to eliminate or minimize associated sensitivity temporarily.

1. Fluorides can be used to precipitate fluoride-rich crystals on the tooth surface.
2. Calcium hydroxide can be burnished into the root surface.
3. Cavity varnishes can be used to cover the tooth surface temporarily and allow for natural resolution.

C. There are toothpastes specifically formulated for desensitizing teeth at home. Toothpastes containing potassium nitrate or strontium chloride as the active ingredient have been demonstrated to provide relief in some patients.

D. An appropriate strategy for managing dentinal hypersensitivity is to warn the patient about the possibility of hypersensitivity before beginning treatment. Before initiating instrumentation, the dental hygienist should provide the patient with the following information regarding dentinal hypersensitivity:

1. If sensitivity resulting from nonsurgical periodontal therapy occurs, it will gradually disappear over a few weeks.
2. *Thorough daily plaque removal is the most important factor in the prevention and control of sensitivity. Without meticulous plaque control, no treatment for dentinal hypersensitivity will be successful.*
3. There is no treatment that will immediately stop the sensitivity. If it occurs, there are several agents that can be professionally applied to reduce sensitivity.

SECTION 3: DECISIONS FOLLOWING NONSURGICAL PERIODONTAL THERAPY

THE RE-EVALUATION APPOINTMENT

1. Re-evaluation refers to a formal step in nonsurgical therapy that is designed to gather information to be used in several critical clinical decisions regarding future care of a patient with chronic periodontitis.
2. **Scheduling.** The patient should be scheduled for a re-evaluation appointment 4 to 6 weeks after completion of nonsurgical periodontal therapy. The steps in a typical re-evaluation appointment include (Box 17-3):

A. Medical status update of the patient
B. Periodontal clinical assessment as described in Chapter 12.
C. A comparison of the results of the initial assessment with the results of re-evaluation.

1. Ideally, the clinical attachment levels have stayed the same or even improved.
2. Nonresponsive sites (unhealthy sites that show continued loss of attachment) will exhibit the clinical signs of inflammation and/or bleeding upon probing.

D. Decision making related to the need for additional nonsurgical therapy, periodontal maintenance, and periodontal surgery.

Steps in a Typical Re-evaluation Appointment

1. Update the medical status of the patient.
2. Perform a periodontal clinical assessment.
3. Compare the data gathered at the initial periodontal assessment with the data at re-evaluation.
4. Make decisions about the need for additional nonsurgical therapy, periodontal maintenance, and periodontal surgery.

CLINICAL DECISIONS DURING RE-EVALUATION

At the time of re-evaluation, several critical clinical decisions need to be made about the future care of the patient. Box 17-4 outlines the decisions that can be made at the re-evaluation step.

1. **Determining the Need for Additional Nonsurgical Therapy**
   A. It is common for the re-evaluation step to indicate the need for additional nonsurgical periodontal therapy by the dental team.
      1. Self-care efforts by the patient may be deemed inadequate for disease control.
      2. Subgingival calculus deposits originally inaccessible because of deep probing depths may now be reachable because of tissue shrinkage.
   B. The patient may be in need of additional smoking cessation counseling.
   C. In response to each of these scenarios, the dental team is obligated again to attempt to address the factor noted in a continuing effort to help the patient bring the periodontitis under control.
2. **Establishing a Program for Periodontal Maintenance**
   A. Periodontal maintenance includes all measures used by the dental team and the patient to keep periodontitis under control. Periodontal Maintenance is discussed in Chapter 23.
   B. The goal of this stage of periodontal treatment is to prevent the recurrence of periodontal diseases.
   C. All patients with chronic periodontitis should be placed on a program of periodontal maintenance following nonsurgical periodontal therapy.
3. **Evaluating the Need for Periodontal Surgery**
   A. The need for some types of periodontal surgery can be determined at the time of the periodontal assessment. Periodontal surgery and its indications are discussed in Chapter 21.
   B. Periodontal surgery to help control chronic periodontitis or to regenerate periodontium lost because of chronic periodontitis, however, is usually best identified at the time of the re-evaluation.

Box 17-4

Critical Clinical Decisions During Re-evaluation

1. Determine the need for additional nonsurgical therapy.
2. Establish a program for periodontal maintenance.
3. Evaluate the need for periodontal surgery.

RECOGNIZING THE NEED FOR REFERRAL TO A PERIODONTIST

1. **Planning for Referral**
   A. Although the general dental team can and should treat most patients with chronic periodontitis, each team must plan ahead for the inevitable time when a patient with periodontitis must be referred to a specialist in periodontics.
   B. The members of the team should discuss this issue in detail to determine the comfort level for treating periodontitis patients within the general dental practice.
   C. Referrals will occur at different points depending on the plan established by the dentist.
2. **General Guidelines for Referral to a Periodontist.** The following guidelines will be helpful for most dental teams.
   A. The dental team of a general dental practice should treat patients with mild or moderate chronic periodontitis when periodontal surgery is not indicated.
   B. Patients with moderate to severe chronic periodontitis who have the need for surical intervention should be referred to a periodontist unless the general dentist has had enough additional training to reach a comfort level with the surgery needed.
   C. Patients with a periodontal diagnosis other than chronic periodontitis, such as aggressive periodontitis, should be referred to a periodontist.
   D. Patients with a need for intravenous sedation to accomplish the indicated periodontal therapy should be referred to a periodontist.
   E. Patients who exhibit continued periodontal breakdown despite thorough nonsurgical therapy should be referred to a periodontist.

RELATIONSHIP BETWEEN NONSURGICAL PERIODONTAL THERAPY AND PERIODONTAL SURGERY

1. **Indications for Surgical Therapy.** Periodontal surgery may play an important role in periodontal therapy for certain patients.
   A. Although periodontal surgery is not a part of nonsurgical therapy, the members of the dental team should be aware of the relationship between nonsurgical and surgical periodontal therapy throughout the treatment planning process.

2. Table 17-1 shows an overview of the relationship of nonsurgical periodontal therapy to surgical periodontal treatment for patients with gingival and periodontal disease.
   A. Gingivitis
      1. For most patients with gingivitis only, the gingivitis can be controlled with nonsurgical therapy alone.
      2. The dental team should be aware that any patient may require surgical therapy, regardless of his or her disease status. For example, a patient with gingivitis could have an area of severe gingival recession that requires surgical correction even though periodontal surgery is not usually indicated for patients with gingivitis.
   B. Slight Periodontitis. For most patients with slight (mild) periodontitis, the periodontitis can be controlled with nonsurgical therapy alone.
   C. Moderate Periodontitis. For some patients with moderate periodontitis, the periodontitis can be controlled with nonsurgical therapy alone. For other patients with moderate periodontitis, control of the periodontitis will require thorough nonsurgical periodontal therapy followed by periodontal surgery.
   D. Severe Periodontitis. For most patients with severe periodontitis, control of the periodontitis will require thorough nonsurgical periodontal therapy followed by periodontal surgery.

Table 17-1. Indications for Nonsurgical and Surgical Therapy

Disease Status	Nonsurgical Therapy	Surgical Therapy
Plaque-associated gingivitis	Always indicated	Usually not indicated
Slight chronic periodontitis	Always indicated	Usually not indicated
Moderate chronic periodontitis	Always indicated	Need varies with patient
Severe chronic periodontitis	Always indicated	Usually indicated

CHAPTER SUMMARY STATEMENT

Nonsurgical periodontal therapy refers to all the educational and treatment measures, other than periodontal surgery, used by the dental team to help bring gingivitis and periodontitis under control. The goals of nonsurgical periodontal therapy are to control the bacterial challenge to the patient, to minimize the impact of systemic risk factors, to eliminate or control local environmental risk factors, and to stabilize the attachment level. The precise steps included in nonsurgical periodontal therapy should depend on the precise needs of each individual patient.

A vital component of all plans for nonsurgical periodontal therapy is nonsurgical instrumentation. Biofilms are resistant to both topical and systemic chemical plaque control; therefore, frequent mechanical periodontal debridement of subgingival root surfaces is an essential component of successful nonsurgical periodontal therapy. Dentinal hypersensitivity may occur in some areas of exposed dentin and is another reason that conservation of cementum should be a goal of nonsurgical instrumentation. Thorough daily plaque removal is the most important factor in the prevention and control of hypersensitivity.

Re-evaluation is an important step in nonsurgical periodontal therapy. During re-evaluation the dental team determines the patient's need for additional nonsurgical therapy and/or periodontal surgery and establishes a program for periodontal maintenance.

SECTION 4: FOCUS ON PATIENTS

CASE 1

A new patient for your dental team has obvious clinical signs of moderate chronic periodontitis and generalized plaque and calculus deposits. When your team outlines a plan for nonsurgical periodontal therapy, the patient objects and wants to know if she can be treated with an antibiotic instead. How should your team members respond?

CASE 2

A 16-year-old patient with advanced attachment loss and severe bone loss comes to your dental team for evaluation and treatment. How should your dental team manage this young patient?

References

1. Bray KK. Innovations in periodontal debridement. *Dental Hyg Connect.* 1996;1:1–7.
2. D'Errico JA, Ouyang H, Berry JE, et al. Immortalized cementoblasts and periodontal ligament cells in culture. *Bone.* 1999;25:39–47.
3. Hirsch RS, Clarke NG, Srikandi W. Pulpal pathosis and severe alveolar lesions: a clinical study. *Endod Dent Traumatol.* 1989;5:48–54.
4. Jansson LE, Ehnevid H. The influence of endodontic infection on periodontal status in mandibular molars. *J Periodontol.* 1998;69:1392–1396.
5. Kobayashi T, Hayashi A, Yoshikawa R, et al. The microbial flora from root canals and periodontal pockets of non-vital teeth associated with advanced periodontitis. *Int Endod J.* 1990;23:100–106.

SECTION 5: CHAPTER REVIEW QUESTIONS

1. Which of the following is NOT a goal of nonsurgical periodontal therapy?
   A. Minimize the bacterial challenge to the patient
   B. Eliminate the need for daily self-care
   C. Stabilize the attachment level on the teeth

2. Successful periodontal debridement always results in the complete removal of cementum from the exposed root surface.
   A. True
   B. False

3. Two rationales for periodontal debridement are (i) to increase the effectiveness of the patient's self-care and (ii) to arrest the progress of periodontal disease.
   A. True
   B. False

4. The end point for tooth root instrumentation is which of the following?
   A. Return of soft tissue health
   B. Increased pigmentation of the gingiva
   C. Decreased need for daily self-care

5. The type of healing that occurs following successful root instrumentation is a long junctional epithelium.
   A. True
   B. False

6. Pain caused by dentinal hypersensitivity can result from mechanical, thermal, or chemical stimuli.
   A. True
   B. False

7. Management of dentinal hypersensitivity can include all of the following EXCEPT:
   A. Meticulous daily plaque control
   B. Using chemicals to occlude (block) dentinal tubules
   C. Applications of cold water to the tooth surfaces

8. Successful treatment for all periodontitis patients always results in probing depths less than 3 mm.
   A. True
   B. False

9. When considering a decision for referral to a specialist in periodontics which of the following types of patients would normally NOT be referred?
   A. Patients with aggressive periodontitis
   B. Patients with chronic periodontitis
   C. Patients with a need for periodontal surgery

Chapter

18 Patient's Role in Nonsurgical Periodontal Therapy

Learning Objectives

- Discuss the role of the patient in nonsurgical periodontal therapy.
- Justify the belief that the patient is a cotherapist in the process of nonsurgical periodontal therapy.
- State the benefits of power toothbrushes.
- In the clinical setting, recommend and teach power brushing to an appropriate patient.
- Give examples of oral conditions that might prompt a dental hygienist to recommend a power toothbrush.
- State the rationale for tongue cleaning.
- In the clinical setting, recommend and teach tongue cleaning to an appropriate patient.
- Explain why interdental care is of special importance for a patient with periodontitis.
- Define the term embrasure space and explain its importance in selecting effective interdental aids.
- Define the term root concavity and explain its importance in selecting effective interdental aids.

■ In a classroom or laboratory setting, explain the criteria for selection and correctly demonstrate the use of the following to an instructor: power toothbrush, standard irrigation tip, subgingival irrigation tip, and all the interdental aids presented in this chapter to an instructor.

■ In a clinical setting, recommend, explain, and demonstrate appropriate interdental aids to a patient with type III embrasure spaces. Assist the patient in selecting an appropriate interdental aid that the patient is willing to use on a daily basis.

■ Discuss the precautions for use of home oral irrigation.

■ Compare and contrast cosmetic mouth rinses and therapeutic mouth rinses.

■ Name the characteristics that an ideal mouth rinse would possess.

■ Name three indications for the use of a therapeutic mouth rinse.

■ Explain why the alcohol content of a mouth rinse is an important consideration when recommending a product for patient use.

■ Name three indications for use of a chlorhexidine mouth rinse.

KEY TERMS

Nonsurgical periodontal therapy
Patient role as cotherapist
Volatile sulfur compounds
Embrasure space
Type I embrasure space
Type II embrasure space
Type III embrasure space
Root concavity
Home oral irrigation

Standard irrigation tip
Subgingival irrigation tip
Chemical plaque control
Efficacy
Stability
Substantivity
Safety Council on Dental Therapeutics
Cosmetic mouth rinses
Therapeutic mouth rinses

SECTION 1: PATIENT-PERFORMED MECHANICAL PLAQUE CONTROL

THE PATIENT'S ROLE IN NONSURGICAL PERIODONTAL THERAPY

Nonsurgical periodontal therapy includes all nonsurgical treatment and educational measures used to help control gingivitis and periodontitis, such as patient self-care, periodontal instrumentation, and chemical plaque control.

1. **Patient as Cotherapist.** Because the primary etiologic factor for periodontitis is bacterial plaque, much of nonsurgical periodontal therapy must be directed toward its daily control by the patient.
   A. Successful nonsurgical periodontal therapy always involves the patient in an intensive program of self-care techniques.
   B. The patient's efforts at self-care are so critical to the control of periodontitis that some dental teams refer to the patient as having the role of **cotherapist** in the process of nonsurgical periodontal therapy.
      1. This concept of the patient as cotherapist is used to underscore the vital role the patient plays in establishing control of periodontitis.
      2. The patient should be actively involved in making decisions about his or her own health care and be willing to make a long-term commitment to meticulous self-care and regular professional care.
2. **Goals of Mechanical Plaque Control.** The goal of mechanical plaque control is the physical removal or disruption of bacteria and their products. Mechanical plaque control includes self-care by the patient on a daily basis and subgingival periodontal instrumentation by the dental hygienist at regular intervals.

TOOTHBRUSHING AND TONGUE CLEANING

1. **Manual Toothbrushing**
   A. Ensuring that the periodontitis patient uses a sulcular brushing technique with a soft bristle brush is central to most self-care programs.
   B. Manual toothbrushing techniques are not covered in detail here because these topics are covered fully in other courses in the dental hygiene curriculum.
2. **Power Toothbrushing.** Power brushes have been in existence for many years. In the past, powered brushes were recommended for those individuals with special needs or a disability. Today, there is a power brush available to fit many multiple needs in a wide range of prices.
   A. Rationale for Recommending a Power Toothbrush
      1. While any individual could benefit from a power toothbrush, patients with poor biofilm control, orthodontic appliances, implants, aesthetic restorations, gingival overgrowth, crown and bridge, or physical disabilities are ideal candidates to use power toothbrush.
      2. Some power brushes feature timers. This feature is particularly beneficial for helping patients increase brushing time.
   B. Description
      1. Brush head configurations vary depending on the manufacturer. Popular shapes are round or elliptical.
      2. Handle designs vary in size and ergonomics.
      3. Power sources may come from rechargeable or replaceable (i.e., AA alkaline) batteries
   C. Benefits
      1. Certain power toothbrushes have been shown to remove plaque and reduce gingivitis better than a manual toothbrush. They may also provide better stain reduction and enhance patient compliance with a self-care regimen.[1]

     2. A recent systematic review of power brushes found that only a rotation oscillation toothbrush was consistently superior to a manual toothbrush.[2]

  D. Technique

     1. Whether manual or power, thorough brushing is dependent on correct technique.

       a. As with a manual toothbrush, the patient needs to angle the power toothbrush properly in the mouth. Once in place, however, the brush head motion on a power toothbrush will do all the work.

       b. Since a power brush generates more strokes per minute than a manual brush, the individual may remove more biofilm in the same amount of brushing time.[3]

     2. Power brushes have a different sound and sensation than a manual brush.

       a. It may take some time for a patient to adjust to a new product.

       b. Additionally, some power brushes may increase the foaming action of toothpaste. Patients should be instructed to use a small amount of toothpaste and to place the brush head in the mouth before turning on the unit.

     3. The dental hygienist should read the manufacturer's users guide prior to recommending and/or demonstrating a power brush to a patient. *Patients should also be counseled to follow the manufacturer's instructions for the best outcome.*

3. Tongue Cleaning. Many patients have coated tongues that make it difficult to maintain fresh breath and cause a lessened sense of taste. Daily tongue cleaning controls halitosis and may help to maintain a healthy periodontal environment.

  A. Rationale for Tongue Cleaning

     1. Emerging research indicates that a clean tongue may play a role in maintaining a healthy periodontal environment. *Studies indicate that a coated tongue may contribute to periodontal disease and to bad breath.*[4]

     2. Daily tongue cleaning removes pathogenic bacteria residing on the dorsum of the tongue, leading to reduced numbers of pathogenic bacteria on the tongue and in the saliva.

     3. Tongue coating also can contribute to a lessened sense of taste. Tongue cleaning should be recommended to geriatric patients who have a low desire to eat due to depressed taste sensation.

     4. Most patients are concerned about controlling halitosis and therefore are receptive to the introduction of tongue cleaning to their self-care routine. The practice of tongue cleaning may not only make a patient feel more confident, but may actually help in maintaining a healthy periodontal environment.

  B. Role of Volatile Sulfur Compounds in Halitosis

     1. **Volatile sulfur compounds (VSC)** are a family of gases that are responsible for halitosis. Oral malodor is not the only problem associated with VSC.

       a. An increasing volume of evidence suggests that even in low concentrations these gases are highly toxic to tissues. VSC may therefore play a role in the pathogenesis of inflammatory periodontitis.

       b. Two members of the VSC family of gases, hydrogen sulfide and methyl mercaptan, are principally responsible for mouth odor. Methyl mercaptan is produced primarily by periodontal pathogens.

     2. Tongue cleaning is recommended because the bulk of bacteria and debris, especially the periodontal pathogens that produce methyl mercaptan, accumulate mostly within the filiform papillae and on the back of the tongue.

     3. Methyl mercaptan gases have been shown to increase the permeability of intact mucosa and stimulate the production of cytokines associated with periodontal disease.

  C. Description

     1. Manual tongue cleaners come in a variety of styles. The two most common types are (i) specialized toothbrushes with a thin brush head and (ii) tongue scrapers (**Fig. 18-1**).

     2. All types of tongue cleaners are designed to allow the patient to reach the back of the tongue. Mechanized tongue cleaners are discussed in Section 2 of this chapter.

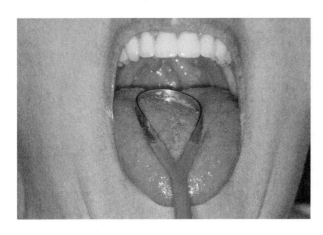

Figure 18-1. Manual Tongue Scraper. Daily tongue cleaning controls halitosis and may help to maintain a healthy periodontal environment.

D. Technique

1. The tongue brush or scraper is positioned as far back on the tongue as possible.

2. Once the brush or scraper is in position, it is pulled forward gently over the tongue. This procedure is repeated two or three times or until the tongue is clean.

3. When first learning tongue cleaning, many patients gag and find the process unpleasant.

a. In the beginning, encourage the patient to place the cleaner wherever it is most comfortable on the tongue.

b. Initially, it is helpful to encourage the patient by reminding him or her of the benefits of tongue cleaning, such as improved breath, improved taste sensation, and of course, better oral health.

c. With regular use, most patients become accustomed to the sensation of the tongue brush or scraper and are able to clean further back on the tongue. Over time, most patients become skilled at tongue cleaning.

INTERDENTAL CARE

1. Importance of Interdental Care

A. For the periodontal patient, interdental plaque control takes on special importance since periodontitis usually damages the interdental tissues first.

B. *Since the importance of interdental plaque control is quite high for the patient with periodontitis, the dental hygienist should be knowledgeable about plaque control measures that can be used to supplement sulcular brushing and flossing.*

1. Indications for the use of interdental aids are summarized in Table 18-1.

2. It is advisable to keep a supply of the various interdental cleaners in the dental office for dispensing to patients. Interdental cleaners often are *not available* at local drug stores or pharmacies.

2. Challenges in Interdental Care for the Periodontitis Patient

A. Embrasure Spaces. The **embrasure space** is the open space apical to the contact area between the proximal surfaces of two teeth.

1. In health, the interdental papilla fills the gingival embrasure space. Dental floss is effective in areas of normal gingival contour.

2. *The tissue destruction characterized by periodontitis usually results in an interdental papilla that is reduced in height or missing, resulting in an open embrasure space. Dental floss is not effective in areas with open embrasure spaces.*

3. Analysis of the embrasure spaces is critical in determining which interdental aid is likely to be most effective in plaque control.

a. Type I embrasure—space filled by the interdental papilla. Dental floss is effective.

   b. **Type II embrasure**—height of interdental papilla is reduced. Interdental brushes, wooden interdental cleaners, and toothpicks are effective.

   c. **Type III embrasure**—interdental papilla is missing. Interdental brushes and end-tuft brushes are effective.

B. Root Concavities. A **root concavity** is a trenchlike depression in the root surface. Root concavities commonly occur on the proximal surfaces of anterior and posterior teeth and the facial and lingual surfaces of molar teeth.

   1. In health, root concavities are covered with alveolar bone and help to secure the tooth in the bone.

   2. Periodontitis results in the apical migration of the junctional epithelium, loss of connective tissue, and destruction of alveolar bone. This tissue destruction results in the exposure of root concavities to the oral environment (either in the presence of tissue recession or, frequently, within a periodontal pocket).

   3. In Figure 18-2A–E, the root of a mandibular canine is covered with a colored powder that represents bacterial plaque on the root surface. This series of figures compares the effectiveness of dental floss and an interdental brush in removing bacterial plaque from the root concavity.

      a. Dental floss is not successful in removing plaque from the root concavity.

      b. The interdental brush is effective in removing bacterial plaque from the root concavity.

   4. Figure 18-3A–C compares the effectiveness of dental floss and an interdental brush in cleaning the root concavity of a maxillary premolar. Note that only the interdental brush is effective in reaching the concave surface of the root concavity.

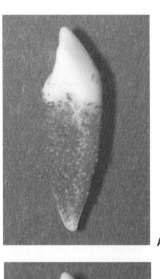

A

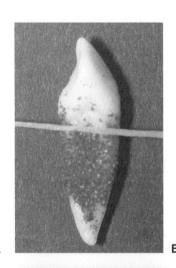

B

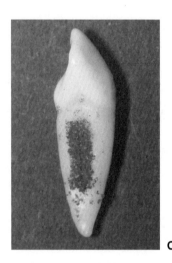

C

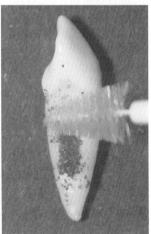

D

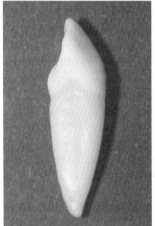

E

Figure 18-2. Plaque Removal from Root Concavity. A: The proximal surface of this mandibular canine is covered with colored powder. B and C: Dental floss is used to clean the proximal surface; the floss is unable to remove the powder from the root concavity. D and E: An interdental brush effectively removes the colored powder from the root concavity.

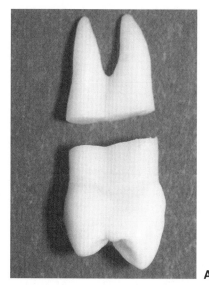
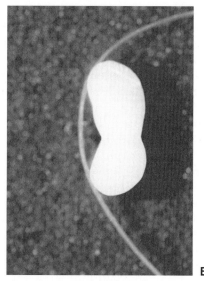
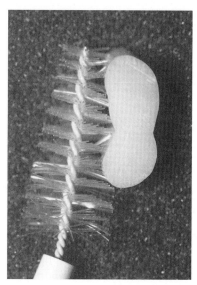

A   B   C

Figure 18-3. Application of Interdental Aids to Root Concavity. A: A maxillary premolar (side view) is cut to expose a cross section of the root. **B:** The root of the same maxillary premolar viewed in cross section; dental floss is unable to clean the root concavity. **C:** The bristles of the interdental brush extend into the root cavity for successful plaque removal.

3. **Dental Floss**
   A. Description. Dental floss is unwaxed or waxed thread made of silk, nylon, or plastic monofilament fibers used to remove dental plaque biofilm from the proximal surfaces of teeth.
   B. Indications
      1. Type I embrasures. Dental floss is effective in removing plaque from tooth crowns and the convex root surfaces in the region of the cementoenamel junction (CEJ) (**Fig. 18-4**).
      2. Recommended for patients with excellent compliance with self-care. Patient compliance with dental flossing is low with many patients being unable or unwilling to perform daily flossing.[5–10]
      3. Power flossing devices may improve patient compliance with daily flossing.
      4. Dental floss is not effective in removing plaque from root concavities and grooves.

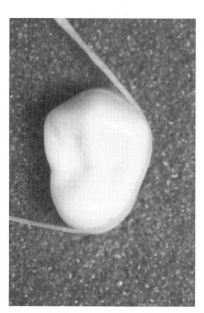

Figure 18-4. Floss Application to Crown.
Floss effectively removes plaque from the convex, rounded surfaces of the crown.

4. **Tufted Dental Floss**
   A. Description. A specialized type of dental floss that has a segment of ordinary floss attached to a thicker, fluffy, yarnlike segment of floss (Fig. 18-5).
   B. Indications
      1. For type II embrasures.
      2. To clean under the pontic of a fixed bridge.
      3. To clean the distal surface of the last tooth in the arch.
      4. To remove plaque from the proximal surfaces of widely spaced teeth.
   C. Technique
      1. For interdental proximal surfaces, the fluffy part of the floss is used interdentally in a C-shape against the tooth, applying pressure with a slight sawing motion against first one proximal surface and then the adjacent proximal tooth surface.
      2. For fixed bridges, the tufted floss is threaded under the pontic and used to clean the undersurface of pontic. Next, the distal surface of the mesial abutment tooth and the mesial surface of the distal abutment tooth are cleaned using the tufted floss.

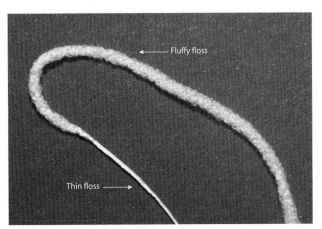

Figure 18-5. Tufted Dental Floss. This aid is a specialized type of floss consisting of a fluffy segment of yarnlike floss attached to a segment of thin floss.

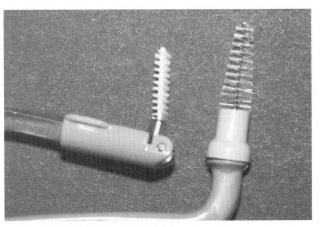

Figure 18-6. Interdental Brushes. Interdental brushes are one of the most useful aids for cleaning root concavities. Examples of two different sizes and designs are shown in this photo.

5. **Interdental Brush**
   A. Description. Tiny conical or pine-tree–shaped nylon bristle brush attached to a handle (Fig. 18-6). Some manufacturers offer brushes in several designs so that the best size and shape of brush can be selected for the embrasure space.
   B. Indications
      1. Useful only when an embrasure space is partially or completely open, since they cannot be used where the interdental papilla fills the interdental space.
      2. One major advantage of these brushes is their use in embrasure spaces adjacent to exposed root surfaces with proximal concavities. *The bristles of an interdental brush can clean root concavities more effectively than any other interdental aid.*
   C. Technique. The brush is inserted into the open interdental space (the brush should insert easily) and moved in and out for several strokes.
6. **End-Tuft Brush**
   A. Description
      1. An end-tuff brush is similar to a standard toothbrush except that the brush head has only a small tuft of bristles (Fig. 18-7).
      2. A standard toothbrush easily can be modified to create a customized end-tuft brush by removing some of the bristles.

B. Indications
 1. Effectively reaches sites around teeth that are difficult for patients to clean, such as the distal surface of the last tooth in the arch, lingual surfaces of mandibular teeth, and crowded or malaligned teeth.
 2. Works well to remove plaque from type III embrasure spaces.
 2. Useful in removing plaque from an exposed furcation area since the small size of the bristle tufts allows them to partially enter the furcation site.
C. Technique
 1. The end of the tuft is directed into the embrasure space or furcation area. Gentle circular strokes are used to clean the area.
 2. For difficult-to-reach mandibular lingual tooth surfaces, the brush is used like a standard brush with a sulcular brushing technique.

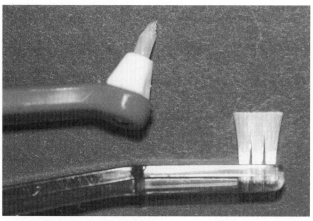

Figure 18-7. End-Tuft Brushes. End-tuft brushes are used to clean areas that are difficult to access with a standard brush.

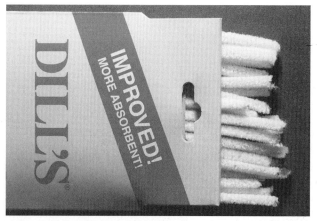

Figure 18-8. Pipe Cleaners. This aid is used to clean type III embrasure spaces.

7. **Pipe Cleaner**
 A. Description. A standard pipe cleaner can be purchased at a shop that specializes in tobacco products and supplies. For purposes of plaque removal, the pipe cleaner should be cut into 3-inch lengths.
 B. Indications for Use of Pipe Cleaners
  1. Effective for type III embrasure spaces.
  2. Can be used between the roots of an exposed furcation area if it can be easily inserted (Fig. 18-8).
 C. Technique
  1. For interproximal plaque removal, the pipe cleaner is inserted into the embrasure space, wrapped around one of the proximal surfaces, and moved back and forth against the proximal surface. Wrap the pipe cleaner around the adjacent proximal surface and repeat.
  2. For exposed furcation areas, the pipe cleaner is inserted carefully through the furcation (do not force).
8. **Wooden Toothpick in a Holder**
 A. Description. This device consists of a round toothpick in a plastic handle.
 B. Indications
  1. Can be used gently along or slightly below the gingival margin for plaque removal.
  2. Effective in type II embrasures if the toothpick is easily inserted between the teeth; however, this aid is not effective in cleaning root concavities unless the teeth are widely spaced.
  3. Can be directed into furcation areas.

C. Technique for Use of a Wooden Toothpick in a Holder
   1. A toothpick is secured in the holder and the long end is broken off flush with the holder so that it will not scratch the inside of the cheek (**Fig 18-9**).
   2. The end of toothpick is moistened with saliva.
   3. The tip is applied at right angles to the gingival margin or directed just beneath the gingival margin at a less than 45° angle. The tip should not be directed against the epithelial attachment. The tip is used to trace the gingival margin around each tooth.
   4. Next, the tip is angled into embrasure spaces or exposed furcation areas and moved gently back and forth to sweep the area free of accumulated plaque.

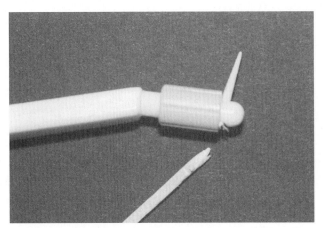

Figure 18-9. Toothpick Holder. To prepare this aid for use, secure a toothpick in the holder and break off the long end so that it is flush with the plastic holder.

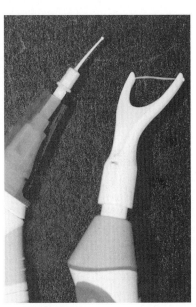

Figure 18-10. Power Dental Flossing Devices. Two examples of power dental flossing devices.

9. **Powered Flossing Devices**
   A. Description. A powered flossing device is a small handheld device for removing plaque biofilm from the proximal surfaces of the teeth. Attachments range from linear tips or picks to floss holders (**Fig. 18-10**).
   B. Benefits of Powered Flossing Devices
      1. In recent research studies, linear tip power flossing devices and those with floss holders have been shown to be as effective as manual flossing in reducing bleeding and gingivitis.[11–13]
      2. Indications for Recommending Power Flossing Devices
         a. In general, a powered device is indicated for patients who have difficulties such as holding the floss correctly, maneuvering floss effectively around teeth, or manipulating the floss through the contact area. Use of power flossing devices has been shown to be preferred by patients over manual flossing.[12]
         b. Patients who are reluctant to place their fingers in their mouth or who are gadget-oriented may find these products user-friendly.
         c. Indications for both types of flossing tips are similar to those for manual dental floss. Additionally, this is a user-friendly product for patients with orthodontic appliances, crown and bridge, or implants.
   C. Directions. Technique is dependent on the type or brand of product. Dental hygienists should read the manufacturer's users guide before recommending and/or demonstrating a powered flossing device to a patient. Patients should be counseled to follow the manufacturer's instructions for the best outcome.

Table 18-1. Aids for Interdental Plaque Removal

Interdental Aid	Description/Example	Indications for Use
Dental floss	Unwaxed or waxed thread made of silk, and nylon, or plastic monofilament fibers	A patient with type I embrasure spaces and excellent compliance to self care regimen
Tufted dental floss	Thickened, yarn-like dental floss (Johnson & Johnson Superfloss)	Type II embrasure spaces, fixed bridges, distal surface of last tooth in the arch, proximal surfaces of widely spaced teeth
Interdental brush	Tiny conical-shaped nylon brushes on a handle (Butler GUM Proxibrush)	Type II or III embrasure spaces Distal surface of last tooth in the arch Exposed furcation areas that permit easy insertion of the brush Embrasure spaces with exposed proximal root concavities
End-tuft brush	Small bristle tuft on a toothbrush-like handle (Butler End-Tuft Brush)	Type III embrasure spaces Distal surface of last tooth in arch Lingual surfaces of mandibular teeth Crowded or malaligned teeth Exposed furcation areas
Pipe cleaner	Standard pipe cleaner cut into 3-inch lengths	Type III embrasure spaces Exposed furcation area that permits insertion
Toothpick in holder	A round toothpick in a plastic handle (Marquis Perio-Aid)	Type II or III embrasure spaces Plaque removal at gingival margin Furcation areas or root concavities
Powered flossers or Interdental cleaners	A powered flossing device (Waterpik Power Flosser and Oral-B Hummingbird)	Type I embrasure spaces Orthodontic appliances with linear tip

SECTION 2: PATIENT-APPLIED HOME IRRIGATION

RATIONALE AND BENEFITS OF ORAL IRRIGATION

1. **Home oral irrigation** involves the use of a pulsating water stream created by a mechanized device to flush an area with water or an antimicrobial agent. Figure 18-11 shows one example of a device used for home oral irrigation.
   A. Pulsating water incorporates a compression and decompression phase that allows debris and bacteria to be efficiently displaced.[14,15]
   B. This pulsation creates two zones of activity.
      1. The area of the mouth where the solution initially contacts is called the **impact zone**.
      2. The subgingival sulcus area that the solution penetrates to is called the **flushing zone**.[16]
   C. **Standard and Subgingival Irrigation Tips.** Irrigation is accomplished using either a standard irrigation tip or a subgingival soft rubber tip.
      1. **Standard irrigation tips** are usually made of a plastic material. The standard tip is used by placing the tip at a 90-degree angle at the neck of the tooth near the gingival margin.
         a. Home oral irrigation devices with standard tips may deliver solution that penetrates 50% or more of the pocket depth.[17]
         b. This type of tip is recommended for generalized, full-mouth irrigation.
      2. **Subgingival irrigation tips** have a soft rubber tipped end.
         a. These tips are used by placing the rubber tip gently beneath the gingival margin. An example of a subgingival irrigation tip is the Pik Pocket subgingival irrigation tip from Waterpik Technologies.
         b. Subgingival placement of the tip allows the water or antimicrobial agent to penetrate deeper into a pocket.
            1) In periodontal pockets 6 mm or less in depth, the subgingival tip may deliver water that penetrates up to 90% of the pocket depth.
            2) In deeper pockets—7 mm or more—depth of penetration is somewhat less at 64% of the depth of the pocket.[18]
   D. Subgingival irrigation tips are recommended for use in areas such as deep pockets, furcation areas, or areas that are difficult to access with a standard tip.

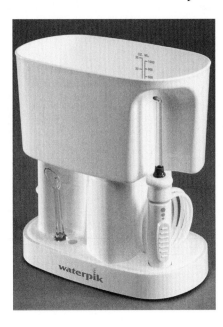

Figure 18-11. Home Irrigation System.
This irrigation unit is an example of a home oral irrigation system that uses a pulsating water stream of water or an antimicrobial agent. (Courtesy of Waterpik Technologies, Ft. Collins, CO.)

2. **Benefits of Home Oral Irrigation.** While previously considered an adjunctive to brushing *and* flossing, new information indicates that home oral irrigation can be considered an effective alternative to daily flossing.[19]
   A. Irrigation is a method of delivering water or antimicrobial agents directly to the periodontal pocket.
   B. Reduction in Bleeding. *Daily home irrigation in combination with manul tooth-brushing has been shown to be more effective in the reduction of gingival bleeding than manual toothbrushing and flossing.*[19–22]
   C. Reduction in Inflammation.
      1. Even though several studies have shown home irrigation to have a minimal effect on plaque removal, significant improvements in inflammation have been demonstrated.
      2. Irrigation may produce these effects by flushing out loosely adherent plaque and toxins or inflammatory substances, although the exact mechanism of action of irrigation is still speculative.
   D. Reduction in Destructive Host Response. Recent studies have shown that home oral irrigation is effective in significantly reducing the inflammatory cytokines—interleukin (IL)-1β and prostaglandin E_2 (PGE_2)—implicated in attachment loss and alveolar bone loss.[23–25]
   E. Patients seem to comply with recommendations to use home irrigators and find it easy to use a standard irrigation tip for supragingival irrigation.[20,27] For subgingival irrigation, it is important to provide patients with clear instructions on its use including the specific areas where the tip should be used.

3. **Indications for Recommending Home Oral Irrigation**
   A. Individuals on Periodontal Maintenance. Home irrigation may have benefits for patients with gingivitis or for those in periodontal maintenance. Studies indicate that home irrigation is an effective means of reducing gingivitis and bleeding on probing; it also has the potential to reduce periodontal pathogens within periodontal pockets.[26–36]
   B. Home irrigation has been shown to be safe and effective for patients with special needs.
      1. Dental Implants. For improving implant health, daily irrigation using the soft rubber tip and 0.06% chlorhexidine (CHX) was superior to rinsing with 0.12% CHX.[32] Although often recommended, the standard jet tip has not been tested on implants.
      2. Individuals with Diabetes. For individuals living with diabetes, twice daily water irrigation using the soft rubber tip improved measures of gingival and systemic health over a 3-month time frame.[37]
      3. Individuals with Orthodontic Appliances. Daily irrigation with water has been demonstrated to provide signfinicant oral health benefits to patients with orthodontic appliances.[38]
      4. Prosthetic Bridgework and Crowns. For individuals with bridgework and/or crowns, daily irrigation produced significant reductions in inflammation.[39]

CONSIDERATIONS FOR IRRIGATOR USE

1. **Precautions For Irrigator Use.** According to the 1997 American Heart Association Recommendations for the Prevention of Bacterial Endocarditis:
   A. Oral irrigator devices used inappropriately or in patients with poor oral hygiene have been implicated in producing bacteremia, but the relationship to bacterial endocarditis is unknown.[40]
   B. Home-use devices pose far less risk of bacteremia in a healthy mouth than the risk presented by ongoing oral inflammation.[40]
      1. Before recommending oral irrigation, practitioners need to consider both the patient's overall medical and oral health status.
      2. A consultation with the patient's physician may be necessary in order to assess the patient's overall risk and execute the best clinical judgment.

2. **Use of Antimicrobial Irrigation Solutions**
   A. *To date, home oral irrigation using antimicrobial agents has NOT been shown to produce superior results than those obtained by home irrigation using water alone.* Therefore, the addition of any antimicrobial agent for home oral irrigation should be considered carefully.
   B. Irrigation Solutions
      1. Chlorhexidine
         a. For home irrigation, chlorhexidine can be diluted with water (Table 18-2). Use of diluted solutions of CHX has been studied in concentrations from 0.02% to 0.06%.
         b. Because of better interproximal and subgingival penetration with irrigation compared to rinsing, a diluted solution of chlorhexidine is acceptable for daily irrigation. In some cases, dilution can minimize staining.
      2. Other Irrigation Solutions
         a. It is best to check with the manufacturer of the irrigation device for information on recommended solutions and dilutions. Some manufacturers do not recommend the use of antimicrobial solutions or mouthwashes as these solutions may damage the device.
         b. Some manufacturers sell premixed solutions for use in their equipment.
3. **Criteria for Equipment Selection.** Selection of an irrigation device is confusing because there are many types on the market. The commercial and scientific claims of all of these devices have yet to be evaluated.
   A. One approach would be to select a device that is ADA-accepted. At this time, the only home irrigation device to receive ADA approval for reducing gingivitis and associated bacteria is the Water Pik Oral Irrigator (Waterpik Technologies).
   B. As each device operates differently in respect to pressure and pulsation, outcomes from studies on one brand of product cannot be transferred to another product brand. Therefore, before recommending any device, it is important to evaluate the research unique to that brand of product.

Table 18-2. Common Dilutions for Chlorhexidine Rinse	
0.02% dilution	5 parts water to 1 part chlorhexidine rinse
0.04% dilution	3 parts water to 1 part chlorhexidine rinse
0.06% dilution	1 part water to 1 part chlorhexidine rinse

TECHNIQUE FOR USE OF IRRIGATION TIPS

1. **General Instructions**
   A. It is important for both dental health care providers and patients to read all instructions thoroughly before using an oral irrigator.
   B. The fluid reservoir can be filled with water, a solution of water and mouthwash, or a solution of an antimicrobial and water.
   C. If using any solution other than water, the irrigation unit should be flushed after use. After using a diluted solution, such as diluted chlorhexidine, clean the unit by filling the reservoir with warm water and holding the handle in the sink. After turning on the unit, run it until the reservoir is empty.
   D. The three basic designs of irrigation tips are the (i) standard jet tip, (ii) soft subgingival tip, and (iii) tongue tip. All tip designs may not be available from all manufacturers. It is important that the dental hygienist give specific instructions for each recommended tip.

2. **Procedure for Use of a Standard Jet Tip**
   A. Adjust the pressure setting to its lowest setting. Over time as the condition of the gingival tissue improves, pressure should be increased to at least the medium setting as this setting is where clinical efficacy has been demonstrated.[15]
   B. The water spray is used to "trace" along the gingival margin with the tip positioned at a 90-degree angle almost touching the gingiva (Fig. 18-12). The tip should be held at each interproximal area for 5 to 6 seconds.

3. **Procedure for Use of a Subgingival Irrigation Tip**
   A. The dental hygienist should determine areas in mouth where use of a subgingival irrigation tip would be beneficial, such as pockets, dental implants, or furcation areas. The patient should be instructed on use of the tip on each area.
   B. The pressure setting is adjusted to its lowest setting. *This tip is designed for use only at the lowest pressure setting.*
   C. The manufacturer's recommendations should be followed for use of the tip. Some tips are placed at the gingival margin, others can be placed 2 mm below the gingival margin.
   D. The tip should be placed at the site prior to starting the irrigation unit. The subgingival tip is directed at a 45-degree angle and placed at the gingival margin or slightly beneath the gingival margin as recommended by the manufacturer (Fig. 18-13).
   E. Once the tip is in place, the irrigation unit is turned on, and the water or solution is allowed to flow for 5 to 6 seconds in the area. After one site has been irrigated, the unit is turned off and the tip is repositioned in the next area of the mouth.

4. **Procedure for Use of a Tongue Irrigation Tip**
   A. The pressure setting is adjusted to its lowest setting. Pressure may be increased over time depending on patient comfort.
   B. The following precautions should be observed for use of a tongue irrigator tip:
      1. Do not use tip if there is an open wound on the tongue.
      2. Do not use tip while wearing any oral jewelry. Remove oral jewelry before use.
   C. The tongue cleaner is placed as far back on the tongue as possible while still maintaining patient comfort. As with manual tongue scrapers, over time the patient will be able to place the tongue tip further back on the tongue without gagging.
   D. Once the tip is in place, the irrigation unit is turned on. The tip is pulled forward, using light pressure. This procedure is repeated until the tongue surface is clean.

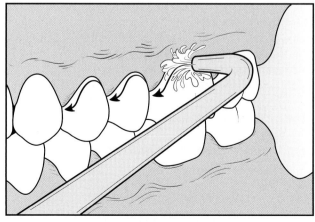

Figure 18-12. Standard Irrigation Tip.

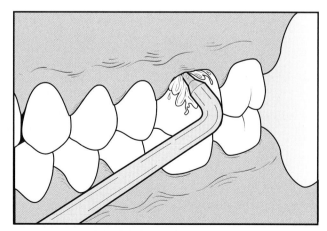

Figure 18-13. Subgingival Irrigation Tip.

SECTION 3: CHEMICAL PLAQUE CONTROL: MOUTH RINSES

Patient applied **chemical plaque control** is the at home use of chemical agents for the control of gingivitis. Therapeutic mouth rinses are primary type of chemical plaque control for at home use.

CRITERIA FOR SELECTION OF A MOUTH RINSE

1. **General Indications**
   A. Mouth rinses are used as adjuncts to mechanical plaque control procedures for controlling *gingivitis* in patients who:
      1. Are unable or unwilling to maintain plaque control.
      2. Have impaired manual dexterity.
      3. Are systemically compromised.
      4. Have just undergone a periodontal surgical procedure.
   B. *It is important for dental hygienists to understand that research studies have **not** documented the effectiveness of mouth rinses in the treatment of periodontitis.*
2. **American Dental Association Seal of Acceptance Program**
   A. The **Council on Dental Therapeutics of the American Dental Association** maintains a seal of acceptance program.
      1. In this program, manufacturers can voluntarily submit documentation demonstrating that their product is both safe and effective.
      2. The documentation submitted by the manufacturer must include multiple long-term studies showing both the safety and the efficacy of the product.
      3. After appropriate evaluation of the documentation, the Council on Dental Therapeutics can award a Seal of Acceptance.
   B. If a product is awarded the **ADA Seal of Acceptance**, the manufacturer must agree to submit advertising copy related to the product to the Council to ensure the absence of false or misleading claims.
   C. Members of the dental team can use the ADA Seal of Acceptance to help guide their recommendations to patients with a high level of confidence.
3. **Types of Mouth Rinses**
   A. **Cosmetic mouth rinses** are products that claim *no therapeutic value.*
      1. Cosmetic products are not included in the acceptance program of the Council on Dental Therapeutics of the American Dental Association.
      2. The routine use of cosmetic mouth rinses by the public is not recommended.
         a. Of concern is the high alcohol content contained in many antiseptic mouth rinses. The alcohol in mouth rinses has no antimicrobial effect, but rather is used as a solution in which to contain the active ingredients of the product.
      3. Patients with certain medical conditions and those recovering from alcohol addiction should avoid mouth rinses with high alcohol content.
   B. **Therapeutic mouth rinses** are products that claim to be beneficial in controlling gingivitis.
      1. *Mouth rinsing is a supragingival procedure; mouth rinses penetrate less than 1 mm into the sulcus.*
      2. Mouth rinses are not effective in the treatment of periodontitis because they cannot reach the base of the pocket.

CHAPTER SUMMARY STATEMENT

The patient plays a vital role in the successful control of periodontal disease. The patient's efforts at self-care are so critical to the control of periodontitis that the patient is regarded as a cotherapist in the process of nonsurgical periodontal therapy. Since the importance of mechanical plaque control is quite high for the patient with periodontitis, the dental hygienist should be knowledgeable about plaque control measures and be prepared to recommend appropriate aids based on the individual needs of each patient.

Interdental plaque control has special importance for the periodontal patient since periodontitis usually damages the interdental tissues first. Interdental aids that are especially useful for patients with type II or III embrasure spaces include interdental brushes and end-tuft brushes. Daily tongue cleaning results in reduced numbers of pathogenic bacteria on the tongue and in the saliva.

Therapeutic mouthrinses may be used as adjuncts to mechanical plaque control procedures; however, they are not effective in the treatment of periodontitis. Home oral irrigation can be a valuable part of a patient's daily self-care routine. Research studies have shown that home irrigation with water provides a reduction of gingivitis, bleeding upon probing, and pocket depths over normal oral hygiene alone in maintenance patients.

SECTION 4: FOCUS ON PATIENTS

CASE 1

A patient with slight (or mild) chronic periodontitis has generalized recession of the interdental gingival papillae. What options would you have for training this patient in interdental plaque control?

CASE 2

You are discussing self-care for plaque removal with a patient with chronic periodontitis. You point out to the patient how the plaque control on the facial and lingual surfaces of his teeth is greatly improved and praise him for this success. The patient comments that he likes using his powered toothbrush and has been brushing longer. Unfortunately, you note that there is heavy plaque on the proximal surfaces of most teeth. The patient tells you that there is, "No way that I am going to use that string. It is just too hard to use." The patient has type II embrasure spaces throughout his mouth. What suggestions might you make for interdental plaque control?

References

1. Jahn CA. Evidence for self-care products: Power brushing and interdental aids. *J Pract Hyg.* 2004;13:24–29.
2. Robinson PG, Deacon SA, Deery C, Heanue M, et al. Manual versus powered toothbrushing for oral health (Cochrane Review). The Cochrane Library, Issue 2, 2005. Chichester, UK: John Wiley & Sons, Ltd.
3. Bakdash B. Current patterns of oral hygiene product use and practices. *Periodonto, 2000.* 1995;8:11–14.
4. Ratcliff PA, Johnson PW. The relationship between oral malodor, gingivitis, and periodontitis: A review. *J Periodontol.* 1999;70:485–489.
5. Kuusela S, Honkala E, Kannas L, et al. Oral hygiene habits of 11-year-old schoolchildren in 22 European countries and Canada in 1993/1994. *J Dent Res.* 1997;76:1602–1609.
6. Lang WP, Ronis DL, Farghaly MM. Preventive behaviors as correlates of periodontal health status. *J Public Health Dent.* 1995;55:10–17.

7. Murtomaa H, Turtola L, Rytomaa I. Use of dental floss by Finnish students. *J Clin Periodontol.*, 1984;11:443–447.

8. Ronis DL, Lang WP, Farghaly MM, et al. Preventive oral health behaviors among Detroit-area residents. *J Dent Hyg.* 1994;68:123–130.

9. Ronis DL, Lang WP, Antonakos, CL, et al. Preventive oral health behaviors among African-Americans and whites in Detroit. *J Public Health Dent.* 1998;58:234–240.

10. Westover W. Results of a seniors' oral health survey in rural Alberta. *Probe.* 1999;33:57–62.

11. Anderson NA, Barnes CM, Russell CM. A clinical comparison of the efficacy of an electro-mechanical flossing device or manual flossing in affecting interproximal gingival bleeding and plaque accumulation. *J Clin Dent.* 1995;6:105–107.

12. Shibly O, Ciancio S, Shostad S, et al. Clinical evaluation of an automated flossing device versus manual flossing. *J Clin Dent.* 2001;12:63–66.

13. Cronin MJ, Dembling WZ, Cugini MA, et al. Safety and efficacy of a novel interdental device [abstract]. *J Dent Res.* 2004;83(Sp Iss):867.

14. Bhaskar SN, Cutright DE, Frisch J. Effect of high pressure water jet on oral mucosa of varied density. *J Periodontol.* 1969;40:593–598.

15. Bhaskar SN, Cutright DE, Gross A, et al. Water jet devices in dental practice. *J Periodontol.* 1971;42:658–664.

16. Cobb CM, Rodgers RL, Killoy WJ. Ultrastructural examination of human periodontal pockets following the use of an oral irrigation device in vivo. *J Periodontol.* 1988;59:155–163.

17. Eakle WS, Ford C, Boyd RL. Depth of penetration in periodontal pockets with oral irrigation. *J Clin Periodontol.* 1986;13:39–44.

18. Braun RE, Ciancio SG. Subgingival delivery by an oral irrigation device. *J Periodontol.* 1992;63:469–472.

19. Barnes CM, Russell CM, Reinhardt RA, et al. Comparison of irrigation to floss as an adjunct to toothbrushing: Effect on bleeding, gingivitis, and supragingival plaque. *J Clin Dent.* 2005;16:71–77.

20. Flemmig TF, Newman MG, Doherty FM, et al. Supragingival irrigation with 0.06% chlorhexidine in naturally occurring gingivitis. 1.6 month clinical observations. *J Periodontol.* 1990;61:112–117.

21. Newman MG, Cattabriga M, Etienne D, et al. Effectiveness of adjunctive irrigation in early periodontitis: Multi-center evaluation. *J Periodontol.* 1994;65:224–229.

22. Macaulay WJ, Newman HN. The effect on the composition of subgingival plaque of a simplified oral hygiene system including pulsating jet subgingival irrigation. *J Periodontal Res.* 1986;21:375–385.

23. Cutler CW, Stanford TW, Abraham C. et al. Clinical benefits of oral irrigation for periodontitis are related to reduction of pro-inflammatory cytokine levels and plaque. *J Clin Periodontol.* 2000;27:134–143.

24. Tsai CC, Ho YP, Chen CC. Levels of interleukin-l beta and interleukin-8 in gingival crevicular fluids in adult periodontitis. *J Periodontol.* 1995;66:852–859.

25. Offenbacher S, Heasman PA, Collins JG. Modulation of host PGE2 secretion as a determinant of periodontal disease expression. *J Periodontol.* 1993;64(5 Suppl):432–444.

26. Jahn CA. Automated oral hygiene self-care devices: Making evidence-based choices to improve client outcomes. *J Dent Hyg.* 2001;75:171–186.

27. Walsh TF, Glenwright HD, Hull PS. Clinical effects of pulsed oral irrigation with 0.2% chlorhexidine digluconate in patients with adult periodontitis. *J Clin Periodontol.* 1992;19:245–248.

28. Brownstein CN, Briggs SD, Schweitzer KL, et al. Irrigation with chlorhexidine to resolve naturally occurring gingivitis: a methodologic study. *J Clin Periodontol.* 1990;17:588–593.

29. Chaves ES, Kornman KS, Manwell MA, et al. Mechanism of irrigation effects on gingivitis. *J Periodontol.* 1994; 65:1016–1021.

30. Ciancio SG, Mather ML. Zambon JJ, et al. Effect of a chemotherapeutic agent delivered by an oral irrigation device on plaque, gingivitis, and subgingival microflora. *J Periodontol.* 1989;60:310–315.

31. Ciancio SG, Lauciello F, Shibly O, et al. The effect of an antiseptic mouthrinse on implant maintenance: Plaque and peri-implant gingival tissues. *J Periodontol.* 1995;66:962–965.

32. Felo A, Shibly O, Ciancio SG, et al. Effects of subgingival chlorhexidine irrigation on peri-implant maintenance. *Am J Dent.* 1997;10:107–110.

33. Fine JB, Harper JP, Gordon JM, et al. Short-term microbiological and clinical effects of subgingival irrigation with an antimicrobial mouthrinse. *J Periodontol.* 1994;65:30–36.

34. Flemmig TF, Epp B, Funkenhauser Z, et al. Adjunctive supragingival irrigation with acetylsalicylic acid in periodontal supportive therapy. *J Clin Periodontol.* 1995;22:427–433.

35. Jolkovsky DL, Waki MY, Newman MG, et al. Clinical and microbiological effects of subgingival and gingival marginal irrigation with chlorhexidine gluconate. *J Periodontol.* 1990;61:663–669.
36. Newman MG, Flemmig TF, Nachnani S, et al. Irrigation with 0.06% chlorhexidine in naturally occurring gingivitis. 11.6 months microbiological observations. *J Periodontol.* 1990;61:427–433.
37. Al-Mubarak S, Ciancio S, Aljada A, et al. Comparative evaluation of adjunctive oral irrigation in diabetics. *J Clin Periodontol.* 2002;29:295–300.
38. Burch J, Lanese R, Ngan P. A two-month study of the effects of oral irrigation and automatic toothbrush use in an adult orthodontic population with fixed appliances. *Am J Orthod Dentofac Orthop.* 1994;106:121–126.
39. Krajewski J, Giblin J, Gargiulo A. Evaluation of a water pressure cleaning device as an adjunct to periodontal treatment. *J Am Soc Periodont.* 1964;2:76–78.
40. Dajani AD, Taubert KA, Wilson W, et al. Prevention of bacterial endocarditis: recommendations by the American Heart Association. *JAMA.* 1997;277:1794–1801.
41. Oyerholser CD, Meiller TF, DePaola LG, et al. Comparative effects of 2 chemotherapeutic mouthrinses on the development of supragingival dental plaque and gingivitis. *J Clin Periodontol.* 1990;17:575–579.

SECTION 5: CHAPTER REVIEW QUESTIONS

1. Who should be involved in determining which devices and aids a patient uses for plaque control?
   A. The dentist
   B. The dental hygienist
   C. The patient
   D. All of the above

2. Power toothbrushes should be recommended ONLY for individuals with a disability.
   A. True
   B. False

3. The technique a patient uses with a power toothbrush is not important since the brush does all of the work.
   A. True
   B. False

4. A coated tongue may contribute to periodontal disease.
   A. True
   B. False

5. Which of the following interdental aids would be recommended for a patient with type I embrasure spaces throughout the mouth?
   A. An interdental brush
   B. Standard dental floss
   C. Tufted dental floss
   D. Toothpick and holder

6. Which of the following might be recommended for plaque removal in an exposed furcation area on a tooth that has experienced gingival recession?
   A. An interdental brush
   B. Standard dental floss
   C. Tufted dental floss
   D. Toothpick and holder

7. Which of the following is the most effective means for cleaning exposed root concavities?
   A. An interdental brush
   B. Standard dental floss
   C. Tufted dental floss
   D. Toothpick and holder

8. Which oral irrigation tip would be most beneficial for use in a deep periodontal pocket?
   A. Standard irrigation tip
   B. Subgingival irrigation tip

Learning Objectives

- Discuss the differences between compliance and adherence.
- List and explain the stages of change.
- Give an example of an intervention strategy for each stage of change.
- Provide examples on how to adopt a patient-centered focus.
- Describe how to assess readiness, importance, and confidence levels in patients.

KEY TERMS

Compliance	Precontemplation stage	Relapse
Adherence	Contemplation stage	Intervention
Health promotion	Preparation stage	Importance
Behavior change	Action stage	Confidence
Stages of Change Model	Maintenance stage	Agenda-setting chart

SECTION 1: LEARNING VERSUS CHANGE

SUCCESSFUL OUTCOMES

1. **Successful Periodontal Therapy Outcomes.** A successful outcome from periodontal treatment and periodontal maintenance hinges on three critical components. Breakdown in any one of these areas can lead not only to untreated or recurrent disease, but also to significant concern and frustration for the healthcare provider.
   A. First, the patient must accept and undergo suggested periodontal therapy to treat the problem.
   B. Second, a strict regimen of self-care must be followed.
   C. Third, there is an ongoing need for periodontal maintenance care on a regular basis.
2. **Compliance versus Adherence.** For a person with periodontal disease, a change in a behavior is necessary for successful management of the disease. These changes include adherence to a daily self-care regimen and keeping regular appointments for professional care.
   A. Compliance refers to the extent to which a patient's behavior is in accordance with the health advice that he or she has received from a healthcare provider. *Compliance simply means that a patient is following the recommendations of a dental professional.*
      1. A major source of frustration for many dental care providers is the lack of compliance by patients to recommended therapy.
      2. Hygienists frequently are baffled by a patient's lack of compliance with oral health care recommendations. For example, any of the following scenarios can be perplexing to the clinician.
         - A patient continually asks about bleaching and ignores advice that periodontal treatment is needed.
         - A patient completes periodontal surgery and returns for 3-month maintenance visits the first year after surgery but is then not seen again for several years.
         - A patient has periodontal surgery and returns regularly for maintenance visits, but has extremely poor self-care habits.
   B. **Adherence.** The term adherence refers to behavior change that is patient-driven (rather than clinician-driven). *Adherence means that a patient has made an informed decision to make a behavior change.*

LEARNING VERSUS BEHAVIORAL CHANGE

1. **The Gap Between What We Do and What We Expect**
   A. The most common approach for motivating a patient is to explain the seriousness of the periodontal problem and the importance of compliance with recommendations for improving periodontal health. Dental health care providers often use a "tell, show, do" approach that may include the following:
      1. Tell: Explaining the problem (gingival bleeding), reasons for the problem (plaque biofilm), and advising what should be done about it (a new approach to daily self-care).
      2. Show: Showing the problem area. This may be accomplished using:
         a. A mirror and visually showing calculus, inflammation, or a deep probing depth
         b. Disclosing solution to highlight plaque and/or a phase contrast microscope to demonstrate plaque organisms
         c. The intraoral camera to bring magnification to the problem
         d. Instruction on how to brush and/or floss
         e. Visuals such as flip charts, tooth models, examples of self-care devices, videos, or CD-ROMs
         f. Brochures or literature for at-home reading

   3. Do: Demonstrating or outlining appropriate behavior for the patient. This may be evidenced by:
      a. Demonstration of proper techniques for the use of an interdental aid.
      b. Explaining the course of action that needs to occur such as scheduling frequent appointments for professional care.
   B. Response to the "Tell, Show, Do" Approach
      1. The "tell, show, do approach"—while an important foundation for patient education—can be "not enough" for some patients and "too much" for others.
      2. Patient responses may range from apathy to defensiveness to anger. It is not uncommon to hear complaints from patients about feeling "yelled at" during a dental appointment.
      3. Conversely, practitioners cannot figure out why "the patient is lazy or doesn't learn."
   C. To elicit more effective behavior change, it is critical to understand the gap that exists between what the practitioner does and the outcome expected. It is reasonable to assume that educational efforts do provide patients with oral health knowledge, but it must be realized that changing behavior is much more difficult and complex.
2. Differentiating Learning and Change
   A. Studies have shown that when asked, patients state they have been informed about their periodontal disease. Yet, like individuals who smoke or are overweight, knowledge about periodontal disease often does not always lead to behavior changes.
   B. Healthcare providers often make the assumption that if a patient is told about periodontal disease and counseled on treatment and therapy, this information will motivate him or her to pursue a course of action. Because dental hygienists often act as the primary health educator in the private practice setting, *it is important to acknowledge and accept that learning often does not motivate a person to change his or her behavior.*
      1. Patients easily understand behavior changes (i.e., "I need to use an interdental aid on a daily basis to remove the dental plaque in my mouth.") but consistent, life-long behavior changes are difficult to maintain.
      2. Failing to maintain a behavior change may cause patients to give up and avoid contact with their hygienist and avoid dental care altogether.
   C. Each adult patient is a unique individual possessing different values, life, cultural, and dental/medical experiences.
      1. For behavior change to occur, a patient must feel the importance or susceptibility of the problem. In other words, not only must the individual understand that periodontal disease may cause tooth loss, he or she must feel that he or she will experience tooth loss.
      2. Life experiences or critical situations often spur behavioral change. Examples might be:
         a. A spouse, relative, or friend loses teeth due to periodontal disease
         b. Loss of tooth function due to pain or mobility makes the possibility of tooth loss seem real to the person
   D. There is no cure for periodontitis.
      1. There is no end point for periodontal patients. For example, with periodontitis, patients can be informed that daily self-care will reduce bleeding. If self-care ceases, however, bleeding begins again.
      2. Additionally, periodontal disease often recurs despite the best efforts. Daily self-care and periodontal maintenance help to control periodontitis, but never cure it.

SECTION 2: THE STAGES OF BEHAVIORAL CHANGE

WHAT WE KNOW ABOUT CHANGE

1. **Research on Change.** Research into alcohol abuse and smoking cessation has given dental health care providers a roadmap for health promotion. **Health promotion**, in the context of periodontics, is the art of helping a person change his or her behaviors to move toward a state of improved periodontal health. The Stages of Change Model provides an important and practical tool for health promotion.
2. Behavior change is the process of identifiable stages through which a patient passes through before adopting a new behavior.
3. The Stages of Change model[1,2] shows that for most persons, a change in behavior occurs gradually (Table 19-1).
   a. The individual moves from being (i) uninterested, unaware, or unwilling to make a change to (ii) considering a change, to (iii) deciding and preparing to make a change.
   b. In the fourth stage, (iv) the patient makes a change, and (v) over time, attempts to maintain the new behavior.

Table 19-1. Stages of Change Model

Stages	Patient Stage
Precontemplation	Not thinking about change, unaware of problem May be resigned to the problem (i.e., bleeding gums, loss of teeth) Feels no control over the problem Denial: does not believe periodontal disease will happen to him or her Believes consequences are not serious or important
Contemplation	Begins to weigh the benefits and costs of behavior change
Preparation	Getting ready for change
Action	Making a change
Maintenance	Maintains new behavior over time
Relapse	Falls back to a previous stage and old behaviors May feel demoralized by this "failure"

THE STAGES OF CHANGE MODEL

1. Precontemplation Stage
   A. Individuals in the precontemplation stage are generally considered resistant to change.
   B. Patients in this stage may think that it is all the other people around them who need to change.
   C. Some of the behaviors that precontemplators may exhibit in a dental office include:
      1. Stating that they *only* came because a spouse, parent, or significant other *made* them
      2. Blaming oral health problems on stress or genetics (something that they do not have to answer for or take control of)
      3. Exhibiting defensiveness about the problem
      4. Rationalizing: "Everyone loses their teeth eventually"
      5. Denying or lacking interest in learning about the causes and treatment of the disease

2. Contemplation Stage

    A. In the contemplation stage, patients begin to recognize there is a problem and start to think about solving it.

    B. At the same time, however, resistance to change is still present.

    C. Clues that a patient may be in the contemplation stage include:

        1. Asking for more information about oral health, periodontal disease, and recommended therapies

        2. More willingness to talk about the problem than in the past

3. Preparation Stage

    A. For individuals in the preparation stage, change is becoming a priority.

    B. In this stage, the person is fixed on making final adjustments that must be made to accomplish the behavior change. It is a time when a patient may go public about the intended change to friends and family.

    C. A person in the preparation change feels increasing confidence about his or her decision to change.

    D. Behaviors to notice in the preparation stage include:

        1. Stating intentions such as, "When I leave this appointment today, I am going to start flossing," or "I am finally ready to get the name of the periodontist I need to see."

        2. Identifying a plan of action. The patient may name an appropriate time to schedule periodontal surgery, such as during an upcoming vacation time.

4. Action Stage. This is the moment everyone has been waiting for; when the patient begins taking actual steps to address or modify the problem at hand. This stage is a hard-won accomplishment on the part of both the patient and the dental team. Some ways the action stage will be obvious are a clinical assessment that shows less plaque and bleeding and appointments for periodontal care are made and kept.

5. Maintenance Stage and Relapse Prevention

    A. In the maintenance stage, individuals strive to turn new actions into lifelong habits.

        1. Unfortunately, it is not uncommon, especially for dental patients, to relapse into old behaviors. Most patients find themselves moving through the stages of change several times before a change becomes truly established.

    B. Cues that a person is about to relapse into old behaviors include:

        1. Mentioning temptations such as a busy lifestyle or being very tired at night as reasons it is difficult to find time for self-care.

        2. Self-blaming for failures; patients need to be reassured that brief lapses do not mean failure. It may help them to know that everyone experiences many stops and starts along the way to behavior change.

INTERVENTIONS TO PROMOTE CHANGE

1. An **intervention** is an approach or strategy that is intended to change a person's knowledge, attitudes, awareness, or behavior in order to improve the periodontal health of the person.

    A. The Stages of Change Model[1,2] is useful for selecting appropriate health promotion interventions. By identifying a person's stage in the change process, dental hygienists can tailor the intervention.

    B. *The focus of the intervention is not to convince a person to change behavior, but rather, to help him or her progress through the stages of change.*

2. Using the structure of the Stages of Change Model, the hygienist's goal should shift away from an unrealistic goal (i.e., getting the patient to change his or her behavior) to a more realistic goal (i.e., identifying the stage of change and involving the person in a process to move to the next stage).

A. **Interventions for the Precontemplation Stage**

1. A person's stage of change can be identified by starting with brief and simple advice, such as, "Changing to a new method for removing plaque from between your teeth would be very helpful in reducing the bleeding."

   a. A person's response to direct advice provides helpful information that the hygienist can use to assess the person's stage of change.

   b. Interventions based on the Stages of Change Model can be tailored to each patient to enhance the chance of success.

      1. For example, a patient responds, "Everyone on my father's side of the family has bleeding gums and they all still have their teeth." The hygienist, who responds by explaining the benefits of using an oral irrigator to reduce gingival bleeding, will most likely be ineffective because this intervention strategy is not matched to the patient's stage of change. The hygienist in this example has jumped to the action stage, while the patient is in the precontemplation stage.

      2. Patient resistance is evidence that the dental hygienist has moved too far ahead of the patient in the change process.

2. Patients in the precontemplation stage can be especially challenging to the hygienist.

   a. Hygienists should engage the patient by developing a positive relationship and asking questions that stimulate patient thinking.

      1. It takes time for a patient to learn to trust that the hygienist is not there to judge or to force him or her into changing.

      2. *The hygienist's role is to support and encourage the person, give advice, provide feedback, and clarify goals. It is not to impose a prescription for change on the patient.*

   b. The goal for the precontemplation stage is to get the patient to begin thinking about changing behavior.

      1. The hygienist should begin by identifying what a patient wants help with. Simple questions can give the hygienist insight into the person's stage of change. For example, "On a scale of 1 to 10 how interested are you in receiving periodontal care?"

   c. Understanding what things are important to the patient—such as cost, avoidance of pain, appearance—can serve as a starting point in the change process.

   d. When dealing with individuals in this stage of change, keep the following in mind:

      1. Resist pushing for action. If the patient is not ready to change, it will not help to keep insisting that he or she learns to how to use an oral irrigation device.

      2. Refrain from the nagging or the "yelling" patients often complain about. If a patient feels chastised at every visit, it can undermine the relationship, and visits may cease.

      3. Keep faith in the individual's ability to eventually change. It is not unusual for a person to remain in the precontemplation stage for years.

      4. Avoid enabling the behavior. Although empathy is important, the patient needs to be informed and understand the consequences of not taking action as well as the general health implications.

      5. Increase frequency of professional care. Disease progression often can be controlled by frequent professional care as a substitute for less than adequate patient self-care.

B. **Interventions for the Contemplation Stage**

1. The contemplation stage may last for quite a while. Effective ways for dealing with contemplators may include:

    a. Refrain from pushing the individual to action. Keep in mind contemplators are thinking about change but still have some resistance. For example, they are considering seeing the periodontist but are not ready just yet.

    b. Provide support, listen, and give feedback. Praise patients for small steps taken. Ask about ways to provide assistance.

  2. Empathy, praise, and encouragement are especially helpful when a patient struggles with uncertainty and doubts about change.[3]

    a. A successful approach is for the hygienist to ask patients about possible strategies to overcome barriers to change.[3] (For example, "What if you scheduled your appointments over your lunch break, so that you would not have to miss so much time from work?")

    b. It is helpful to ask patients about previous methods or attempts to improve their oral health. This approach can open up an avenue for further discussion.

C. Interventions for the Preparation Stage

  1. When a person experiments with changing a behavior, such as cutting down on smoking, he or she is moving toward more decisive action. The hygienist should encourage the person to identify barriers to full-fledged action. For example, "What is the biggest barrier that is keeping you from stopping smoking?" Such a discussion provides opportunities for the hygienist to recommend strategies for change. For example, "I can give you the telephone of the Smoking Quit line. This line provides, among other things, a person to talk to when you have a craving for a cigarette."

  2. Ways to support the patient during the preparation stage include:

    a. Guide the patient to begin with small steps. For example, the patient may state his intention to begin daily flossing, oral irrigation, and use of an interdental aid. The hygienist can gently guide the patient to begin with one behavior at a time.

    b. Continue with encouragement. Explore ways to offer support during the first few days of the change such as reinforcing telephone calls or e-mails.

D. Interventions for the Action Stage

  1. During the action stage, the hygienist should ask the patient about successes and difficulties (i.e., "Do you ever have difficulty getting the interdental brush in this area?").

  2. Action takes energy and commitment, and it is easy to lose momentum for the chosen behavior. Ways to keep patients motivated in this stage include:

    a. Praise. Be generous with praise and admiration.

    b. Reminders. Help the patient remember to floss by suggesting placement of several small containers of it throughout the house.

    c. Rewards. Praise the patient for tremendous progress made. Suggest ways that he or she can reward himself or herself for remembering to floss every day for a week.

E. Interventions for the Maintenance and Relapse Prevention. There are many ways that the dental hygienist can reinforce the maintenance period. These include:

  1. Give credit to the patient. Help the patient feel good by acknowledging what a difficult task they have accomplished.

  2. Continuing to provide support. It is common to offer support during the stages up to and through action, but it is easy to forget that maintenance also requires commitment and energy. Continue to support the patient each time he or she comes in for an appointment.

  3. Continue to ask the patient about successes and difficulties.

    F. Relapse from Changed Behavior. Relapse is common when an individual makes a behavior change.

        1. The hygienist can help by explaining that even though a relapse has occurred that the person has learned something new about himself or herself and about the process of change. For example, a patient may have learned that she does not have enough time to brush and use an interdental brush in the morning since mornings are a hectic time in her household. She might find it easier to use the interdental brush in the evening after the children are asleep.

        2. The hygienist should focus the patient's attention on his or her successes. For example, "Mary, you have learned how to use the interdental brush skillfully and now you have a better plan for finding time to use the interdental brush in your daily schedule."

SECTION 3: ADOPTING A PATIENT-CENTERED FOCUS

Rather than the *dental professional* advising the patient what to do, a **patient-centered approach** focuses on what the *patient* thinks or is *ready* to do.

PATIENT-CENTERED BEHAVIORAL CHANGE

    1. Is the Patient Ready for Change?

        A. The first step in facilitating a patient-centered behavior change is to assess the readiness of the patient to change.

        B. There are two important issues to consider in determining a person's readiness to change. These are (i) importance of the situation to the person and (ii) the individual's confidence in his or her ability to change.[4]

        C. Periodontal patients often have multiple behaviors that need changing, such as smoking cessation, periodontal therapies, and adoption of a new self-care regimen. Simply asking the patient what issue is most important to him or her helps to establish both rapport and a patient-centered focus.

        D. A review of the person's typical day is another tool that can facilitate behavior change. Reviewing a typical day can point out times when a new behavior, such as daily self-care, might fit into the person's schedule.

    2. How Important Is Change to the Patient?

        A. Importance is the value or interest that a person assigns to a behavior.

        1. The change may have a low-level of importance, a high-level of importance, or anywhere in between for the patient.

        2. Just because the dental hygienist feels that daily self-care is important does not mean the patient will (despite being given adequate information on its benefits). In the context of the patient's life, there may be higher priorities.

B. There are several strategies for exploring importance with a patient.[1,2]

    1. Do little more. If the behavior is a very low priority for the patient, do not push for action or a decision. Explore whether there are other issues he would rather discuss.

    2. Rate it on a scale of 1 to 10. If the hygienist senses that the behavioral change holds some importance to the patient, ask the patient to rank the importance on a scale of 1 to 10. From there, it is okay to explore why that number was chosen and what could be done to raise it.

    3. Examine the pros and cons. This is useful when a person is uncertain about change.

    4. A hypothetical look over the fence. This involves asking the patient to "suppose" they have made a change. For example, "How would you feel if you made that first visit to the periodontist?" This approach works well when the change is a high priority for the patient.

3. How Confident Is the Patient?

    A. Confidence is a person's belief or self-assurance in his or her ability to succeed. It is not uncommon for patients to understand health problems but lack the motivation to do anything about them. In fact, research has shown that patients commonly believe that flossing is very important for good oral health, but lack confidence that they can to do it correctly.

    B. The strategies recommended[1,2] for exploring and improving confidence include:

        1. Do little more. This approach is appropriate for those with low confidence. Refrain from pushing the issue and allow the patient time to think about it at home.

        2. Rate it. Assess confidence on a scale of 1 to 10 and explore the reasons for the number and ways to raise it.

        3. Brainstorm solutions. Rather than advise patients on how to change the behavior, encourage them to find ways to do it. For example, there are more ways to floss than just wrapping the string around your fingers. Explore other possibilities including having a selection of alternative powered devices the patient can touch and feel.

        4. Reviewing past successes and failures. This can go hand in hand with brainstorming. Build on things that have worked and evaluate the reason some things have failed. For example, if a person likes using a power toothbrush, he also might like using a powered flossing device.

        5. Reassess confidence. Focus on the strategies that seem to bring the most enthusiasm and confidence to the patient.

AGENDA SETTING BY THE PATIENT

An **agenda-setting chart** is a useful tool when multiple behavior changes are recommended for long-term management of periodontal disease.[5,6] A sample agenda-setting chart is shown in Figure 19-1. The steps in this process are:

1. The hygienist draws boxes on a piece of paper and fills in behavior changes that have been shown to affect periodontal disease. The hygienist also draws some blank boxes on the piece of paper. For example, "toothbrushing," "interdental aids," "quitting smoking," and "frequent professional care" may each occupy a square.

2. The hygienist spends a few minutes *briefly* explaining these ways to improve periodontal health.

3. The hygienist asks the patient what things he or she might like to add to the boxes. For example, the patient might wish to add "get teeth fixed for improved appearance" and "have better smelling breath" in the blank boxes.

4. The hygienist asks the patient to identify which goal he would like to start with. For example, the patient may wish to begin by learning and using a new toothbrushing method.

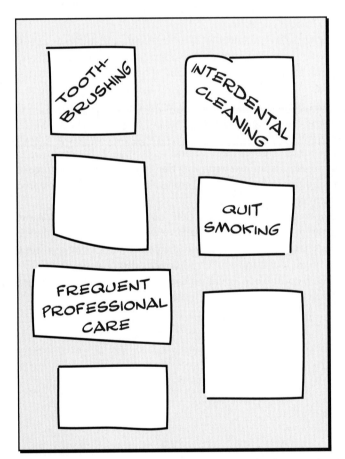

Figure 19-1. Agenda-Setting Chart. Shown here is an example of an agenda-setting chart. Agenda-setting charts are useful tools in helping a patient move into the action stage of behavior change.

CHAPTER SUMMARY STATEMENT

Dental hygienists need to develop skills to assist patients who will benefit from behavior change. The Stages of Change Model provides an important and practical tool for health promotion. For most persons, a change in behavior occurs gradually. An individual moves from being (i) uninterested, unaware, or unwilling to make a change (precontemplation stage) to (ii) considering a change (contemplation), to (iii) deciding and preparing to make a change (preparation).

In the fourth stage (action), (iv) the patient makes a change, and (v) over time, attempts to maintain the new behavior (maintenance).

SECTION 4: FOCUS ON PATIENTS

CASE 1

Mr. Jones, a 58-year-old nonsmoker, has been a long-time patient in the practice. His family comes regularly, but he is very sporadic in his visits and usually states that his wife "nagged" him to come. It has been 3 years since his last visit. At that time, he had progressed to a state of generalized 5-mm pocketing in the posterior teeth. You had strongly recommended periodontal debridement and a daily routine of brushing, flossing, and home irrigation. He scheduled the periodontal debridement appointment but did not show up. When you called him about the missed appointment, he said he was very busy with work and, "Hey, everybody he knows has 'gum' problems. It's part of getting old." When you ask if he had at least implemented the recommended self-care routine, he says "I just told you, I'm busy."

At today's visit with Mr. Jones, he states that he was diagnosed with type 2 diabetes about 6 months ago. He has been working on his diet, and his condition is well-controlled through oral medication. He tells you he knew he was a few pounds overweight and out of shape, but he never thought he would get diabetes. He also states that the doctor told him that diabetes could affect many parts of the body including teeth. So far, he says, he has no additional complications, but he does remember the last time he was in that he "was supposed to have some work done on his gums."

1. What stage of change do you believe Mr. Jones is in? Why?
2. What opening statement might you make to Mr. Jones?
3. Create an agenda setting chart for Mr. Jones, and with a classmate, assume the roles of Mr. Jones and the R.D.H., and role-play through the strategy.
4. Based on what you heard from the agenda setting, what do you recommend next for Mr. Jones?

CASE 2

Sue Smith, a 42-year-old, periodontally healthy, nonsmoker has not been in for a prophylaxis since she became a first-time mother (to twins) nearly 1 year ago. Uncharacteristically, she is late for her appointment. When she does arrive, she appears frazzled, and before she even gets to the chair she says, "You're going to be mad at me; I haven't flossed in a year! I'm mad at myself." Sue had started coming to your office about 5 years ago after she married her husband, who was already a patient in the practice. At that time, she had some early gingivitis and admitted that she did not floss regularly because "the string always broke." After finding a type of floss compatible with her mouth, she had turned into one of your most motivated and oral health conscious patients.

1. What stage of change do you believe Sue is in? Why?
2. What is your response to her opening statement, that you will be mad at her?

3. With another classmate, assume the roles of Sue and the R.D.H., and take 5 minutes to go through a typical day for Sue.
4. Based on what you have heard about Sue's day, what strategies might you recommend to help Sue get back into flossing?

CASE 3

Your last patient of the day is Jane Davis. She is a 50-year-old former smoker who had periodontal surgery about 3 years ago. She is faithful to her 3-month maintenance visits but still has problems with her daily self-care regimen. The first thing she says to you when you seat her is, "I do just great for the first few weeks after my appointment, and then I start to forget. What can I do to stay on track?"

1. With a classmate, assume the roles of Jane and the R.D.H., and role-play the strategies of assessing importance and confidence regarding home self-care for Jane.
2. Based on your findings, would you target importance or confidence as the area needing the most attention? Why?
3. What strategies would you use to increase either importance or confidence?

CASE 4

Jake, a 17-year-old junior in high school, has been a patient in the practice since he was 3-years-old. He comes in every 6 months and is a faithful brusher. He completed orthodontic treatment 1 year ago and is feeling confident about his smile. He is quiet and doesn't ask many questions. He thinks his mouth is doing and feeling great. When asked about flossing he states, "The gums bleed once in a while when I do floss so I don't like to floss very often." He is more concerned about white teeth and fresh breath.

1. What stage of change do you believe Jake is in regards to flossing? Why?
2. How important is flossing to Jake? How could you assess importance?
3. Which item would you begin talking with him about?
4. What would be your opening question?
5. Based on Jake's comments, what strategies would you use to increase importance and readiness?

References

1. Prochaska JO, DiClemente CC, Norcross JC. In search of how people change. *Am Psychol*,.1992;47:1102–1104.
2. Prochaska JA, Norcross DiClemente CC. *Changing for Good: A Revolutionary Six-Stage Program For Overcoming Bad Habits and Moving Your Life Positively Forward*. New York: Avon Books; 1994.
3. Smith DE, Heckemeyer CM, Kratt PP, et al. Motivation interviewing to improve adherence to a behavioral weight-control program for older obese women with NIDDM. A pilot study. *Diabetes Care*. 1997;20:50–54.
4. Stewart JE, Wolfe GR, Maeder L, et al. Changes in dental knowledge and self-efficacy scores following interventions to change oral behavior. *Patient Educ Couns*. 1996;**27**:269–277.
5. Miller RW, Rollnick S. *Motivational Interviewing*. New York: Guilford Press; 2002.
6. Scott NC, Rees M, Rollnick S, et al. Professional responses to innovation in clinical method: Diabetes care and negotiating skills. *Patient Educ Couns*. 1996;29:67–73.

ACKNOWLEDGMENT

The author would like to acknowledge Carol A. Jahn for her contribution as author of this chapter in the previous edition.

SECTION 5: CHAPTER REVIEW QUESTIONS

1. The extent to which a person's behavior is in accordance with the health advice that he or she has received from a healthcare provider?
   A. Adherence
   B. Compliance

2. A behavior change that is patient-driven is termed:
   A. Adherence
   B. Compliance

3. Explaining the causes of periodontal disease and recommending changes in the patient's behavior usually results in a change in the patient's behavior.
   A. True.
   B. False.

4. A person who believes that periodontal disease has no important consequences for him is in which of the Stages of Change?
   A. Preparation
   B. Precontemplation
   C. Action
   D. Maintenance

5. A person who is experimenting with small changes in behavior is in which of the Stages of Change?
   A. Preparation
   B. Precontemplation
   C. Action
   D. Maintenance

6. A person who has been using an interdental brush on a daily basis for 5 years is in which of the Stages of Change?
   A. Preparation
   B. Precontemplation
   C. Action
   D. Maintenance

7. A person who is ready to make a change in his behavior is in which of the Stages of Change?
   A. Preparation
   B. Precontemplation
   C. Action
   D. Maintenance

8. An agenda-setting chart is a useful tool for determining which behavior change a patient would like to work on first.
   A. True.
   B. False.

Chapter

20 Nutrition and Periodontal Disease

Learning Objectives

- Discuss how good nutrition benefits oral health.
- List nutrients necessary to build healthy periodontal tissues and explain the function of each one.
- List nutrients that assist the body with wound healing and explain the function of each one.
- Explain the benefits to periodontal tissues of including chewy/crunchy foods with each meal.
- Create a meal plan including foods that keep oral tissues healthy.

KEY TERMS

Ascorbic acid-deficiency gingivitis

Osteoporosis

Recommended daily allowance (RDA)

SECTION 1: THE INFLUENCE OF DIET AND NUTRITION ON THE PERIODONTIUM

RELATIONSHIP BETWEEN NUTRITION AND THE ORAL CAVITY

The human body requires daily nourishment to carry out all body functions. Each of us gets nourishment from food and drink but our diet preferences are as unique as we are. There is a wide range of food choice practices in the human population, dictated by cultural, religious, economic, and geographical influences. A person who increases the number of behaviors that promotes overall good health, like exercise, staying smoke-free, and eating a healthy diet have a lowered incidence of periodontal disease.[1]

1. **Relationship Between Healthy Food Choices and the Oral Cavity.** Most people are aware that a well-nourished body performs optimally and maintains a strong immune system, but few recognize the relationship between healthy food choices and a healthy oral cavity. There are two major diseases that affect the dentition: dental caries and periodontal disease.
   A. Dental Caries. The relationship between diet and dental caries is clear and well documented, establishing a simple equation: plaque bacteria plus carbohydrates equals acid that demineralizes enamel.
   B. Periodontal Disease
      1. Scientists have searched for a specific connection between diet and periodontal disease.[2,3]
         a. It has not been established that a nutrient deficiency alone can cause a periodontal infection or that nutritional supplements or diet alone can prevent the progression of periodontal disease.
         b. The overall nutritional status of an individual can secondarily affect a person's susceptibility to periodontal disease and may influence disease progression.
      2. *If one statement can be made about the relationship between diet and periodontal disease, it is that poor nutrition will not cause periodontal disease, but it will exacerbate an already existing condition.*
2. **Effects of Nutrient Deficiencies on the Periodontium** (Table 20-1)
   A. Vitamin A Deficiency. Vitamin A works to promote cell differentiation, allowing each cell to mature to perform a specific function.
      1. If Vitamin A is deficient then the cell differentiation and maturing process can be affected. In animal studies a deficiency of Vitamin A altered epithelial integrity and caused keratinization of nonkeratinized mucosa.
      2. For humans, there needs to be continued research in this area for an association of periodontal disease and a deficiency of Vitamin A.
   B. Vitamin B Complex Deficiency. Oral changes common to B complex deficiencies include glossitis (inflammation of the tongue), gingivitis, angular cheilosis (fissuring at the corners of the mouth), and inflammation of the entire oral mucosa.
   C. Vitamin C Deficiency
      1. The epidemiologic data from the Third National Health and Nutrition Examination Survey suggest that diets low in vitamin C plus the habit of smoking produce an increased risk for periodontal disease.
      2. Vitamin C deficiency increases the permeability of the sulcular epithelium.
      3. **Ascorbic acid-deficiency gingivitis** is a sign of a severe vitamin C deficiency called scurvy.
         a. This type of gingivitis is characterized by bleeding gums and petechiae— tiny red spots under the mucosa that are the result of the escape of a very small amount of blood into the tissue.
         b. Vitamin C deficiency appears to be a secondary factor that can exaggerate *existing* inflammation of the periodontium.

D. Vitamin D Deficiency

1. **Osteoporosis** is a condition of decreased bone mass. Osteoporosis leads to fragile bones that are at an increased risk for fractures. "Porosis" means spongy, which describes the appearance of osteoporosis bones when they are broken in half and the inside is examined. Normal bone marrow has small holes within it, but a bone with osteoporosis will have much larger holes.

2. With osteoporosis, bone density is lost primarily from skeletal bones, but alveolar bone loss has been documented in persons with osteoporosis. Bone loss increases if periodontitis is present in conjunction with osteoporosis.

Table 20-1. Oral Deficiency Symptoms

Vitamin	Oral Symptom of Deficiency
A	Xerostomia Oral Leukoplakia Hyperkeratosis Hyperplastic gingival tissue
B	Red swollen lips with vertical fissures and chelosis Smooth, red, burning tongue (glossitis) Red, ulcerated, burning gingival tissues Angular cheilosis (fissuring at the corners of the mouth)
C	Purplish red, swollen, bleeding gingival tissues Loose teeth Slow gingival healing time
D	Inadequate healing of bone Loss of alveolar bone Thinning of the latticelike bone filling the interior of the alveolar process
K	Poor blood clotting, failure of wounds to stop bleeding

Adapted from Sroda R. *Nutrition for a Healthy Mouth.* Philadelphia: Lippincott Williams & Wilkins; 2006:70.

BUILDING HEALTHY PERIODONTAL TISSUES

1. **Nutrition's Role in Maintaining Oral Health.** Like the rest of the body, the hard and soft tissues of the periodontium have nutritional needs for development and maintenance. **Table 20-2** summarizes the beneficial functions of nutrients and minerals in the oral cavity.

Table 20-2. Functions of Nutrients and Minerals in the Oral Cavity

Nutrient/Mineral	Function
Vitamin A	Builds and maintains healthy gingival epithelial tissues Aids in health of host immune system
B-Complex	Forms new cells Aids in health of host immune system
Vitamin C	Aids with wound healing Helps the host resist infection
Vitamin D	Aids with calcium absorption
Protein	Promotes growth, maintenance, and repair of tissues
Calcium	Builds and maintains the alveolar process
Iron	Forms collagen in connective tissues Aids in wound healing Regulates inflammatory responses
Zinc	Forms collagen in connective tissues Aids in wound healing Regulates inflammatory responses
Copper	Aids in wound healing
Selenium	Prevents harm to cells
Magnesium	Works with vitamin D and calcium to build and maintain the alveolar process

Adapted from Sroda R. *Nutrition for a Healthy Mouth.* Philadelphia: Lippincott Williams & Wilkins; 2006:152.

2. **Recommended Daily Allowance.** The **recommended daily allowance (RDA)** is the amounts of nutrients and calories an individual is recommended to consume daily.
   A. Sulcular epithelium has a turnover rate of 3 days, one of the fastest of all body tissue. To help the body continually generate healthy sulcular epithelium, one should consume the recommended daily allowance of protein, vitamins A, B complex, D, and the minerals calcium and magnesium.

B. Together, the recommended nutrients build and maintain healthy gingival tissue and strong alveolar bone.

1. Protein. Protein is a major nutrient that is needed for growth, maintenance, and repair. Adequate protein intake will provide the body with nutrients needed to synthesize new epithelial cells.

2. Vitamin A. Eating foods rich in vitamin A will assist in building healthy sulcular lining and enhance the immune system. If the body is depleted of vitamin A, there may be an altered response to infection, and a diseased sulcus may take longer to repair itself.

3. B-complex Vitamins. Thiamin, riboflavin, niacin, pyroxidine, cobalamin, folic acid, biotin, and pantothenic acid work together as cofactors. They are vital to the formation of new cells and in keeping the immune system strong.

4. Vitamin D. This vitamin enhances the absorption of calcium and magnesium, giving strength to the alveolar process that supports the dentition. Decreased dietary intake of calcium results in poorly calcified alveolar process and more severe periodontal disease.

3. **Assisting the Periodontium with Repair**

A. A periodontal infection is a "wound" that the body needs to heal and inadequate nutrition may cause impairment of the repair process.

B. Certain nutrients will assist the body with the repair (Box 20-1).

1. Protein is the major nutrient that maintains and repairs diseased or wounded tissue. Antibodies are made from protein that target and destroy specific disease causing invaders.

2. Vitamin C assists the body in making collagen, a substance that helps with the repair of wounds. The vitamin C deficiency disease is scurvy and manifests as purplish-red, swollen, bleeding gingival tissues.

3. Minerals iron, zinc, and copper assist with collagen formation.

Box 20-1

Nutrients Needed to Repair Damaged Tissue

- Protein
- Vitamin C
- Iron
- Zinc
- Copper

FIBROUS FOODS PROMOTE PERIODONTAL HEALTH

1. Eating crunchy, fibrous foods can have a beneficial effect on the periodontium.

A. The process of chewing textured foods increases salivary production. Saliva has antibacterial properties that can protect gingival tissues.

B. The physical effect of chewing exercises the periodontal ligament space and creates stronger periodontal fiber attachment. Bone development is denser allowing for a stronger support of teeth.

C. Including one crunchy food with each meal brings more saliva into the oral cavity to help with oral clearance of the food.

2. A diet consisting mainly of soft sticky food will:

A. Take longer to clear the oral cavity

B. Cause accumulation of more plaque

SECTION 2: INCLUDING NUTRITIONAL COUNSELING IN TREATMENT

COUNSELING PATIENTS

1. **Nutritional Counseling in Periodontal Care.** Ideally, nutritional counseling should be part of the treatment plan for every patient with periodontal disease.
   A. Just as you would counsel a patient to eliminate foods that contribute to dental caries, patients should be informed about foods that keep their immune system healthy and foods that contain nutrients that promote healing.
   B. A 7-day diet diary provides an accurate account of food selection. A 3-day diet diary can reveal important information also, as long as it includes at least one weekend day.
2. **Making Healthy Food Choices.** Unhealthy lifestyle choices, disease, and medications can increase a person's risk for periodontal disease. Although a patient cannot change the fact that he or she has a disease or takes medication, he or she can learn to make a change in their food choices.
   A. Nutritional recommendations for periodontal health are the same for overall health:
      1. Follow the USDA Food Guide Pyramid http://www.nal.usda.gov/fnic/Fpyr/pyramid.html
      2. Follow the 2005 Dietary Guidelines for Healthy Americans http://www.healthierus.gov/dietaryguidelines
      3. Take a daily multivitamin that contains the recommended daily allowance for all vitamins and minerals
      4. Include at least one fibrous, crunchy food with each meal
      5. Eat foods rich in vitamins A, B complex, D, protein, and minerals like calcium, magnesium, iron, zinc, copper, and selenium.
   B. Refer to **Table 20-3** for food choice suggestions for a healthy oral cavity.

Table 20-3. Nutrient Rich Foods to Keep the Oral Cavity Healthy

Nutrient	Food Sources
Vitamin A	Carrots, yellow and orange fruits and vegetables, spinach, broccoli, liver, eggs, butter, and fortified foods
B Complex	Fortified cereals, whole grains, dairy products, meats, poultry, fish, vegetables, fruits
Vitamin C	Kiwi, citrus fruits, cantaloupe, strawberries, leafy green vegetables, and cruciferous vegetables
Vitamin D	Liver, egg yolks, fish oil (the body manufactures from sun)
Protein	Meat, milk, eggs, fish, crustaceans, legumes, peas, beans, grains
Calcium	Dairy products, tofu, broccoli, and legumes
Iron	Meat, fish, poultry, egg yolks, leafy greens, legumes
Zinc	Meat, poultry, fish
Copper	Liver, whole grains, nuts, legumes, vegetables, fruits
Selenium	Grains, vegetables, meats
Magnesium	Leafy green vegetables, nuts, meats, legumes, grains

WHERE DOES NUTRITIONAL COUNSELING FIT?

The following topics are suggestions for integrating nutrition/diet information as a routine part of patient education:

1. With *pregnant women and parents*, discuss the following points:
   A. Adequate nutrition throughout pregnancy to ensure fetal development and oral structure development
   B. Prevention of early childhood caries by weaning the baby off of the bottle to a cup by the first birthday
   C. Fluoride as an essential nutrient for developing teeth systemically
   D. Dietary sources of iron since it is a common nutrient deficiency
   E. Snacking habits of children, frequency of carbohydrate intake, hidden sugars
   F. Consumption of bottled water by children—are they missing out on fluoridated water?
2. With *children*, discuss the following points:
   A. Snacking habits, healthy food choices, hidden sugars
   B. Cariogenicity of foods, stickiness, frequency
   C. Sugar substitutes for caries control
   D. Sources of systemic and topical fluoride, not swallowing toothpaste
   E. Calcium, vitamin D intake for developing bones and teeth
3. With *adolescents*, discuss the following points:
   A. Healthy overall nutrition for remaining growth and development/calcium intake
   B. Food independence, influence of peers
   C. Healthier fast food choices
   D. Fad dieting, eating disorders and oral manifestations
   E. Physical activity, athletic performance and nutritional status
   F. Reading food labels, identifying nutrient quality of food
4. With *adults*, discuss the following points:
   A. Food variety using the Food Guide Pyramid
   B. Adequate vitamin/mineral intake for periodontal health
   C. Chewing problems for edentulous or surgery patients, liquid/soft diets
   D. Carbohydrate intake and risk for root caries
   E. Decreased sense of taste, smell, possible effects on appetite and overall health
   F. Adequate dietary calcium and prevention of osteoporosis
   G. Diabetes and periodontal disease, wound healing
   H. Nutrient and drug interactions
5. With *post-surgical patients*, suggest:
   A. Patients undergoing periodontal surgery may need suggestions for soft or liquid diets on a short-term basis when chewing is uncomfortable.
   B. A soft or liquid diet can be recommended to patients who have no special therapeutic dietary needs. Those persons already following therapeutic or diabetic meal plans who need suggestions for soft or liquid diets may need to consult a registered dietitian for diet modification.

CHAPTER SUMMARY STATEMENT

Educating patients that oral health is interdependent with general health is an important part of periodontal treatment. Nutrition and dietary choices can be modified to improve both oral and general health. The challenge is to integrate current nutrition information in the periodontal treatment plan to help reduce oral disease.

SECTION 3: FOCUS ON PATIENTS

CASE 1

A new patient in your practice is a 29-year-old female with a history of gestational diabetes during her second pregnancy last year. She presents with moderate gingivitis, generalized moderate calculus, and posterior pocket depths of 4 to 5 mm. She complains about wanting to lose the extra 20 pounds she did not lose after the second pregnancy. She is also tired of her gums bleeding when she brushes. What are the implications for your treatment plan?

CASE 2

A 42-year-old recall patient returns to your office for a routine visit. He has not been seen for about a year. He is noticeably thinner than the last time you saw him, and he reports that he has a new sales job and travels frequently. He admits his "quit smoking" plan has not worked, and that driving and smoking are part of his busy routine. His blood pressure is slightly elevated and he presents with moderate subgingival calculus interproximally. Upon probing you find pocket depths that were 4 mm are now 5 mm. What are the implications for your treatment plan?

CASE 3

A 52-year-old male is new to your practice and presents with generalized 6- to 7-mm pockets in mandibular and maxillary posteriors. Tissues are marginally red with generalized slight to moderate bleeding upon probing. Oral examination reveals a bright red shiny tongue, extraction of all third molars and large carious lesions on three posterior teeth. He reports eating a soft diet due to broken carious teeth and is a practicing vegetarian. His last dental visit was over 10 years ago. Evaluation of oral hygiene practices reveals ineffective daily plaque removal with the 30-minute random toothbrushing method and no interproximal cleaning. What can be deducted about the relationship between his diet and oral condition, and what would you recommend during diet counseling?

References

1. Al-Zaharani MS, Borawaski EA, Bissada NF. Periodontitis and three health-enhancing behaviors: Maintaining normal weight, engaging in recommended level of exercise, and consuming a high-quality diet. *J Periodontol*. 2005;76:1362–1366.
2. Al-Zahrani MS, Bissada NF, Borawski EA. Diet and periodontitis. *J Int Acad Periodontol*. 2005;7:21–26.
3. Neiva RG, Steigenga J, Al-Shammari KF, et al. Effects of specific nutrients on periodontal disease onset, progression and treatment. *J Clin Periodontol*. 2004;30:579–896.
4. Boyd LD, Madden TE. Nutrition, infection, and periodontal disease. *Dent Clin North Am*. 2004;47:337–354.
5. Sroda R. Nutrition for a healthy mouth. In: *Diet, Nutrition, and Periodontal Disease*. Balitmore: Lippincott, Williams and Wilkins; 2006.

SECTION 4: CHAPTER REVIEW QUESTIONS

1. A deficiency of protein in the diet will cause periodontal disease.
   A. True
   B. False

2. Which of the following vitamins enhances the absorption of calcium and magnesium?
   A. Vitamin A
   B. Vitamin B complex
   C. Vitamin C
   D. Vitamin D

3. Which of the following minerals aids with wound healing?
   A. Copper
   B. Selenium
   C. Magnesium
   D. Calcium

4. Chewing fibrous foods will remove plaque at the gingival margin, thereby reducing the incidence of periodontal disease.
   A. True
   B. False

5. A healthy immune system decreases the incidence of periodontal disease.
   A. True
   B. False

Chapter

21 Periodontal Surgical Concepts for the Dental Hygienist

Refer to the CD packaged with this book for full color versions of the clinical photographs in this chapter.

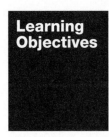
Learning Objectives

- List the objectives for periodontal surgery.
- Explain the term relative contraindications for periodontal surgery.
- Define the terms repair, reattachment, new attachment, and regeneration.
- Explain special considerations for the dental hygienist for the following types of periodontal surgery:
  - Periodontal flap for access
  - Bone replacement grafts
  - Guided tissue regeneration
  - Apically positioned flap with osseous surgery
  - Mucogingival surgery/periodontal plastic surgery
  - Crown lengthening surgery
  - Gingivectomy
  - Dental implant surgery
- List three general guidelines for suture removal.
- List four general guidelines for periodontal dressing management.
- Explain the important topics that should be covered in postsurgical instructions.
- List the eight steps in a postsurgical visit.

KEY TERMS

Elevation
Osseous defect
Osseous surgery
Relative contraindications
Repair
Long junctional epithelium
Reattachment
New attachment
Regeneration
Resective
Periodontal flap
Flap for access
Bone replacement graft

Autograft
Guided tissue regeneration
Apically positioned flap with osseous surgery
Mucogingival surgery
Periodontal plastic surgery
Soft tissue graft
Connective tissue graft
Free gingival graft
Crown lengthening surgery
Dental implant
Gingivectomy
Gingival curettage

SECTION 1: INTRODUCTION TO PERIODONTAL SURGERY

As a member of the dental team, a dental hygienist must be able to respond to patients' questions and concerns about periodontal surgery and communicate with other health care providers about this important topic. The objective of this chapter is to provide the dental hygienist with foundation information related to understanding periodontal surgery. Since this textbook is written specifically for the dental hygienist, this chapter does not include details for surgical techniques; these details are readily available in most standard periodontal textbooks.

1. **Historical Perspective.** Historically periodontal surgery has evolved dramatically over several decades.
    A. Originally periodontal surgery was used primarily to remove damaged tissues that were thought to be diseased.
    B. Modern periodontal surgery has evolved to a level of sophistication and scope that makes this modality an integral part of most aspects of dental care.
2. **Benefits of Modern Periodontal Surgery.** All busy general dental practices encounter many patients that can benefit from periodontal surgery.
    A. In most instances, as the severity of periodontitis increases, controlling the disease becomes more difficult and the need for periodontal surgery as part of comprehensive patient care becomes more likely.
    B. Modern periodontal surgery can be used to support other aspects of patient care such as (i) enhancing restorative procedures, (ii) improving patient appearance, and (iii) preparing a patient for implant supported prostheses.

INDICATIONS FOR PERIODONTAL SURGERY

Periodontal surgery is necessary when the periodontium is unhealthy and cannot be repaired with nonsurgical treatment. Box 21-1 outlines some of the indications for periodontal surgery. The scope of periodontal surgery has evolved to include most aspects of comprehensive dental care. Indications for periodontal surgery are discussed briefly below, and subsequent sections of this chapter provide more details about the various types of periodontal surgery.

Box 21-1

Indications for Periodontal Surgery

- To provide access for improved root surface debridement
- To reduce pocket depths
- To provide access for treatment of periodontal osseous defects
- To resect or remove tissues
- To regenerate the periodontium lost due to disease
- To graft bone or bone stimulating materials into osseous defects
- To improve the appearance of the periodontium
- To enhance prosthetic dental care
- To allow for placement of a dental implant

---

1. **To Provide Access for Improved Periodontal Instrumentation of Root Surfaces**
    A. As probing depths increase, it becomes more and more difficult to access root surfaces for thorough periodontal instrumentation.

    B. Carefully planned incisions through the gingiva can allow for temporary **elevation**—lifting of the soft tissue off the tooth surface. Elevation of the soft tissue provides improved access to root surfaces in deeper periodontal pockets. More details about this type of surgery are presented under flaps for access in the Descriptions of Surgery section of this chapter.

2. To Reduce Pocket Depths

    A. As a pocket depth increases, it becomes too deep to clean with daily at home self-care and plaque biofilms thrive in the environment of the deep pocket.

    B. Surgical procedures reduce the pocket depths so that a combination of daily self-care and professional care increases the chance of maintaining the teeth.

3. To Provide Access to Periodontal Osseous Defects

    A. An **osseous defect** is a deformity in the alveolar bone.

        1. As periodontal disease advances, bone loss results in changes in the normal shape and structure of the alveolar bone.

        2. The pattern of bone loss can vary from one tooth to the next and on different aspects of the same tooth.

    B. Periodontal surgery to modify the bone level or shape is called **osseous surgery**.

        1. Bone defects can be managed surgically through a variety of techniques.

        2. Information about how osseous defects can be managed using periodontal surgery is presented under the topics apically positioned flap with osseous surgery, bone replacement graft, and guided tissue regeneration in the Descriptions of Surgery section of this chapter.

4. To Resect or Remove Tissue

    A. Enlarged gingival tissues can be unsightly and can also interfere with proper oral hygiene measures. In some patients, enlarged gingiva can even interfere with comfortable mastication.

    B. Periodontal surgery can be used to remove and reshape enlarged gingiva. Additional information on this type of periodontal surgery is found in the Descriptions of Surgery section under gingivectomy.

5. To Regenerate the Periodontium Lost Due to Disease

    A. One of the long-range goals in periodontics is to be able to regenerate the periodontium lost because of disease. The term regenerate implies growing back lost cementum, lost periodontal ligament, and lost alveolar bone.

    B. Regenerative procedures can reverse some of the damage by regenerating lost bone and tissue. Although it is not possible to regenerate the periodontium in all instances, it is possible to achieve this regeneration in many sites using some sophisticated periodontal surgical techniques. Information on periodontal surgery that can be expected to regenerate the periodontium is presented under guided tissue regeneration in the Descriptions of Surgery section.

6. To Graft Bone or Bone-Stimulating Materials Into Osseous Defects

    A. Some periodontal osseous defects offer the opportunity for the periodontal surgeon to graft either bone or bone-stimulating materials into the defects.

    B. Although this surgery may seem quite similar to regeneration surgery, grafting bone does not necessarily imply regeneration of other parts of the periodontium such as cementum and periodontal ligament. More information on this interesting topic is located under bone replacement graft in the Descriptions of Surgery section of this chapter.

7. To Improve the Appearance of the Periodontium

    A. Some patients have gingival levels or gingival contours that result in an unattractive smile. Periodontal surgery includes a variety of techniques for improving the appearance of the gingiva and improving the quality of a patient's smile.

    B. There are, of course, many restorative techniques for improving the appearance of the teeth themselves, but in many patients alteration of the appearance of the gingiva is also needed to achieve a truly pleasing appearance. More information on this topic is found in the Descriptions of Surgery section under mucogingival surgery/periodontal plastic surgery and crown lengthening surgery.

8. **To Enhance Prosthetic Dental Care**
   A. Modern prosthetic dental care can create the need for a variety of periodontal surgical procedures such as altering alveolar ridge contours, lengthening tooth crowns, or augmenting the amount of gingiva actually present.
   B. Modern periodontal surgery includes many procedures directed toward enhancing some aspect of restorative dentistry, and enhancing prosthetic dental care may involve combinations of all types of periodontal surgery. In the Descriptions of Surgery section, the topic of crown lengthening surgery discusses one important aspect of enhancing prosthetic care with periodontal surgery.
9. **To Allow for the Placement of a Dental Implant**
   A. Replacement of missing teeth is an option that must be considered when natural teeth are lost. This topic of dental implants is discussed in Chapter 24, but is listed here as one of the indications for periodontal surgery for completeness of this list of indications.
   B. Periodontal surgery can also be used to prepare sites for dental implants.
      1. One the basic tenets of dental implant placement is that the implant must be surrounded by sound alveolar bone.
      2. It is not at all unusual for edentulous sites—where implants are to be placed—to be deficient in the amount of alveolar bone needed to surround the implant. Such sites require some type of bone grafting procedure prior to implant placement.

CONTRAINDICATIONS FOR PERIODONTAL SURGERY

1. **Contraindications for Surgery Are Relative**. Most contraindications for periodontal surgery are **relative contraindications**. The term relative contraindication is used to convey the idea that each patient is different from all others.
   A. Certain conditions may make periodontal surgery inadvisable for some patients when the conditions or situations are severe or extreme. These same conditions, however, may not be contraindications in other patients when the conditions are mild.
   B. An example of this concept might be patients with hypertension (high blood pressure). A patient with uncontrolled hypertension would not be a candidate for periodontal surgery as long as the blood pressure remains severely elevated. At the same time, a patient with only mildly elevated blood pressures may be a suitable candidate for periodontal surgery.
2. Box 21-2 outlines a list of the more common *relative contraindications* for periodontal surgery; each of these relative contraindications is discussed briefly below.

Box 21-2

Relative Contraindications for Periodontal Surgery

- Patients who have certain systemic diseases or conditions
- Patients who are totally noncompliant with self-care
- Patients who have a high risk for dental caries
- Patients who have unrealistic expectations for surgical outcomes

A. Patients who have certain systemic diseases or conditions

1. Systemic diseases or conditions that are relative contraindications for periodontal surgery include conditions such as the following:

    a. Recent history of myocardial infarction (heart attack)

    b. Uncontrolled hypertension

    c. Uncontrolled diabetes

    d. Certain bleeding disorders

    e. Kidney dialysis

    f. History of radiation to the jaws

    g. HIV infection

2. It should be noted that consultation with a patient's physician is always indicated if there is any doubt about the patient's health status and how that status might affect any planned periodontal surgical intervention.

B. Patients who are totally noncompliant with self-care

1. The outcomes of many types of periodontal surgery are, in part, dependent upon the level of plaque control maintained by the patient's daily efforts at self-care.

2. Lack of compliance with self-care instructions can be a relative contraindication for some types of periodontal surgery if that lack of compliance precludes acceptable periodontal surgical outcomes.

C. Patients who have a high risk for dental caries

1. Some types of periodontal surgery result in exposure of portions of tooth roots. In a patient with uncontrolled dental caries where the risk for dental caries will remain quite high, it would not be wise to perform some types of periodontal surgery due to the potentially devastating effect of rampant root caries.

2. Thus, a high risk for dental caries can be a relative contraindication for some types of periodontal surgery.

D. Patients who have unrealistic expectations for surgical outcomes

1. Periodontitis damages the tissues that support the teeth, and surgical correction of that damage does not always result in a perfectly restored periodontium even when performed by the most skilled periodontal surgeon.

2. If a patient cannot understand the nature of periodontal surgery and cannot develop realistic expectation for the outcomes of any planned surgery, it would not be wise to proceed with any plan for periodontal surgery. Thus, patient expectations can also be a relative contraindication for periodontal surgery.

SECTION 2: TERMINOLOGY USED TO DESCRIBE HEALING FOLLOWING PERIODONTAL SURGERY

The dental hygienist needs to have an accurate understanding of four terms that are used in describing the healing of the periodontium following periodontal surgery: repair, reattachment, new attachment, and regeneration. These terms are used with precision in periodontics textbooks and articles when describing the results of periodontal surgery.

1. Healing by *REPAIR*
   A. **Repair** is healing of a wound by formation of tissue that does not truly restore the original architecture or original function of the body part.
      1. An example of repair is the formation of a scar during the healing of an accidental cut involving the finger.
      2. Certainly the healing is complete following formation of the scar, but the scar tissue is not precisely the same tissue in appearance or function that existed on that part of the finger before the wound.
   B. Repair is a perfectly natural type of healing for many wounds, including some wounds created by periodontal surgery.
      1. An example of repair in the periodontium is the healing that occurs following periodontal instrumentation.
         a. The usual healing of this wound results in a close readaptation of epithelium to the tooth root.
         b. This readaptation of epithelium has been referred to as formation of a **long junctional epithelium**. The long junctional epithelium is illustrated in Figure 17-1 of Chapter 17.
      2. A long junctional epithelium is a perfectly legitimate type of healing, but does not duplicate the precise periodontal tissues that were originally anatomically close to the tooth root. For example, with the formation of a long junctional epithelium there is no formation of new bone, cementum, or periodontal ligament during the healing process that occurs after periodontal debridement.

2. Healing by *REATTACHMENT*
   A. **Reattachment** is the reunion of the connective tissue and root that have been separated by incision or injury but ***not by disease.***
   B. Frequently it is necessary to move *healthy tissue* away from the tooth root or bone temporarily during some types of periodontal surgery. For example, moving the tissue may be necessary to allow access to damaged parts of the periodontium on adjacent teeth. The expected healing for this type of incision is healing by reattachment.

3. Healing by *NEW ATTACHMENT*
   A. **New attachment** is a term used to describe the union of a *pathologically exposed root* with connective tissue or epithelium.
   B. New attachment occurs when the epithelial and connective tissues are newly attached to a tooth root ***where periodontitis had previously destroyed this attachment.***
   C. New attachment differs from reattachment because new attachment must occur in an area formerly *damaged by disease*, whereas reattachment occurs when tissues are separated in the *absence of disease*.

4. Healing by *REGENERATION*
   A. **Regeneration** is the biologic process by which the architecture and function of lost tissue is *completely* restored.
   B. Regeneration results in the regrowing of the precise tissues that were present before the damage or disease occurred.
   C. For healing of the periodontium to be described as regeneration, the healing would have to result in the reformation of lost cementum, lost periodontal ligament, and lost alveolar bone.
   D. Unfortunately, the periodontium *cannot be regenerated predictably* with current periodontal surgical techniques.

SECTION 3: OVERVIEW OF COMMON TYPES OF PERIODONTAL SURGERY

This section discusses broad categories of periodontal surgery to provide the dental hygienist with an overview of some terminology used in both the modern and the historical application of periodontal surgery. The terms used in the descriptions below are important for each member of the dental team to understand and to be able to use with precision.

1. **Historical Perspectives.** Various types of periodontal surgery have been recommended for patients with advanced periodontitis and other periodontal conditions for many years.
   A. Historically, periodontal surgery was recommended mainly to remove what was thought to be dead or infected tissue in the periodontium. Thus, these early periodontal surgical procedures were mainly **resective** (i.e., designed to remove damaged periodontal tissues).
   B. Resective surgical procedures have limited use (i.e., gingivectomy) or are not recommended (i.e., gingival curettage) as a part of modern periodontal therapy.
2. **Modern Periodontal Surgical Techniques**
   A. During the past few decades, as more research data became available, a refinement of both the goals and techniques for periodontal surgery has taken place.
   B. *The emphasis in periodontal surgery has shifted from the resective types of surgery to surgical procedures that attempt to regenerate lost periodontal tissues.*

PERIODONTAL FLAP

1. **Procedure Description**
   A. A **periodontal flap** is a surgical procedure in which incisions are made in the gingiva around the necks of the teeth and the underlying soft tissues are **elevated** (lifted away) from the tooth roots and the alveolar bone.
   B. **Figure 21-1** shows a series of drawings that illustrate the incisions involved in performing a periodontal flap.
2. **Indications for a Periodontal Flap**
   A. Most modern periodontal surgical procedures require performing periodontal flaps.
   B. The flap elevation is done to provide access for some treatment either to tooth roots or to the alveolar bone, or to both of these structures.
      1. Periodontal flaps can be elevated simply to provide access to tooth surfaces for meticulous periodontal instrumentation (scaling and root planing). Use of a periodontal flap for improved access is discussed in more detail on the following page.
      2. Periodontal flaps also may be used to provide access to reshape or treat alveolar bone defects resulting from periodontitis. In the following sections of this chapter, the topic of apically positioned flaps with osseous surgery provides an example of this type of procedure.

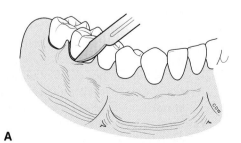

Figure 21-1. Performing a Periodontal Flap.
A: Making an incision to separate the soft tissue from the roots of the teeth.   **A**

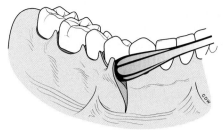

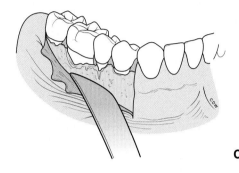

B   B: Elevating (or lifting) the soft tissue flap from the roots of the teeth and alveolar bone.

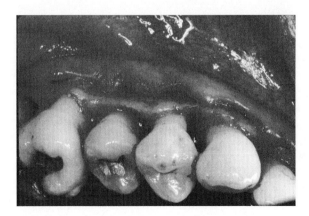

C   C: With the soft tissue moved away, the tooth roots and alveolar bone are exposed.

PERIODONTAL FLAP FOR ACCESS

1. **Procedure Description**
   A. **Flap for access** surgery (or modified Widman flap surgery) is used to provide access to the tooth roots for improved root preparation. In this surgical procedure the gingival tissue is incised and temporarily elevated (lifted away) from the tooth roots (**Fig. 21-2**).
   B. The tissues are elevated only long enough to allow good access for debridement of the tooth roots. Following root treatment (that may involve root surface debridement or the application of chemicals), the gingival tissue is replaced at its original position and sutured in place.

Figure 21-2. Flap for Access Periodontal Surgery. Note that the flap surgery has provided good access for both visualization and instrumentation of the tooth roots.

2. **Healing After Flap Surgery**
   A. The healing expected from the flap for access surgery is *healing by repair* and usually involves formation of a *long junctional epithelium*.
   B. Research shows that flap for access surgery can result in a stable dentogingival unit that can be maintained in health with periodontal maintenance by the dental team and proper self-care by the patient.

3. **Special Considerations for the Dental Hygienist**
    A. During periodontal instrumentation, it may not be possible to perform thorough calculus removal if the pocket depths are deeper than 5 to 7 mm. Flap for access surgery allows for improved access to root surfaces within deep pockets.
    B. Even in patients where flap for access surgery is planned, every effort should be made to control chronic periodontitis with nonsurgical therapy prior to the surgical intervention.
        1. The dental hygienist plays an important role in promoting patient understanding of how nonsurgical and surgical treatment are related.
        2. Thorough and meticulous nonsurgical therapy can reduce the extent of any planned periodontal surgical treatment, and is always an important part of patient care.

BONE REPLACEMENT GRAFT

1. **Procedure Description**
    A. Bone replacement graft is a surgical procedure used to encourage the body to rebuild alveolar bone that has been lost as a result of periodontal diseases.
    B. This procedure involves (i) elevation of a periodontal flap to gain access to the alveolar bone and tooth roots, (ii) cleaning of granulation tissue from alveolar bone defects, (iii) treatment of the tooth roots as needed, and (iv) placement of grafting material into the bone defect. The periodontal flap is then returned to its original position, sutured in place, and allowed to heal. **Figure 21-3** shows an alveolar bone defect exposed during a periodontal surgical procedure. This type of defect is ideally suited for bone replacement graft.

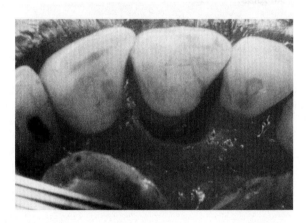

Figure 21-3. Exposure of an Alveolar Bone Defect During a Periodontal Surgical Procedure. Note the extensive alveolar bone loss around one of the central incisor teeth. This type of bone defect would be an ideal site for bone replacement graft.

2. **Materials Used for Bone Replacement**
    A. It is common to use bone harvested (taken) from part of the patient's jaw for bone replacement graft. When bone is grafted from one area of the patient's jaw to another, the graft is referred to as an **autograft**.
    B. Natural bone is not always the material used for grafting since donor sites in a patient's mouth are not always readily available. Materials other than bone from the patient's jaw can also be used, and include treated bone from cadavers and other species (such as bovine bone) or artificial materials that stimulate bone regrowth.
    C. Table 21-1 provides an overview of materials used for bone replacement grafts.
3. **Healing After Bone Grafting**
    A. Final healing expected from bone grafting includes a partial or complete rebuilding of alveolar bone lost because of periodontitis.
    B. Bone grafting can result in rebuilding of some bone lost due to disease.
        1. It is not known, however, if bone grafting always results in the reformation of cementum, periodontal ligament, and alveolar bone.

   2. The reformed bone may not actually be attached to the cementum by periodontal ligament fibers.

  C. Research has shown that a successful bone graft combined with good plaque control and thorough periodontal maintenance can result in retaining a severely compromised tooth over time.

4. Special Considerations for the Dental Hygienist

  A. The site of a bone replacement graft should be left undisturbed for many months and not be probed until an appropriate interval has elapsed. The dental hygienist should consult with the dentist to determine when a grafted site may be probed safely.

  B. Meticulous plaque control in the site is critical. In the early stages of the healing, the dental team maintains some of the responsibility for plaque control at the site, because the patient may temporarily be unable to perform adequate self-care.

Table 21-1. Materials Used for Bone Replacement Grafts

Type	Description	Example of Material
Autograft	Bone taken from patient's own body	Bone removed from the jaw
Allograft	Bone taken from another person	Treated bone harvested from cadavers
Xenograft	Bone taken from another species	Treated bovine (cow) bone
Alloplast	Synthetic bone material	Hydroxyapatite mineral or ceramic

GUIDED TISSUE REGENERATION

1. Procedure Description

  A. Guided tissue regeneration is a surgical periodontal procedure that attempts to regenerate lost periodontal structures (i.e., regrow lost cementum, periodontal ligament, and alveolar bone).

    1. As the name implies, this surgical procedure can result in a true regeneration of the periodontium and is currently in widespread use.

    2. *Although regeneration of the cementum, periodontal ligament, and alveolar bone is one of the ultimate goals of periodontal therapy, regeneration of the periodontium is not completely predictable with techniques in use today.*

  B. Guided tissue regeneration involves (i) elevation of a periodontal flap, (ii) cleaning of alveolar bone defects, (3) treatment of tooth roots, and (4) placement of barrier materials to control the usually rapid growth of epithelium into the wound.

    1. Figure 21-4 illustrates the placement of a barrier during an attempt at guided tissue regeneration.

    2. Some of the barrier materials in current use require removal, so their use necessitates a second surgical procedure to remove the barrier material.

2. Healing After Guided Tissue Regeneration

  A. The healing expected from guided tissue regeneration is *regeneration* of part or all of the periodontium that was destroyed by periodontitis.

  B. As already mentioned, guided tissue regeneration requires the use of a barrier material.

    1. During surgery, a barrier material is placed under the flap to stop the rapidly growing epithelium from migrating along the root surface and interfering with the connective tissue regrowth on the root. (It is the connective tissue components from the periodontal ligament space that actually provide the cells needed to regrow cementum, periodontal ligament, and alveolar bone.)

2. It is important to note that if a barrier material were not used, the epithelial tissue would regrow very rapidly, covering the tooth root and blocking access to the root by the slower growing connective tissue. The epithelial growth covering the root blocks the connective tissue cells of the periodontal ligament from making contact with the root surface.

C. Bone graft materials can be used in conjunction with barrier materials to encourage the body to regrow alveolar bone during the process of regenerating the periodontium.

Figure 21-4. Placement of a Barrier During an Attempt at Guided Tissue Regeneration.

A: Flap elevated to expose the alveolar bone defect on the facial surface of the first molar.

B: Barrier material sutured over the bone defect

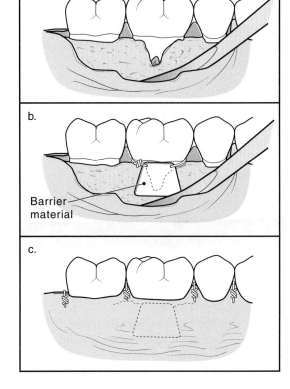

C: Flap replaced around the teeth and sutured, covering the barrier material.

3. **Special Considerations for the Dental Hygienist**
   A. During the surgical procedure, every effort is made to close the wound to completely cover the barrier material.
      1. If exposure of part of the barrier material is noted at any of the post-surgical visits, measures should be instituted to minimize bacterial contamination of the barrier material.
      2. For example, a patient with exposed barrier materials may need special self-care instructions for the topical application of antimicrobials.
   B. Sites treated by guided tissue regeneration should not be probed for several months following the procedures. The dental hygienist should consult with the dentist to determine when the site can be probed safely.

APICALLY POSITIONED FLAP WITH OSSEOUS SURGERY

1. **Procedure Description**
    A. An **apically positioned flap with osseous surgery** is a periodontal surgical proce-dure designed specifically to eliminate or minimize pocket depths.
        1. This procedure involves (i) elevation of a periodontal flap, (ii) removal of granu-lation tissue, (iii) treatment of tooth roots, and (iv) correction of bone contours to mimic the contours of healthy alveolar bone (**periodontal osseous surgery**).
        2. Following contouring of the alveolar bone, the flap is sutured at a position that is more apical to its original position (**apically positioned flap**).
    B. This periodontal surgical procedure is ideal for minimizing periodontal pocket depths in patients with moderate periodontitis. **Figure 21-5** illustrates the results of an apically positioned flap. Note that the gingival margin is apical to (below) the cemento-enamel junction. The reduced pocket depth will facilitate plaque control by the patient and the dental team.

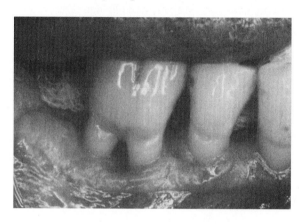

Figure 21-5. Results of an Apically Positioned Flap. Note that the gingival margin as sutured leaves the cementoenamel junction coronal to the gingival margin.

2. **Healing of an Apically Positioned Flap**
    A. Research has shown that an apically positioned flap combined with periodontal osseous surgery can result in a stable dentogingival junction that can be main-tained in health.
    B. Outcomes of this type of surgery (as with most types of periodontal surgery) depend in part upon meticulous patient self-care combined with periodontal maintenance provided by the dental team.
    C. Final healing of this type of surgery results in a normal attachment (both junc-tional epithelium and connective tissue attachment) at a position more apical on the tooth root.
3. **Special Considerations for the Dental Hygienist**
    A. During surgery to minimize periodontal pockets, it is common for the gingival margin to be positioned against the teeth at a more apical level than it originally occupied.
        1. This apical positioning results in exposure of a portion of the root to the oral cavity.
        2. The exposure of a portion of the root may be an esthetic concern for the patient.
    B. Temporary dentinal hypersensitivity is a frequent patient postsurgical complaint. As discussed in other chapters, dentinal hypersensitivity diminishes over time if the patient maintains good plaque control.
    C. Before surgery, the members of the dental team should inform the patient about the changes in appearance and potential for dentinal hypersensitivity. The dental hygienist should also assure the patient that if sensitivity does occur, measures can be taken to help deal with it.

MUCOGINGIVAL SURGERY / PERIODONTAL PLASTIC SURGERY

1. **Procedure Description**
    A. The most common variation of **mucogingival surgery** is designed to alter components of the attached gingiva.
        1. Gingiva lost because of disease or trauma can be restored to a tooth surface through these periodontal surgical procedures. During the past few years some of these techniques have been referred to as **periodontal plastic surgery** by many authors.
        2. Mucogingival surgery also includes other techniques designed to provide for other outcomes such as removal of an aberrant frenulum or deepening of a vestibule.
        3. Many of these types of procedures alter the appearance of the tissues. Most patients want to have a beautiful smile. Because the gingiva is readily visible in many patients, patients frequently seek improvements in the appearance of the gingiva. An example of such a problem is an unsightly area of gingival recession.
        4. Some of these procedures improve function. Function can be compromised, since a lack of any attached gingiva on a tooth can limit the options for restoration of a tooth by contraindicating the placement of restoration margins subgingivally.
    B. Types of Mucogingival Surgery
        1. **Soft tissue grafts** are used to cover roots and replace absent gingival tissue due to excessive recession. Recession may occur for a variety of reasons (aggressive toothbrushing, oral habits, periodontal disease). Once the contributing factor for recession has been identified and controlled, a soft tissue graft procedure will repair the defect and help prevent additional recession.
        2. Two of the more common mucogingival surgical procedures that can replace lost gingival tissues (such as seen in areas of gingival recession) include connective tissue grafts and free gingival grafts.
            a. A **connective tissue graft** is a type of mucogingival surgery that requires harvesting a donor section of *connective tissue,* usually from the palate. The connective tissue graft can be placed partially under a flap created at the site to be grafted. This flap helps supply nutrients to the grafted tissue during the critical phase of healing.
            b. A **free gingival graft** is a type of mucogingival surgery that requires harvesting a donor section of tissue, also usually from the palate. This donor tissue includes both the *surface epithelium and some of the underlying connective tissue.* **Figure 21-6** shows a free gingival graft placed on the facial surface of a tooth root.
            c. Both connective tissue grafts and free gingival grafts result in two oral wounds—one where the graft tissue is harvested and one where the graft tissue is placed.

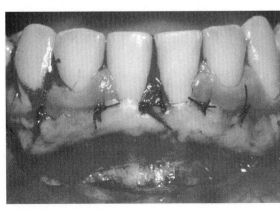

Figure 21-6. Free Gingival Graft on the Facial Surface of Tooth Root. The graft is placed over an area of root previously exposed because of advanced gingival recession.

2. **Healing After Mucogingival Surgical Procedures**
   A. Expected healing of these mucogingival surgical procedures would be *new attachment* of the grafting material (donor tissue) to the tooth root.
   B. Both free gingival grafts and connective tissue grafts can be used to replace lost gingival tissues, but the connective tissue grafts result in a more natural tissue color in the healed tissues and in a more esthetic final result.
3. **Special Considerations for the Dental Hygienist**
   A. Mucogingival surgical procedures usually result in two oral wounds. For example, the free gingival graft requires harvesting donor tissue from some site in the mouth, usually the palate. During healing, these donor sites can bother the patient more than does the actual site of the gingival grafting, since some of these donor sites leave an open wound that can require some time to heal.
   B. The dental hygienist should discuss postsurgical discomfort with the patient and alert the dentist if the patient reports protracted discomfort from these wounds.
   C. In addition, it is critical that the grafted sites not be disturbed during the early stage of healing. The members of the dental team should caution the patient against disturbing the tissue during the early phase of healing.
   D. It is the responsibility of the members of the dental team to help the patient maintain good plaque control during the early phase of healing since mechanical plaque control must be restricted to avoid movement in the grafted tissues.

CROWN LENGTHENING SURGERY

1. **Procedure Description**
   A. **Crown lengthening surgery** is designed to create a longer clinical crown for a tooth by removing some of the gingiva and by removing some alveolar bone from the necks of the teeth.
      1. Crown lengthening can be used to improve the esthetics (appearance) of the gingiva, especially on anterior teeth.
         a. An individual's smile may be unattractive because the height or symmetry of the gingiva surrounding the teeth. Although the crowns are the correct length, they appear to be short because too much gingival tissue covers the teeth.
         b. During this procedure, the gingival tissues are reshaped to expose more of the natural crown of the tooth.
      2. Crown lengthening is also used to make a restorative dental procedure possible. Crown lengthening surgery is necessary when a tooth is decayed or broken below the gingival margin or has insufficient remaining tooth structure for a restoration.
         a. When a badly damaged tooth is to be restored, the dentist will evaluate the tooth and surrounding tissues to determine if the final restoration of the tooth will damage the soft tissue attachment.
         b. If such damage can be predicted, crown lengthening surgery is usually indicated prior to the restoration placement.
   B. The actual procedure followed in crown lengthening surgery usually involves an apically positioned flap with osseous surgery. Unlike the typical apically positioned flap with osseous surgery, a crown lengthening surgery may be indicated in the presence of a perfectly healthy periodontium simply to allow for restoration of a badly damaged tooth or for improvement of the esthetics.
2. **Healing After Crown Lengthening Surgery**
   A. Healing of crown lengthening surgery is similar to that described for the apically positioned flap with osseous surgery.
   B. Final healing of crown lengthening surgery results in a normal attachment (both junctional epithelium and connective tissue attachment) at a position more apical on the tooth root.

3. **Special Considerations for the Dental Hygienist**
   A. Since crown lengthening surgery usually involves an apically positioned flap and exposure of additional tooth surface to the oral environment, temporary dentinal hypersensitivity is also a common result of this type of periodontal surgery. It is imperative for the dental team to warn patients in advance that they may experience dentinal hypersensitivity following crown lengthening surgery.
   B. As already discussed, when dentinal hypersensitivity results, the dental hygienist may need to institute measures to help the patient deal with the sensitivity.
   C. Control of dentinal hypersensitivity requires meticulous plaque control during the healing phase, and this can be a problem since mechanical plaque control must be restricted following most surgical procedures. It is the responsibility of the dental team to aid the patient in this plaque control until healing allows the patient to resume routine self-care.

DENTAL IMPLANT PLACEMENT

1. **Procedure Description**
   A. A **dental implant** is an artificial tooth root that is placed into the alveolar bone to hold a replacement tooth or prosthesis (denture or bridge). Most dental implants in current use are endosseous implants that are placed in alveolar bone and protrude through the mucoperiosteum. See Chapter 24 for a more complete description of the dental implant.
      1. Dental implant placement usually requires exposure of alveolar bone using flap surgery, drilling a precise hole in the alveolar bone, and insertion of a metallic implant into the site.
      2. There are a variety of dental implants in current use including various lengths, diameters, and designs. Many types of dental implants even have threads much like a screw has threads.
   B. Some dental implants are designed to be covered with gingiva during healing, and others are designed to leave a portion of the implant exposed in the oral cavity during healing. Those that are covered require a second surgical procedure following healing to expose the top of the implant.

2. **Healing**
   A. Healing following placement of a dental implant results in bone growth in such close proximity to the implant surface that the implant is stable enough to support a tooth shaped restoration or a dental prosthetic appliance.
   B. It should be noted that though dental implants are not surrounded by cementum and periodontal ligament (as are natural teeth), these implants are subject to periodontal disease that can result in the loss of supporting bone just like the natural tooth.

3. **Special Considerations for the Dental Hygienist**
   A. Patient self-care following placement of a dental implant is critical, and the members of the dental team must assume responsibility for helping the patient with plaque control during the critical healing period.
   B. Once an implant site heals, the gingiva surrounding the implant can be maintained in health using self-care techniques similar to what is required to keep gingiva around a natural tooth healthy.
   C. Implant maintenance and the role played by the dental hygienist is discussed in detail in Chapter 24.

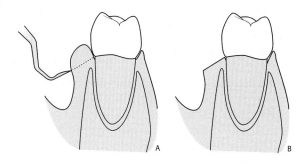

Figure 12-7. Gingivectomy.
A: The placement of a special gingivectomy knife to incise the excess gingival tissue.
B: The excess tissue is removed.

GINGIVECTOMY

1. **Procedure Description**
   A. The **gingivectomy** is a surgical procedure designed to excise or to remove gingival tissue and was used for many years in periodontics as a primary treatment modality.
   B. **Figure 21-7** shows a series of drawings that illustrate the incisions involved in performing a gingivectomy.
2. **Indications for Gingivectomy**
   A. Before the development of modern periodontal flap techniques, the gingivectomy was in widespread use in the treatment of periodontitis patients.
   B. In modern periodontal therapy, the gingivectomy is usually limited to removing enlarged gingiva to improve esthetics or to allow for better access for self-care in isolated sites, though it can be used to reshape more extensive areas of enlarged gingiva as might be seen in gingival overgrowth in response to certain medication use. **Figure 21-8** shows the gingivectomy used to reshape an area of enlarged gingiva.
   C. As a surgical technique, gingivectomy has several disadvantages:
      1. One disadvantage to gingivectomy is that it leaves a large open connective tissue wound that results in a somewhat slower surface healing than most other periodontal surgical procedures. This generally results in the expectation of more discomfort for the patient during the healing phase.
      2. Another disadvantage of gingivectomy is the resulting longer appearance of the tooth due to the excision of some of the gingiva. Despite this disadvantage, the gingivectomy is still a useful surgical procedure in selected sites.

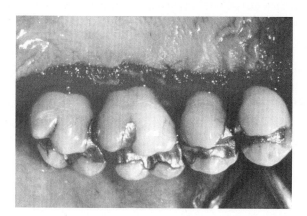

Figure 21-8. Gingivectomy Used to Reshape an Area of Enlarged Gingiva. Note that the gingivectomy results in a rather large wound that exposes connective tissue. This large wound usually results in protracted healing since healing requires that the epithelium grow across the wound created by the gingivectomy.

3. **Healing After a Gingivectomy**
   A. The final healing of the wound created by a gingivectomy is a normal attachment of the soft tissues to the tooth root, but at a level that is more apical in position than the original level.
   B. Following a gingivectomy, the teeth in the surgical area will appear to be longer since more of the root is exposed where the tissue was excised. Of course, if this is the desired result of the procedure—because of enlarged gingiva—then, this procedure can result in an acceptable outcome. However, if more tooth structure being exposed is not desirable, another surgical approach may be indicated.

4. **Special Considerations for the Dental Hygienist**
   A. As already mentioned, the gingivectomy wound leaves a broad connective tissue surface exposed that can be very uncomfortable for the patient during the healing phase.
   B. Postsurgical discomfort can be managed by placing a periodontal dressing (bandage material) over the wound and by prescribing analgesics (pain medications) for use following surgery.
   C. At the time of the first postsurgical visit, the dental hygienist may need to replace the periodontal dressing to enhance wound comfort until total epithelialization of the wound has occurred.
   D. Healing of the wound created by a gingivectomy procedure progresses in a predictable manner. Research studies have shown that oral epithelium grows across the exposed connective tissue at an approximate rate of 0.5 mm per day. Thus it is possible for the alert clinical team to predict healing times; this of course is useful when counseling patients about what to expect during the postsurgical phase.

GINGIVAL CURETTAGE

1. **Procedure Description**
   A. **Gingival curettage** is an older type of periodontal surgical procedure that involves an attempt to scrape away the lining of the periodontal pocket usually using a periodontal curet, often a Gracey curet.
      1. *Gingival curettage normally is not a part of modern periodontal therapy.* The procedure is discussed here briefly because the dental hygienists will encounter many patients who have undergone this procedure in the past and a few dentists who still recommend some variation of this procedure.
      2. Research has demonstrated that the same benefits from gingival curettage can be derived from thorough periodontal instrumentation and meticulous plaque control. Thus, curettage is no longer a recommended periodontal surgical procedure.
   B. Although the gingival curettage is no longer recommended as a periodontal surgical procedure, some clinicians advocate performing gingival curettage with chemicals or lasers that destroy the pocket lining. At present, these types of gingival curettage are not part of mainstream periodontal therapy, but much more research on the use of lasers in periodontal therapy is needed to clarify this confusing area.

2. **Indications.** *Gingival curettage is not recommended as part of modern periodontal therapy.*

SECTION 4: MANAGEMENT OF THE PATIENT FOLLOWING PERIODONTAL SURGERY

This section discusses components of the postsurgical visit including suture removal, periodontal dressings, postsurgical instructions, and postsurgical visits. The dental hygienist can play a major role in postsurgical management.

SUTURE PLACEMENT AND SUBSEQUENT REMOVAL

1. **Suture Placement**
   A. Many periodontal surgical procedures require the placement of sutures to stabilize the position of the soft tissues during the early phases of healing. A **suture** is a stitch taken to repair an incision, tear, or wound.
   B. In general two types of suture material are used: nonresorbable and resorbable. **Figure 21-9** illustrates a typical suture material.
      1. **Nonresorbable suture material** does not dissolve in body fluids and must be removed by the dental team.
      2. **Resorbable suture material** is designed to dissolve slowly in body fluids, but it sometimes does not dissolve well in saliva.
   C. Suture placement for some periodontal surgical procedures is quite complex, however, **Figures 21-10, and 21-11** illustrate some typical suture placement that might be needed following flap surgery. These drawings are included to give the dental hygienist some idea about what might be encountered at the time of the postsurgical visit.

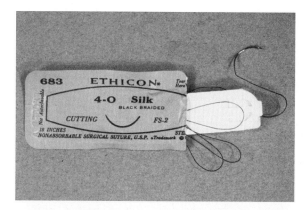

Figure 21-9. Typical Suture Material.

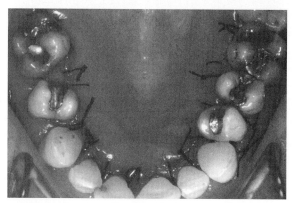

Figure 21-10. Interrupted Interdental Sutures.
Interrupted interdental sutures on the maxillary arch. (Courtesy of Dr. John S. Dozier, Tallahase, FL.)

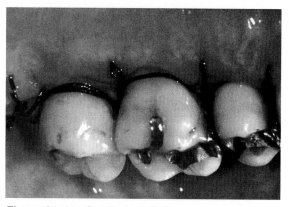

Figure 21-11. Continuous Suture. Continuous suture on the maxillary arch. (Courtesy of Dr. Don Rolfs (Periodontal Foundations, Wenatchee, WA.))

2. **Suture Removal**
   A. Nonresorbable sutures placed during surgical procedures are removed as part of the routine postsurgical visits. Remnants of resorbable sutures can also be removed at the routine visits to avoid unnecessary tissue inflammation caused by retained suture material.
   B. Guidelines for removal vary, but in general, sutures should be removed when wound healing has progressed to the point at which the sutures are loose in the tissues. Most sutures are loose at the time of the 1-week postsurgical visit.
   C. Most sutures should not be left in place longer than 2 weeks because they can act as irritants if left in the tissue too long.

3. **General Suture Removal Guidelines.** Each periodontal surgical procedure is unique, however, listed below are some general guidelines for suture removal.
   A. Guideline 1. The number and type of sutures placed is a routine part of the chart entry for periodontal surgery. Knowing the number of sutures placed can help the dental hygienist confirm that all sutures have been located and removed.
   B. Guideline 2. Reading chart entries related to suture placement can seem confusing at first, since abbreviations and sutures sizes are usually entered in the chart.
      1. Typical suture sizes used in periodontal surgery are 3-0, 4-0, and 5-0.
         a. In this sizing system, the 3-0 size is larger than the 4-0 size, and 4-0 is larger than 5-0.
         b. In the mouth, 5-0 can be a little more difficult to locate than a 4-0 size, especially in the posterior part of the mouth.
      2. The dental hygienist should learn the precise abbreviations used in the chart entries in the individual clinical setting. A typical example of an abbreviation would be "4-0 BSS". This would mean the size of the suture is 4-0, and BSS stands for black silk suture, a commonly used nonresorbable suture material.
   C. Guideline 3
      1. Sutures should be removed by cutting the suture material near the knot and grasping the knot with pliers.
      2. When the suture is gently pulled from the tissue, care should be taken not to force the knot itself through the tissue. This technique is illustrated in **Figure 21-12**
      3. It should be noted that suture removal is rarely painful for the patient if care is taken not to create unnecessary tissue movement.

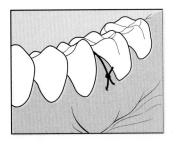 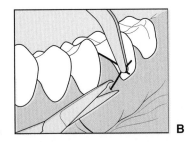 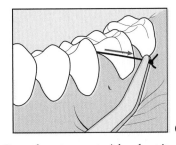

Figure 21-12. Suture Removal. A: Suture in place. B: Grasp the suture material and cut it near the knot. C: Gently pull the suture material from the tissue.

PERIODONTAL DRESSING PLACEMENT

1. **Definition.** Periodontal surgical wounds are sometimes covered with a protective bandage called **periodontal dressing**
2. **Types of Periodontal Dressings**
   A. One type requires the mixing of materials from two tubes to form a puttylike consistency. This type of periodontal dressing usually contains zinc oxide, mineral oils, rosin plus a bacteriostatic or fungicidal agent. Each of the various brands of these dressings requires familiarization prior to mixing and placing.

    B. A second type of periodontal dressing in use is a light-cured gel that contains polyether urethane dimethacrylate resin.

    C. The dental hygienist should study the manufacturer's instructions with care and practice placement of the dressing on a typodont (model) before using it in a patient's mouth.

3. General Guidelines for Management of Periodontal Dressings

    A. The periodontal dressing does not adhere to the teeth or gums and is retained by pushing some of the material into embrasure spaces to lock the dressing around the necks of the teeth.

    B. Less periodontal dressing is better. The proper amount of dressing is only enough to cover the wound. **Figure 21-13** illustrates the proper amount of dressing covering a periodontal surgical wound.

    C. The dressing should be placed so that there is no contact between the dressing and the teeth in the opposing arch. Occlusal contact with teeth in the opposing arch will quickly dislodge the dressing.

    D. Suture material can become trapped within the periodontal dressing. When removing dressings, it might be necessary to loosen the dressing slightly and cut the suture before completely removing the dressing from the necks of the teeth.

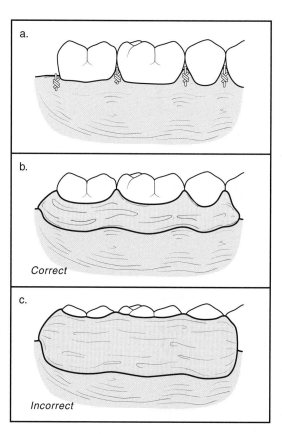

Figure 21-13. Periodontal Dressing Placed Over a Surgical Wound.

A: Flap sutured in place.

B: Correctly placed periodontal dressing. Note the dressing does not extend near the occlusal surfaces of the teeth.

C: Incorrectly placed periodontal dressing. Note that the dressing extends to near the occlusal surface of the teeth and is likely to be dislodged when the patient bites down.

POSTSURGICAL INSTRUCTIONS FOLLOWING PERIODONTAL SURGERY

Postsurgical instructions following periodontal surgery should be given to the patient by the members of the dental team. Most dental teams provide both written and verbal instructions to minimize confusion and to help ensure patient compliance. Typical postsurgical instructions are outlined in Box 21-3. If sedation was required for periodontal surgery, the companion who accompanied the patient should be included when postsurgical instructions are given. The primary elements covered in most postsurgical care instructions are outlined below.

1. **Modifying efforts at self-care:** Most periodontal surgical procedures require some restriction on mechanical plaque control, especially during the early phase of healing. It is common practice to prescribe 0.12% chlorhexidine mouthrinse to be used twice daily to aid with self-care until the patient can resume mechanical plaque control.
2. **Managing postoperative medications:** Patients should be encouraged to take medications as prescribed. If systemic antibiotics are prescribed, it is particularly important for the patient to understand that all of this prescribed medication should be taken. Commonly, postsurgical medications include either nonsteroidal or narcotic pain medications, but usually, these pain medications should only be taken as needed.
3. **Chewing food following periodontal surgery:** Chewing food is always a concern following a periodontal surgical procedure. Many of these procedures require that the surgical site be undisturbed for an extended period of time. Frequently, chewing must be limited to areas not involved by the surgery until healing has progressed to an acceptable level. Recommendations for a soft diet for 24 to 48 hours are routine following most periodontal surgical procedures.
4. **Dealing with facial swelling:** It is common for the patient to experience some facial swelling following some types of periodontal surgery. Swelling can arise from the tissue trauma incurred during the procedure and can even occur during the second and third day following the surgery. Although this swelling can be disconcerting to the patient, it is usually not a sign that healing is compromised. Swelling can be minimized by the intermittent use of ice packs for the first 8 to 10 hours following the surgery.
5. **Allaying concerns about bleeding:** Some bleeding following periodontal surgery is to be expected. Patients should be reassured that minor bleeding is not a cause for alarm. Postsurgical instructions should be clear, however, that if excessive bleeding occurs the emergency number should be contacted immediately.

Box 21-3

Typical Postsurgical Instructions

1. If you have questions or concerns, call the office or the office emergency number right away. Office: 555-1111; emergency 555-2222.
2. *Do* take medications as prescribed. Report any problems with the medications immediately.
3. *Do* take it easy for several days. Limit your activity to mild physical exertion.
4. *Expect* some bleeding following the procedure. If heavy bleeding persists, call the office emergency number.
5. *Expect* some swelling. Use of an ice pack on the face in the area of the surgery can minimize swelling.
6. Diet Recommendations:
   a. Soft food only on the day of the surgery
   b. No hot beverages on the day of surgery
   c. Avoid chewing on the surgical site
7. Self-care:
   a. Rinse with recommended mouth rinse starting the day after surgery
   b. If dressing was placed, it may also be brushed lightly

POSTSURGICAL VISITS

It is the dentist's responsibility to manage postsurgical problems, such as extreme pain or infection. The dental hygienist, however, performs much of the routine postsurgical management. Following periodontal flap surgery, the patient is most often reappointed in 5 to 7 days for the first postsurgical visit. Postsurgical care for the various types of periodontal surgery varies; however, steps to be followed at a typical postsurgical visit are outlined below.

1. **Step 1.** An interview is conducted with the patient to determine what he or she experienced during the days following the surgery. The patient interview should be detailed enough to provide the dental hygienist with an overview of possible problems to investigate and solve at this visit. The following are some of the items that would normally be included in this interview. It is imperative that the dental hygienist alerts the dentist if any unusual conditions are observed during the postsurgical visit or reported by the patient.

    a. Analgesics. Following periodontal surgery, analgesics (pain control medications) are used to control patient discomfort. The patient should be asked if he or she used the pain medication, the current level of discomfort, and if another prescription is needed.

    b. Antibiotics. If antibiotics were needed following a surgical procedure, remind the patient that all of the antibiotic tablets should be taken. It is also important to find out if the patient experienced any unusual reactions to the antibiotic.

    c. Antimicrobial mouth rinse. An antimicrobial mouth rinse such as 0.12% chlorhexidine gluconate may have been prescribed for the patient to use during healing, since mechanical plaque control is difficult following periodontal surgery. Ask about the amount of mouth rinse remaining. During the course of the visit, it may be necessary to give the patient another prescription for this mouth rinse.

    d. Swelling. Following periodontal surgery, it is common for the patient to experience some facial swelling. Remember that although this swelling can be disconcerting to the patient, it is common and usually not a sign that healing is compromised.

    e. Postsurgical bleeding. Inquire about postsurgical bleeding. It is common for patients to experience a little bleeding following periodontal surgery, but heavy bleeding should not occur following the procedure.

    f. Sensitivity to cold. Sensitivity to cold following root exposure during periodontal surgery is quite common. Although this is an annoying postsurgical occurrence, the sensitivity normally disappears within the first few weeks following the surgery if excellent plaque control is maintained. Dentinal hypersensitivity is discussed in other chapters in this textbook.

2. **Step 2.** The patient's vital signs including blood pressure, pulse, and temperature are assessed. An elevated temperature at the first postsurgical visit can indicate a developing infection.

3. **Step 3.** Any periodontal dressing is removed so that the surgical site can be examined. The surgical site is rinsed with warm sterile saline and cotton-tipped applicators are used to remove any debris adherent to the teeth, soft tissues, or sutures. Tissue swelling or exudate such as pus can indicate a developing infection.

4. **Step 4.** The sutures are cut and removed using sterile scissors.

5. **Step 5.** All plaque from the teeth is removed in the area of the surgery. It is usual that patients cannot perform perfect plaque control during the first days following periodontal surgery, so plaque accumulation is likely. Part of the responsibility of the dental team is to help the patient with plaque control during the critical stage of healing.

6. **Step 6.** If indicated, the periodontal dressing is replaced. For most surgical procedures, the periodontal dressing should be discontinued as soon as the patient can resume some mechanical plaque control. In a few instances the tissues will not be well adapted to the necks of the teeth, and replacement of the periodontal dressing should be considered to protect the healing wound.

7. **Step 7.** The patient is instructed in self-care. Mechanical plaque control should be resumed as soon as possible following periodontal surgery, but special instructions may be necessary during the first few weeks following the surgery.
   a. Special tools such as brushes with very flexible bristles may be required during early stages of healing.
   b. During postsurgical healing, it is frequently necessary to modify the patient's plaque control techniques as the tissues heal and mature. Gingival margin contours are usually altered to some degree by the surgery, and this may necessitate the introduction of additional self-care aids. Monitoring and modification of the patient's self-care efforts during the healing phase is one of the most important responsibilities of the dental team and can help assure success of the surgical procedure.
8. **Step 8.** The patient is reappointed for the second postsurgical visit. This second visit should occur 2 to 3 weeks following the surgery.

CHAPTER SUMMARY STATEMENT

There are several types of periodontal surgery that can be used to help control periodontitis and to rebuild lost periodontal tissues. Reasons for performing periodontal surgery include (i) providing access for improved treatment of root surfaces, (ii) reducing the depths of periodontal pockets and creating tissue contours to facilitate patient self-care, (iii) encouraging regeneration of periodontal tissues, (iv) augmenting the gingival tissues, and (v) placing dental implants. Dental hygienists are often called on to discuss periodontal surgery with patients and to provide routine postsurgical care.

SECTION 5: FOCUS ON PATIENTS

CASE 1

During nonsurgical periodontal therapy for chronic periodontitis, a dental hygienist encounters multiple sites where the probing depths exceed 5 mm. During periodontal debridement (scaling and root planing), the hygienist is unable to instrument the root surfaces thoroughly in the areas of the deeper pockets. What should the dental hygienist tell the patient related to this observation?

CASE 2

During nonsurgical periodontal therapy, a patient with chronic periodontitis informs you that the dentist had previously discussed the possibility of periodontal surgery. The patient expresses deep concern and fear over the thought of periodontal surgery. The patient tells you about an aunt who had periodontal surgery many years ago and had many problems following the surgery. How should you respond?

CASE 3

At the time of the 1-week postsurgical visit, a patient who had undergone flap for access surgery has a temperature of 100.5°F and a pulse rate of 70 beats per minute. Clinical examination of the surgical site reveals that the sutures are in place but that there appears to be some swelling of the flap. How should you proceed?

Suggested Readings

Anthony JM. Advanced periodontic techniques. *Clin Tech Small Anim Pract.* 2000;15:237–242.

Drisko CH. Trends in surgical and nonsurgical periodontal treatment. *J Am Dent Assoc.* 2000;131(suppl):31S–38S.

Flores-de-Jacoby L, Mengel R. Conventional surgical procedures. *Periodontol 2000.* 1995;9:38–54.

Heard RH, Mellonig JT. Regenerative materials: An overview. *Alpha Omegan.* 2000;93:51–58.

Lang NP, Loe H. Clinical management of periodontal diseases. *Periodontol 2000.* 1993;2:128–139.

Scabbia A, Cho KS, Sigurdsson TJ, et al. Cigarette smoking negatively affects healing response following flap debridement surgery. *J Periodontol.* 2001;72:43–49.

Trieger N. Surgical treatment of periodontal infections. *Atlas Oral Maxillofac Surg Clin North Am.* 2000;8:27–34.

Wolff LF. Guided tissue regeneration in periodontal therapy. *Northwest Dent.* 2000;79:23–28, 40.

SECTION 6: CHAPTER REVIEW QUESTIONS

1. One of the indications for periodontal surgery is to provide access for improved root surface debridement.
   A. True
   B. False

2. One relative contraindication for periodontal surgery can be a high risk for dental caries.
   A. True
   B. False

3. The term healing by repair means that the architecture and function of lost tissue is completely restored.
   A. True
   B. False

4. In bone replacement graft procedure, using an autograft means that the graft material is taken from the patient.
   A. True
   B. False

5. A connective tissue graft is a type of mucogingival/periodontal plastic surgery.
   A. True
   B. False

6. Crown lengthening surgery results in longer clinical crowns for the teeth.
   A. True
   B. False

7. The suture size 4-0 is smaller than the suture size 3-0.
   A. True
   B. False

8. When placing periodontal dressing, the main guideline is to place as much dressing as possible over the wound surface.
   A. True
   B. False

9. Facial swelling following periodontal surgery is always a sign that healing will not occur.
   A. True
   B. False

10. During postsurgical visits it is important to remind patients to take all prescribed antibiotic tablets.
    A. True
    B. False

Chapter

22 Chemical Agents in Periodontal Care

 Refer to the CD packaged with this book for full color versions of the clinical photographs in this chapter.

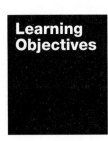

Learning Objectives

- Describe the difference between systemic delivery and local delivery of chemical agents.
- Describe three examples of mouth rinse active ingredients that can help control gingivitis.
- Explain why toothpastes are nearly ideal delivery mechanisms for chemical agents.
- List 4 active ingredients that can be added to toothpastes to benefit patients and explain what conditions the ingredients can help.
- Define the term systemic antibiotic.
- Explain why systemic antibiotics are not usually used to treat patients with plaque-associated gingivitis and with chronic periodontitis.
- Define the term controlled-release delivery device.
- Summarize research findings that relate to using irrigation to deliver chemicals to periodontal pockets.
- Explain the term host modulation as it relates to periodontitis patients.

KEY TERMS

Systemic delivery
Local delivery
Antibiotic resistance
Therapeutic mouth rinses
Efficacy
Stability
Substantivity

Safety
Active ingredient
Inactive ingredient
Essential oils
Controlled-release delivery device
Systemic antibiotics
Host modulation

SECTION 1: INTRODUCTION TO CHEMICAL AGENTS IN PERIODONTAL CARE

Gingival and periodontal diseases are caused by bacterial infections. Over the years, many bacterial infections that have affected mankind have been brought under control using various medications or chemicals to attack specific germs that cause diseases. It is quite natural for researchers and clinicians alike to search for medications or chemicals to help control periodontal diseases.

1. **Mechanisms for Delivery of Chemical Agents**
    A. **Systemic Delivery**—chemical agents, such as antibiotics, delivered in the form of a tablet or capsule.
    B. **Local Delivery**—chemical agents delivered locally in the mouth in the form of mouth rinses, dentifrices, subgingival irrigation solutions, or controlled-release devices.
2. **Resistance of the Dental Plaque Biofilm to Local Delivery of Chemical Agents**
    A. The surface of the dental plaque biofilm is covered by a slime layer.
    B. The protective nature of the slime layer limits the extent to which chemical agents delivered locally to the oral cavity can be expected to control plaque and therefore control gingivitis.
3. *At this point, there is no chemical agent that can halt periodontitis, but there are a number of different chemical agents that can be used as part of a comprehensive treatment plan for patients with either gingivitis or periodontitis.* An overview of the types of chemical agents that have been suggested for use in periodontal patients is presented in **Table 22-1**.
4. **Considerations Regarding the Use of Antibiotic Agents.** Antibiotics are drugs that fight infections caused by bacteria.
    A. **Antibiotic resistance** is the ability of a bacterium to withstand the effects of an antibiotic. Antibiotic resistant strains of bacteria survive and continue to cause more tissue damage.
    B. Dental health care providers must weigh the benefits and disadvantages when considering the use of antibiotic drugs or chemicals for the treatment of periodontal infections.

Table 22-1. Delivery Systems for Chemical Agents

Influence	Delivery System	Uses
Oral: *supra*gingival	Therapeutic mouth rinses	Reduce the severity of gingival inflammation
	Therapeutic dentifrices	Reduction in dentinal hypersensitivity Reduction in gingival inflammation Reduction of supragingival calculus deposits Reduction in surface stains on teeth
Oral: *sub*gingival	Professional irrigation	Disruption and dilution the bacteria and their products from within periodontal pockets
	Controlled-release delivery devices	Subject subgingival bacteria to therapeutic levels of a drug for a period of a week or longer
Systemic	Tablets, capsules	Aggressive periodontitis Acute oral infections

SECTION 2: MOUTH RINSES AS AIDS IN CONTROLLING GINGIVITIS

1. **Cosmetic versus Therapeutic Mouth Rinses**
   A. Cosmetic mouth rinses have been marketed for many, many decades.
      1. Many of the early mouth rinses were used primarily simply to cover up or mask the odors of halitosis (bad breath).
      2. Those early mouth rinses contained chemicals that made temporary improvement in odors arising from the mouth, but were not helpful in actually controlling oral disease such as gingivitis.
   B. Therapeutic Mouth Rinses. **Therapeutic mouth rinses** are products that claim to be beneficial in controlling gingivitis (**Fig. 22-1**). Over the last few decades, researchers have been searching for chemicals that can be added to mouth rinses that might actually help reduce plaque build up on the tooth surface and thereby help control gingivitis or periodontitis.

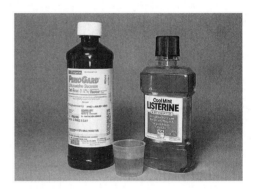

Figure 22-1. Therapeutic Mouth Rinses. Two examples of therapeutic mouth rinses. The mouth rinse pictured on the left has chlorhexidine gluconate as the active ingredient. The mouth rinse pictured on the right has essential oils as the active ingredients.

2. **Characteristics That an *Ideal* Mouth Rinse Should Possess**. Investigations into chemical plaque control have not yet produced a plaque control mouth rinse that can be used as a substitute for mechanical plaque control. However, these investigations have indeed produced mouth rinses that can be useful components of a comprehensive program of patient self-care. An *ideal mouth* rinse would possess these four characteristics.
   A. **Efficacy**—the agent should inhibit or kill periodontal pathogens.
   B. **Stability**—the agent should be stable at room temperature and have a reasonable shelf life.
   C. **Substantivity** (sub-stan-tiv-ity)—the agent should be retained in the oral cavity and be released slowly over time with continued antimicrobial effect.
   D. **Safety**—the agent should not produce any harmful effects on the local tissues or systemically to the patient.

3. **Ingredients**
   A. Products such as mouthwashes and dentifrices contain both active ingredients and inactive ingredients.
      1. An **active ingredient** is a component in a mouthwash that is expected to produce some benefit for the patient (such as a reduction in gingivitis).
      2. An **inactive ingredient** is included simply to add color, improve the taste, act as a preservative, or keep components in a liquid state.
   B. Many chemicals—that might be placed in mouth rinses—have been investigated for their effect against plaque and gingivitis.
      1. Chemicals that reduce plaque formation to only a minor degree usually have no clinically significant effect against gingivitis, and therefore are not useful in controlling a disease such as gingivitis. Many mouth rinses marketed today fall into this category.

2. Three mouth rinse ingredients that have some effect against gingivitis have been studied extensively.
   a. Essential oils
   b. Chlorhexidine gluconate
   c. Cetylpyridinium chloride

4. **Mouth Rinses Containing Essential Oils** (e.g.,. Listerine)
   A. A group of chemicals called **essential oils** has been used as an active ingredient in mouth rinses for many years. Chemical agents included in the group of chemicals called essential oils include thymol, menthol, eucalyptol, and methyl salicylate.
   B. Availability. These mouth rinses are available over-the-counter (without a prescription).
   C. Efficacy
      1. This group of chemicals can indeed help control plaque and have received the Seal of Acceptance from the American Dental Association for their effect against *gingivitis*.
      2. Investigations have demonstrated that the overall severity of gingivitis can be reduced by approximately 35% using these rinses.
      3. Mouth rinses containing essential oils are less effective than chlorhexidine gluconate mouth rinses. However, these mouth rinses are much less expensive than chlorhexidine gluconate mouth rinses and can be purchased without a prescription.

5. **Mouth Rinses Containing Chlorhexidine Gluconate**
   A. Availability. Currently available only through prescriptions, mouth rinses containing chlorhexidine gluconate as the active ingredient have also been demonstrated to reduce the severity of gingivitis. In the United States the concentration of chlorhexidine gluconate used in prescription mouth rinses is 0.12%, but it should be noted that a slightly higher concentration is used in some other countries.
   B. Efficacy. The American Dental Association Council on Dental Therapeutics has accepted chlorhexidine as an antimicrobial and antigingivitis agent.
      1. Investigations have demonstrated that the overall severity of *gingivitis* can be reduced by approximately 50% when patients use these rinses as recommended.
      2. *Chlorhexidine is the most effective antimicrobial agent for long-term reduction of plaque and gingivitis.* For this reason, it is often regarded as the standard against which all other topical chemical plaque control agents are judged.
      3. The effectiveness of chlorhexidine gluconate mouth rinses is due to these characteristics:
         a. Efficacy—chlorhexidine is bactericidal against gram-positive and gram-negative bacteria and yeasts (such as those responsible for oral candidiasis).
         b. Substantivity—chlorhexidine binds with hard and soft oral tissues and is slowly released over time in a concentration that will kill bacteria.
         c. Safety—chlorhexidine seems to have a very low level of toxicity and shows no permanent retention in the body.
   C. Use. Recommendations for use of this mouth rinse are to rinse with one-half ounce for 30 seconds twice daily.
      1. Special Needs Patients. The use of a chlorhexidine mouth rinse is suggested for specific groups of patients, such as patients with immunodeficiencies and patients who are unable or unwilling to perform plaque control.
      2. Postsurgical Care. In periodontal treatment, chlorhexidine is used for postoperative rinsing and as an adjunct to mechanical plaque control. Use of a chlorhexidine mouth rinse immediately following periodontal surgery, for 4 to 6 weeks, is effective in facilitating postsurgical healing.
      3. Control of *Candida* Infections. Chlorhexidine can be used effectively as a disinfectant for dentures in patients with *Candida* infections.

4. Control of Dental Caries. Chlorhexidine is also effective against the bacteria responsible for dental caries. Patients at increased risk for root caries include those with moderate to severe bone loss, geriatric patients, and patients with removable partial dentures. Daily or weekly rinsing with a chlorhexidine mouth rinse reduces the counts of mutans streptococci, Lactobacillus, and Candida.

5. Oral Piercing After Care. Chlorhexidine mouth rinses are also recommended for tongue piercing after-care.

6. **Mouth Rinses Containing Cetylpyridinium Chloride** (e.g.,. Cepacol, Pro-Health, Scope)

   A. Some mouth rinses currently marketed contain cetylpyridinium chloride.

   B. Investigations have shown that this chemical can reduce the severity of gingivitis but the level of reduction is less than either chlorhexidine gluconate or the essential oils.

   C. Currently these products do not have the American Dental Association Seal of Acceptance.

7. **Problems with Mouth Rinse Ingredients**

   A. No chemicals are completely safe for all patients, and all mouth rinses have produced unwanted side effects in some patients. Reported side effects for some of the active ingredients discussed above are outlined in Box 22-1 and Box 22-3.

   B. In addition to the active ingredients, mouth rinses contain inactive ingredients such as flavoring agents and preservatives that can create problems for some patients.

      1. Alcohol. Some mouth rinses have rather high levels of alcohol content, and these should be avoided in patients addicted to alcohol.

      2. Salt. Some mouth rinses have rather high levels of sodium, making them questionable for use in certain patients with hypertension (high blood pressure).

Box 22-1

Possible Side Effects of Essential Oils

- Burning sensation in the mouth
- Bitter taste
- Drying out of mucous membranes

Box 22-2

Possible Side Effects for Chlorhexidine Gluconate

- Allergic reaction
- Extrinsic staining of teeth
- Discoloration of tongue
- Alterations of taste
- Increase in calculus formation

SECTION 3: DENTIFRICES AS DELIVERY MECHANISMS FOR CHEMICAL AGENTS

Dentifrices such as toothpastes and gels would appear to be nearly ideal delivery mechanisms for ingredients that might benefit patients, since most patients use these products. Originally dentifrices were simply aids to brushing deposits off tooth surfaces, but today there are a variety of chemical agents that can be added as active ingredients to toothpastes that may actually benefit some patients in other ways.

1. **Categories of Toothpastes.** The American Dental Association loosely classifies toothpastes as falling into one of the following categories:
   A. Antitartar activity
   B. Caries prevention
   C. Cosmetic effects
   D. Gingivitis reduction
   E. Plaque formation reduction
   F. Reduction of tooth sensitivity
2. **Active Chemical Ingredients.** This classification of toothpastes underscores the broad range of benefits that can be derived from active ingredient chemical agents added to some toothpastes.
   A. A broad range of chemical agents added to some of these toothpastes imparts the special characteristics. For example, a chemical agent added to some pastes is responsible for the antitartar or anticalculus activity of the paste.
   B. See **Table 22-2** for some examples of the chemical agents that can be used as active ingredients in toothpastes.
   C. Toothpastes appear to be ideal delivery mechanisms for chemical agents that might be expected to control certain oral conditions, such as gingival inflammation. It is reasonable to expect that additional research in this area will result in additional toothpaste formulations that target periodontal conditions such as gingivitis.

Table 22-2. Toothpaste Active Ingredients

Ingredient	Action
Potassium nitrate, sodium citrate, strontium chloride	Reduces dentinal hypersensitivity
Pyrophosphates, triclosan, zinc citrate	Reduces *supragingival* calculus
Triclosan, stannous fluoride	Reduces gingival inflammation
Peroxides, sodium tripolyphosphate, sodium hexametaphosphate	Removes surface stains on teeth

SECTION 4: SUBGINGIVAL IRRIGATION WITH ANTIMICROBIAL CHEMICALS

1. **Description of Subgingival Irrigation. Professional subgingival irrigation** is the in-office flushing of pockets performed by the dental hygienist or dentist using one of three systems:
   A. A blunt-tipped irrigating cannula that is attached to a hand-held syringe
   B. Ultrasonic unit equipped with a reservoir
   C. A specialized air-driven handpiece that connects to the dental unit airline
2. **Rationale For Subgingival Irrigation**
   A. The purpose of subgingival irrigation is the disruption and dilution the bacteria and their products from within periodontal pockets.
   B. Studies have been conducted on the extent of irrigant penetration achieved using various types of equipment.
      1. With Hand-Held Syringe (**Fig 22-2**): One study reported penetration of 90% for sites 6 mm or less in depth and penetration of 64% for pockets 7 mm or deeper when the tip was inserted 1 to 2 mm into the pocket. When positioned 3 mm within periodontal pockets the syringe provides a means of reaching the apical subgingival plaque border with the irrigating solution.
      2. With Mechanized Pulsed-Jet Irrigator: This device was found to be even more effective than a hand-held syringe.
      3. With Precision-Thin Ultrasonic Tips (**Fig 22-3**): Infiltration of the irrigant has been shown to be equal to the depth reached by the ultrasonic tip.

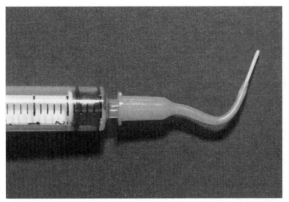

Figure 22-2. Hand-Held Syringe. Close-up view of the tip of a hand-held syringe used for subgingival irrigation. The tip is positioned subgingivally for delivery of an antimicrobial solution.

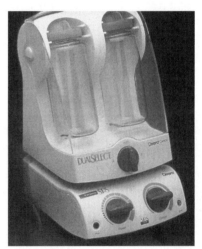

Figure 22-3. Hand-Held Syringe. This ultrasonic device has a dispensing system for antimicrobial solutions while using an ultrasonic tip for calculus removal. (Courtesy of Dentsply Cavitron, Dentsply International, York, PA.)

3. **Irrigant Solutions.** Solutions used for subgingival irrigation include chlorhexidine gluconate, povidone-iodine and water, stannous fluoride, tetracycline, or Listerine. Chlorhexidine gluconate and essential oil mouth rinses can be used full-strength. Povidone-iodine can be diluted as 1 part povidone-iodine to 9 parts water. Stannous fluoride is diluted as 1 part stannous fluoride to 1 part water.
4. **Benefits of Subgingival Irrigation**
   A. A single application of in-office subgingival irrigation with an antimicrobial agent has been shown to have only limited or no beneficial effects over periodontal instrumentation alone.

1. There is no long-lasting substantivity of the antimicrobial agent in the periodontal pocket due to the continuous flow of gingival crevicular fluid from the pocket, and the presence of serum and proteins in the pocket.
2. A substantive antimicrobial agent, such as chlorhexidine gluconate, would have to be retained in the pocket and be released slowly over a period of time to interfere with the repopulation of bacteria within the pocket.
3. Most experts do not recommend routine in-office subgingival irrigation. Although irrigation initially does reduce the number of bacteria, the bacteria are not eliminated and their numbers return to the original levels in a short period of time.
B. *The majority of research studies concluded that irrigation with water provided an equally beneficial effect as irrigation with an antimicrobial agent. These results suggest that it may be the physical flushing of the pocket that may produce any benefits from subgingival irrigation.*
C. Subgingival irrigation performed before periodontal instrumentation may reduce the incidence of bacteremia and reduce the number of microorganisms in aerosols.

SECTION 5: CONTROLLED-RELEASE OF ANTIMICROBIAL CHEMICALS

1. **Overview of Controlled-Release Mechanisms**
   A. A **controlled-release delivery device** is placed directly into the periodontal pocket and is designed to produce a steady release of an antimicrobial agent over a period of several days within the periodontal pocket.
   B. Antimicrobial agents currently used in controlled-release delivery devices include chlorhexidine and antibiotic drugs. In the future, other drugs may be used for this purpose.
   C. The antimicrobial agent may be incorporated in a variety of delivery devices including fibers, chips, or gels.
2. **Rationale for Use.** The goal of these devices is to subject subgingival bacteria to therapeutic levels of a drug for a sustained period of up to a week or longer.
3. **Benefits of Controlled-Release Delivery Devices**
   A. Use of controlled-release delivery devices has been shown to result in some small increase in attachment level in a periodontal pocket.
   B. Unfortunately, very few controlled studies are available to guide dental health care providers in the appropriate use of these new devices.
      1. *Based on information currently available, it appears that most of these devices do not produce the therapeutic results of periodontal instrumentation.*
      2. Controlled-release devices may be indicated for use in localized sites that are nonresponsive after thorough nonsurgical and surgical periodontal therapy.
      3. Currently most clinicians use these devices in combination with periodontal debridement rather than as a substitute for periodontal debridement.
4. **Controlled-Release Mechanisms.** Several controlled-release delivery products have been introduced in the United States over the last few years, and it is likely that more will be available within the next few years.
   A. **Tetracycline HCL Fibers**
      1. Tetracycline-containing fibers that are inserted into the periodontal pocket to deliver a high concentration of tetracycline to the site.
      2. Application.
         a. A gingival retraction cord-packing instrument is used to insert the fibers. Insertion is time consuming and an adhesive is needed to retain the fibers.
         b. The fiber is placed under the gingival margin around the entire tooth.
         c. The entire pocket is filled by layering the fiber back and forth upon itself (**Fig. 22-4**). The pocket should be filled with the fiber up to 1 mm below the gingival margin.
         d. Finally, adhesive is applied along the gingival margin to affix the fiber.

3. Patient Instructions
   a. Avoid brushing, flossing, or chewing at the site treated with the fibers.
   b. Call the office if the fiber falls out, so that a new fiber can be placed in the site.
   c. Return to the dental office after 10 days to have the fibers removed.
4. Adverse Reactions. Adverse reactions that have been reported include discomfort on fiber placement, oral candidiasis, possible allergic response, severe gingival inflammation, and throbbing pain. The use of antibiotic preparations may result in the development of resistant bacteria.
5. Contraindications for Use.
   a. This product should not be used in patients who are hypersensitive to any tetracycline.
   b. Administration of tetracycline during pregnancy may cause permanent discoloration of the teeth of the fetus.
   c. Because of the potential for serious adverse reactions from tetracycline in nursing infants, this product should not be used in nursing women.

B. **Minocycline Hydrochloride Microspheres**
   1. Another example of a controlled-release mechanism delivers the antibiotic minocycline hydrochloride in a powdered microsphere form. Minocycline hydrochloride is a broad-spectrum, semisynthetic tetracycline derivative that is bacteriostatic for up to 14 days.
   2. Application
      a. A cannula tip is used to expel the microspheres into the pocket (**Fig. 22-5**).
      b. Over time, the powdered microspheres completely dissolve, so there is nothing to remove from the pocket.
   3. Adverse Reactions. Possible adverse reactions include oral candidiasis and a possible allergic response. The use of antibiotic preparations may result in the development of resistant bacteria.
   4. Contraindications for Use. This product is a tetracycline derivative, and therefore, should not be used in patients who are hypersensitive to any tetracycline or with woman who are pregnant or nursing.

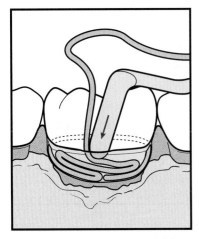

Figure 22-4. Fibers Inserted into the Pocket. The tetracy-cline-containing fiber is inserted into the periodontal pocket. The entire pocket is filled by layering the fiber back and forth upon itself.

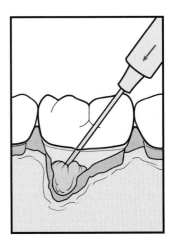

Figure 22-5. Products Expelled into the Pocket. The minocycline hydrochloride microspheres and the doxycycline gel are examples of products that are expelled into the periodontal pocket using a cannula tip.

C. **Doxycycline Hyclate Gel**
  1. This product is a gel system that delivers the antibiotic doxycycline (a tetracycline derivative) to the periodontal pocket.
  2. Application
     a. The gel is expressed into the pocket with a cannula after which the gel solidifies into a waxlike substance.
        1) The cannula tip is placed near the pocket base and gel is expressed using a steady pressure until the gel reaches the top of the gingival margin (**Fig. 22-5**).
        2) A problem with this delivery system is that the gel tends to cling to the cannula when it is withdrawn from the pocket. This problem can be reduced by using a moistened dental hand instrument to hold the gel in place while slowly withdrawing the cannula tip from the pocket.
     b. In clinical trials, a periodontal dressing was used to retain the gel in the pockets.
     c. The gel is biodegradable (it dissolves) so there is nothing to remove from the pocket, however, if a periodontal dressing is used, the patient will have to return for a second visit to remove the dressing.
  3. Adverse Reactions
     a. Possible adverse reactions include oral candidiasis and a possible allergic response.
     b. The use of antibiotic preparations may result in the development of resistant bacteria.
  4. Contraindications for Use. This product is a tetracycline derivative, and therefore, should not be used in patients who are hypersensitive to any tetracycline or with women who are pregnant or nursing.

D. **Chlorhexidine Gluconate Chip**
  1. Another example of a controlled-release device is a tiny gelatin chip containing the antiseptic chlorhexidine that is inserted into periodontal pockets 5 mm or greater in depth (**Fig. 22-6**).
  2. Application
     a. The gelatin chip is inserted into the periodontal pocket.
     b. The gelatin chip can be difficult to insert into some pockets due to the size and shape of the chip.
     c. The gelatin chip is bioabsorbed so there is no need to have it removed after placement.
  3. Adverse Reactions. *Since chlorhexidine is not an antibiotic, there is no risk of antibiotic resistance with use of the chlorhexidine gluconate gelatin chip.*

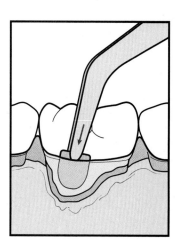

Figure 22-6. Gelatin Tip Inserted into Pocket. The gelatin chip is inserted into periodontal pockets 5 mm or greater in depth.

SECTION 6: SYSTEMIC ANTIBIOTICS IN PERIODONTAL CARE

1. **Antibiotics** are medications used to help fight infections either because they kill bacteria or because they can inhibit the growth of bacteria. **Systemic antibiotics** refer to those that can be taken orally and are in widespread use in fighting bacterial infections. Systemic antibiotics that have been investigated for use as part of periodontal care are listed in Box 22-4.

2. **Use for Treatment of Gingivitis and Chronic Periodontitis.** *The use of systemic (oral) antibiotics is not normally a part of nonsurgical periodontal therapy for patients with plaque-associated gingivitis or with chronic periodontitis.*

3. **Patient Education.** Even though these drugs are not normally used for these diseases, systemic antibiotics are discussed here because periodontal patients will often ask why antibiotics are not being recommended for them.

   A. This question often arises when the patient learns that periodontitis is a bacterial infection. This is a natural question for a patient to ask given the widespread use of antibiotics in fighting infections of all sorts.

   B. When confronted with a question from a patient about why antibiotics are not being recommended, the dental hygienist should explain the following:

      1. Most cases of gingivitis and periodontitis can be readily controlled without the use of systemic antibiotics.

      2. In the mouth, bacteria grow so quickly and so readily that to control diseases such as periodontitis with an antibiotic would require that the drug be taken for many, many years for these chronic diseases.

      3. Overuse of antibiotics often results in the development of antibiotic-resistant strains of bacteria, simply compounding a complex problem.

      4. **Use for Treatment of Aggressive Periodontitis.** *Even though systemic antibiotics are not normally used to treat patients with chronic periodontitis, they are frequently used by the periodontist in management of patients with some of the rarer forms of periodontitis such as aggressive periodontitis* (Box 22-4).

      5. **Use for Treatment of Acute Oral Infections.** In addition, systemic antibiotics are frequently used when treating acute oral infections such as a periodontal abscess.

Box 22-4

Systemic Antibiotics Commonly Used in Periodontal Care

- Penicillin and amoxicillin
- Tetracyclines
- Erythromycin
- Metronidazole
- Clindamycin

SECTION 7: HOST-MODULATION DRUGS IN PERIODONTAL CARE

1. **Host modulation** refers to altering the defense mechanisms used by the human body to help keep infections such as periodontitis under control. Modulation of host defenses is an important focus for periodontal research, and host modulation will undoubtedly play a larger part in nonsurgical therapy in the future.

2. **Enzyme-Suppression Therapy.** Currently, there is one systemic medication (in tablet form) that can indeed alter the host response to the bacterial challenge.

   A. Low-Dose Doxycycline
      1. This medication contains *low-doses* of a drug called doxycycline. At higher doses, doxycycline is actually an antibiotic used to treat a variety of infections.
      2. Doxycycline has other effects besides its antibiotic effect.
         a. *If this medication is given at low doses (below that needed for any antibacterial effect), it decreases the effects of the enzyme collagenase.*
         b. The enzyme collagenase plays a part in destruction of certain parts of the periodontium in periodontitis. Since collagen is one of the building blocks of the periodontium, prevention of its destruction could inhibit the progress of periodontitis.
         c. Since doxycycline at low doses alters the body defenses by inhibiting part of the destruction that can occur in periodontitis, it is considered one example of a host modulation.

   B. Future Host-Modulation Drugs. Members of the dental team should expect additional host-modulation products to appear on the market. Careful evaluation of each of the products will be needed.

SECTION 8: FOCUS ON PATIENTS

CASE 1

A patient shows you a bottle of mouth rinse and asks you if it would be all right to use this mouth rinse instead of brushing and flossing so frequently. You study the label on the bottle of mouth rinse and find that the active ingredients are the essential oils. How should you respond to this patient about substituting this rinse for brushing and flossing?

CASE 2

A patient being treated by the members of your dental team has generalized moderate chronic periodontitis. Following your thorough explanation of the nature of chronic periodontitis and your emphasis that this disease is indeed a bacterial infection, the patient asks this question, "If periodontitis is an infection, can you get the dentist to give me a prescription for an antibiotic?" How should you respond to this patient's question?

CASE 3

A new patient being seen by your dental team has recently moved into your city. She has previously been treated for chronic periodontitis and has been on periodontal maintenance for several years. She is experiencing some tooth sensitivity that has been diagnosed as mild dentinal hypersensitivity. What measures can you recommend that might help reduce the patient's dentinal hypersensitivity?

Suggested Readings

American Academy of Periodontology. Chemical agents for control of plaque and gingivitis. Committee on Research, Science and Therapy. Position Paper. Chicago: The Academy, 1994.

American Academy of Periodontology. The role of controlled drug delivery for periodontitis. *J Periodontol.* 2000;71:125–140.

Anwar H, Strap J, Costerton J. Establishment of aging biofilms: Possible mechanism of bacterial resistance to anti-microbial therapy. *Antimicrob Agents Chemother.* 1992;36:1347–1351.

Banting D, Bosma M, Bollmer B. Clinical effectiveness of a 0.12% chlorhexidine mouthrinse over two years. *J Dent Res.* 1989;68:1716.

Braun RE, Ciancio SG. Subgingival delivery by an oral irrigation device. *J Peridontol.* 1992;63:469–472.

Caton JG, Ciancio SG, Blieden TM, et al. Treatment with subantimicrobial dose doxycycline improves the efficacy of scaling and root planing in patients with adult periodontitis. *J Periodontol.* 2000;71:521–532.

Christersson LA, Norderyd OM, Puchalsky CS. Topical application of tetracycline-HCL in human periodontitis. J Clin Periodontol. 1993;20:88–95.

Ciancio SG. Agents for the management of plaque and gingivitis. *J Dent Res.* 1992;71:1450–1454.

Ciancio S. Expanded and future uses of mouthrinses. *J Am Dent Assoc.* 1994;125(Suppl 2):29S–32S.

Cubells AB, Dalmau LB, Petrone ME, et al. The effect of a triclosan/copolymer/fluoride dentifrice on plaque formation and gingivitis: A six-month study. *J Clin Dent.* 1991;2:63–69.

DeSalva SJ, Kong BM, Lin YJ. Triclosan: A safety profile. *Am J Dent.* 1989;2:185–196.

Drisko C, Cobb C, Killoy R, et al. Evaluation of periodontal treatments using controlled-release tetracycline fibers. Clinical response. *J Periodontol.* 1995;66:692–699.

Drisko CH. Review: Non-surgical periodontal therapy: Pharmacotherapeutics. In: *Annals of Periodontal Therapy 1996 World Workshop in Periodontics.* Chicago: 1996, American Academy of Periodontology; 1996:493–506.

Drisko CH. Nonsurgical periodontal therapy. *Periodontology 2000.* 2001;25:77–88.

Garrett S, Johnson L, Drisko CH, et al. Two multi-center clinical studies evaluating locally delivered doxycycline hyclate, placebo control, oral hygiene, and scaling and root planing in the treatment of periodontitis. *J Periodonto.l* 1999;70:490–503.

Gilbert P, Das J, Foley I. Biofilm susceptibility to antimicrobials. *Adv Dent Res.* 1997;11:160–167.

Gjermo P. Chlorhexidine and related compounds. *J Dent Res.* 1989;68:1602.

Golub LM, Ramamurthy N, McNamara TF, et al. Tetracyclines inhibit tissue collagenase activity. A new mechanism in the treatment of periodontal disease. *J Periodont Res.* 1984;19:651–655.

Goodson JM, Cugini MA, Kent RL, et al. Multi-center evaluation of tetracycline fiber therapy. I. Experimental design, methods, and baseline data. *J Periodont Res.* 1991;26:361.

Goodson JM, Cugini MA, Kent RL, et al. Multi-center evaluation of tetracycline fiber therapy: II. Clinical response. *J Periodont Res.* 1991;36:371.

Goodson JM. Pharmacokinetic principles controlling efficacy of oral therapy. *J Dent Res.* 1989:68:1625–1632.

Gordon JM, Lamster IB, Seiger MC. Efficacy of Listerine antiseptic in inhibiting the development of plaque and gingivitis. *J Clin Periodontol.* 1985;12:697.

Greenstein G, Lamster I. Efficacy of subantimicrobial dosing with doxycycline. Point/Counterpoint. *J Am Dent Assoc.* 2001;132:457–466.

Greenstein G. Povidone-iodone's effects and role in the management of periodontal diseases: A review. *J Periodontol.* 1999;70:1397–1405.

Grossman E, Reiter G, Sturzenberger OP, et al. Six-month study on the effects of a chlorhexidine mouthrinse on gingivitis in adults. *J Periodont Res.* 1986;21:33.

Haffajee AD, Socransky SS, Gunsolley JC. Systemic antiinfective periodontal therapy. A systematic review. *Ann Periodontol.* 2003;8:115–181.

Hardy JH, Newman, HN, Strahan JD. Direct irrigation and subgingival plaque. *J Clin Periodontol.* 1982;9:57–65.

Henke CJ, Villa KF, Aichelmann-Reidy ME, et al. An economic evaluation of a chlorhexidine chip for treating chronic periodontitis: The CHIP (chlorhexidine in periodontitis) study. *J Am Dent Assoc.* 2001;132:1557–1569.

Hanes PJ, Purvis JP. Local anti-infective therapy: Pharmacologic agents. A systematic review. *Ann Periodontol.* 2003;8:79–98.

Itic J, Serfaty R. Clinical effectiveness of subgingival irrigation with a pulsated jet irrigator versus syringe. *J Periodontol.* 1992;63:174–181.

Jeffcoat M, Bray KS, Ciancio SG, et al. Adjunctive use of a sub-gingival controlled release chlorhexidine chip reduces probing depth and improved attachment level compared with scaling and root planing alone. *J Periodontol.* 1998;69:989–997.

Kinane DF, Radvar M. A six-month comparison of three periodontal local antimicrobial therapies in persistent periodontal pockets. *J Periodontol.* 1999;70:1–7.

Killoy WJ. The clinical significance of local chemotherapies. *J Clin Periodontol.* 2002;29:22–29.

Killoy WJ, Polson AM. Controlled local delivery of antimicrobials in the treatment of periodontitis. *Dent Clin North Am.* 1998;42:263.

Krust KS, Drisko CL, Gross K, et al. The effects of subgingival irrigation with chlorhexidine and stannous fluoride. A preliminary investigation. *J Dent Hyg.* 1991;65:289–295.

Lamster IB, Alfano MC, Seiger MC, et al. The effect of Listerine antiseptic on reduction of existing plaque and gingivitis. *Clin Prev Dent.* 1983;5:12.

Lang NP, Brecx MC. Chlorhexidine digluconate—an agent for chemical plaque control and prevention of gingival inflammation. *J Periodont Res.* 1986;21(suppl):74–89.

Lobene RR, Lovene S, Soparker PM. The effect of cetylpyridinium chloride mouthrinse on plaque and gingivitis. *J Dent Res.* 1977;56:595.

Macaulay WJ, Newman HN. The effect on the composition of subgingival plaque of a simplified oral hygiene system including pulsating jet subgingival irrigation. *J Periodontal Res.,* 1986;21:375–385.

Newman JC, Kornman KS, Doherty FM. A 6-month multicenter evaluation of adjunctive tetracycline fiber therapy used in conjunction with scaling and root planing in maintenance patients: Clinical results. *J Periodontol.* 1994;65:685.

Nosal G, Scheidt MJ, O'Neal R, et al. The penetration of lavage solution into the periodontal pocket during ultrasonic instrumentation. *J Periodontol.* 1991;62:554–557.

Perlich MA, Bacca LA, Bollmer BW, et al. The clinical effect of a stabilized stannous fluoride dentifrice on plaque formation, gingivitis, and gingival bleeding: A six month study. *J Clin Dent.* 1995;6:54–58.

Quirynen M, Mongardini C, De Soete M, et al. The role of chlorhexidine in the one-stage full-mouth disinfection treatment of patients with advanced adult periodontitis. *J Clin Periodontol.* 2000;27:578–589. 2000.

Quirynen M, Teughels W, De Soete M, et al. Topical antiseptics and antibiotics in the initial therapy of chronic adult periodontitis: Microbiological aspects. *Periodontol 2000* 2002;28:72–90.

Radvar M, Pourtaghi N, Kinane DF. Comparison of 3 periodontal local antibiotic therapies in persistent periodontal pockets. *J Periodontol.* 1996;67:860–865.

Rahn R. Review presentation on povidone-iodine antisepsis in the oral cavity. *Postgrad Med J.* 1993;69:S4–S9.

Rams TE, Feik D, Listgarten MA, et al. Peptostreptococcus micros in human periodontitis. *Oral Microbiol Immunol.* 1992;7:1–6.

Scheie AAA. Modes of action of currently known chemical antiplaque agents other than chlorhexidine. *J Dent Res.* 1989;68:1609.

Slots J. Selection of antimicrobial agents in periodontal therapy. *J Periodont Res.* 2002;37:389–398.

Slots J, Ting M. Systemic antibiotics in the treatment of periodontal disease. *Periodontol 2000.* 2002;28:106–176.

Socransky SS, Haffajee AD. Dental biofilms: Difficult therapeutic targets. *Periodontol 2000.* 2002;28:12–55.

Soskolne WA, Heasman PA, Stabholz A, et al. Sustained local delivery of chlorhexidine in the treatment of periodontitis: A multicenter study. *J Periodontol.* 1997;68:32–38.

Southard SR, Drisko CL, Killoy WJ, et al. The effect of 2% chlorhexidine digluconate irrigation on clinical parameters and the level of Bacteroides gingivalis in periodontal pockets. *J Periodontol.* 1989;60:302–309.

Systemic antibiotics in periodontics. *J Periodontol.* 1996;67:831–838.

Thomas J, Walker C, Bradshaw M. Long-term use of subantimicrobial dose doxycycline does not lead to changes in antimicrobial susceptibility. *J Periodontol.* 2000;71:1472–1483.

van der Ouderaa FJG. Anti-plaque agents. Rationale and prospects for prevention of gingivitis and periodontal disease. *J Clin Periodontol.* 1991;18:447–454.

van Steenberghe D, Bercy P, Kohl J, et al. Subgingival minocycline hydrochloride ointment in moderate to severe chronic adult periodontitis: A randomized, double-blind, vehicle-controlled, multicenter study. *J Periodontol.* 1993;64:637–644.

van Steenberghe D, Rosling B, Soder PO, et al. A 15 month evaluation of the effects of repeated subgingival minocycline in chronic adult periodontitis. *J Periodontol.* 1999;70:657–667.

Watts EA, Newman HN. Clinical effects on chronic periodontitis of a simplified system of oral hygiene including subgingival pulsated jet irritation with chlorhexidine. *J Clin Periodontol.* 1986;13:666–670.

Wennstrom JL, Heijl L, Dahlen G, et al. Periodic subgingival antimicrobial irrigation of periodontal pockets (I). Clinical Observations. *J Clin Periodontol.* 1987;14:541–550.

Wennstrom JL, Dahlen G, Grondahl K, et al. Periodic subgingival antimicrobial irrigation of periodontal pockets II. Microbiological and radiographical observations. *J Clin Periodontol.* 1987;14:573–580.

Wennstrom JL, Newman HN, MacNeil SR, et al. Utilization of locally delivered doxycycline in non-surgical treatment of chronic periodontitis. A comparative multi-center trial of 2 treatment approaches. *J Clin Periodontol.* 2001;28:753–761.

Williams RC, Paquette DW, Offenbacher S, et al. Treatment of periodontitis by local administration of minocycline microspheres: A controlled trial. *J Periodontol.* 2001;72:1535–1544.

SECTION 9: CHAPTER REVIEW QUESTIONS

1. Which of the following explains why mouth rinses cannot cure gingivitis completely?
   a. Many bacteria that cause gingivitis are protected within a biofilm
   b. Bacteria cannot be killed with any mouth rinse active ingredient
   c. Prescription mouth rinses are too expensive for patients

2. Which of the following active ingredients is the MOST EFFECTIVE against gingivitis?
   a. Essential oils
   b. Chlorhexidine gluconate
   c. Cetylpyridinium chloride

3. Which of the following is a common side effect for mouth rinses containing chlorhexidine gluconate?
   a. Increased tooth mobility
   b. Extrinsic tooth stain
   c. Dryness of the mouth

4. Examples of the benefits of chemical agents that can be added to toothpastes are that they can (i) reduce dentinal hypersensitivity, (ii) reduce supragingival calculus formation, (iii) or reduce gingivitis.
   a. True
   b. False

5. Active ingredients that can be incorporated into controlled-release delivery mechanisms include chlorhexidine gluconate, doxycycline, and minocycline.
   a. True
   b. False

6. A single application of in-office subgingival irrigation with an antimicrobial agent has been shown to:
   a. Cure both gingivitis and periodontitis in the vast majority of patients
   b. Be superior to periodontal instrumentation done by skilled professionals
   c. Have limited or no more beneficial effects than periodontal instrumentation

7. Which of the following mediations can be both an antibiotic and a host-modulation drug?
   a. Essential oils
   b. Doxycycline
   c. Potassium nitrate

23 Periodontal Maintenance

Refer to the CD packaged with this book for full color versions of the clinical photographs in this chapter.

Learning Objectives

- Define the term periodontal maintenance.
- List the objectives of periodontal maintenance.
- List components of periodontal maintenance.
- Explain treatment procedures that may be needed at a maintenance visit.
- Describe an appropriate maintenance interval.
- Define the term recurrence as it applies to periodontitis.
- List clinical signs of recurrence of periodontitis.
- Explain reasons for recurrence of periodontitis.
- Define the term compliance.
- List strategies that can be used to improve patient compliance.
- In a clinical setting, develop a periodontal maintenance strategy for a patient with periodontitis.

KEY TERMS

Baseline data
Clinical periodontal assessment
Compliance
Comprehensive periodontal therapy
Nonsurgical periodontal therapy

Periodontal maintenance
Recurrence
Re-evaluation
Root caries

SECTION 1: INTRODUCTION TO PERIODONTAL MAINTENANCE

OVERVIEW OF PERIODONTAL MAINTENANCE

1. The **periodontal maintenance** phase of treatment includes all measures used by the dental team and the patient to keep periodontitis under control.
    A. Periodontal maintenance is an essential element of successful periodontal therapy.
        1. Without regular periodontal maintenance, patients exhibit a decrease in self-care and a recurrence of periodontitis.[1]
        2. With good periodontal maintenance, most periodontitis patients can retain their teeth in function and comfort for many years.[2]
    B. Following nonsurgical periodontal therapy or nonsurgical periodontal therapy plus periodontal surgery, periodontitis patients are placed in program of periodontal maintenance. The goal of this stage of treatment is to prevent the recurrence of periodontal diseases.
2. **Rationale for Periodontal Maintenance**
    A. Periodontitis is a chronic disease that cannot be totally cured with the therapies currently available to the dental team.
        1. Periodontitis can be *controlled*, however, in the vast majority of patients.
        2. Among those patients treated for periodontitis, the disease tends to recur, and constant vigilance is needed on the part of the dental team to keep periodontitis under control.
        3. *In most dental teams the dental hygienist is the primary health care provider for this phase of treatment.*
    B. Objectives of Periodontal Maintenance (Box 23-1)
        1. Control inflammation in the periodontium by controlling etiologic factors.
            a. The primary risk factor for inflammatory periodontal diseases is bacterial plaque.
            b. Secondary risk factors include plaque-retentive areas (such as calculus or restorations with overhangs), smoking, and systemic factors.
        2. Preserve attachment levels.
        3. Preserve alveolar bone levels.
3. **Periodontal Maintenance Is a Team Effort**
    A. Periodontal maintenance requires considerable effort from the patient in sustaining meticulous self-care and regular professional periodontal maintenance care throughout his or her life.
    B. Periodontal maintenance requires considerable effort on the part of the dental health team for professional assistance at regular intervals, for renewal of motivation, instruction in plaque control, and elimination or reduction of primary and secondary risk factors.

Box 23-1

Objectives of Periodontal Maintenance

- Control inflammation of the periodontium
- Preserve tooth attachment levels
- Maintain alveolar bone levels

The expected outcome of achieving these objectives would be to maintain the dentition throughout the life of the patient.

4. **Terminology.** Many terms have been used to describe this phase of care.
    A. In 2000, the Board of Trustees of the American Academy of Periodontology approved the term periodontal maintenance as the preferred terminology for the care recommended for patients who have completed periodontal treatment.[3]
    B. Other terms for periodontal maintenance are:
        1. Supportive periodontal treatment (SPT)
        2. Recall maintenance or periodontal recall
        3. Continuing care
5. Appropriate Use of the Term
    1. *The term periodontal maintenance is used to describe the office treatment provided to patients who have been previously treated for periodontitis.*
    2. *It is normally not appropriate to use the term periodontal maintenance for patients treated for gingivitis.*
6. **Components of Comprehensive Treatment.** The phases of **comprehensive periodontal therapy** are summarized in Figure 23-1.
    A. **Clinical Periodontal Assessment**—data gathered during this phase result in a periodontal diagnosis and a plan for initial periodontal therapy.
    B. **Nonsurgical Periodontal Therapy**—during this phase of treatment, the dental team performs all the necessary nonsurgical measures to bring the existing periodontal disease under control.
    C. **Reevaluation**—at the end of the initial periodontal therapy, the results of the initial treatment are re-evaluated.
        1. Based on the findings of this reevaluation, additional therapy such as periodontal surgery might be recommended.
        2. At the reevaluation, the dental team also must decide what periodontal maintenance care will be needed.
    D. **Periodontal Maintenance**—this phase of periodontal treatment begins at the close of the nonsurgical periodontal therapy, and in some patients, periodontal maintenance can run concurrently with the periodontal surgical intervention.

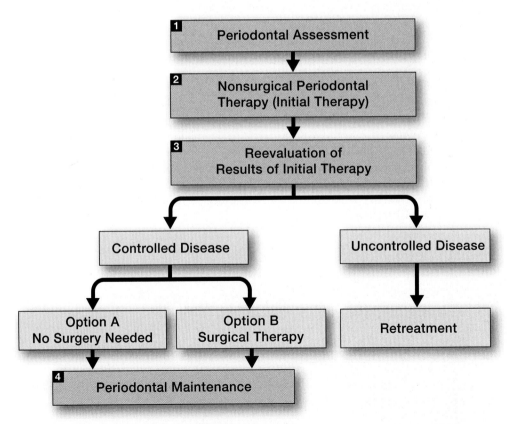

Figure 23-1. Phases of Periodontal Therapy. This flow chart outlines the normal sequence of periodontal therapy for a patient and illustrates where periodontal maintenance falls in this sequence.

SECTION 2: COMPONENTS OF PERIODONTAL MAINTENANCE

Successful periodontal maintenance requires the active participation of the patient, dentist, and dental hygienist. Periodontal maintenance should be adjusted to fit the needs of the individual patient. A typical patient office visit for periodontal maintenance includes steps such as an update of the medical and dental histories, a clinical examination, periodontal assessment, radiographic examination, plaque-control evaluation, periodontal debridement, recommendations and referrals, and an outcomes assessment. Typical components of periodontal maintenance are summarized in Table 23-1.

Table 23-1. Typical Components of Periodontal Maintenance

Procedure	Indicators or Risk Factors for Disease
Medical and dental history	New illnesses Change in medical status Changes in medications Smoking
Clinical examination Extraoral and intraoral examination Dental examination	Tooth loss since last charting Oral lesions Overhangs, poorly contoured restorations; tissue damage from removable prosthesis
Radiographic examination	Progressing radiographic evidence of boneloss
Periodontal examination Inspection of tissues Probing depths Attachment loss Bleeding upon probing Levels of plaque and calculus Furcation involvement Tooth mobility Gingival recession Mucogingival involvement Occlusal analysis	 Inflammation Deepening probing depths Increased loss of attachment Presence of bleeding Extent and distribution Presence of furcation involvement Increasing mobility Progressive recession Minimal keratinized gingiva Occlusal contributing factors
Plaque-control evaluation	Lack of manual dexterity Discontinued use of self-care methods Type II or III embrasure spaces
Treatment Periodontal debridement Counseling Reinstruction in self-care Application of fluorides Prevention of root caries Adjunctive therapy	Noncompliance with recommended maintenance intervals
Planning Recommendations for treatment needs Referrals Determination of maintenance interval Scheduling of next maintenance visit	Noncompliance with recommended maintenance intervals
Outcomes assessment	Recurrence of periodontitis

UPDATES AND EXAMINATIONS DURING PERIODONTAL MAINTENANCE

1. **Review and Update of Medical, Social, and Dental Histories.** Changes in the medical, social, or dental status of the patient should be documented. The following factors should be evaluated:
   A. Social History
      1. Age of the patient
      2. Changes in social history or life changes, such as birth of a child, bereavement, change in job status, or unemployment
   B. Medical History
      1. New illnesses or a change in medical status (referral or consultation with a physician may be indicated)
      2. Current medications
   C. Presence of Local Risk Factors
      1. Risk factors that contribute to periodontal disease, such as smoking, medications (phenytoin, cyclosporine, calcium channel blockers), stress, and systemic disease
      2. Appropriate counseling about risk factors should be provided.
   D. Restorative Needs. New restorative treatment completed since the last visit should be noted on the patient chart. All restorations should be examined.

2. **Clinical Examination.** Results of the clinical, periodontal, and radiographic examinations should be compared with previous baseline data. **Baseline data** are clinical data gathered at the beginning of the periodontal treatment. Data gathered at subsequent appointments are compared with baseline data. Baseline values are first established during the initial assessment phase and again following initial periodontal therapy. The clinical examination usually includes the steps below.
   A. Extraoral and Intraoral Examination
   B. Dental Examination
      1. Caries assessment
      2. Restorative and prosthetic assessment
      3. Tooth loss since last charting
   C. Radiographic Examination
      1. Examination should include an evaluation of bone level, tooth, and periodontal ligament space.
      2. The most recent set of radiographs should be compared with radiographs taken at the current maintenance appointment.

3. **Periodontal Examination**
   A. Inspection of the Tissues
      1. Clinical signs of inflammation include changes in color, texture, or consistency.
      2. The presence of gingival recession increases the risk for dentinal hypersensitivity and root caries. Patients may be concerned about the aesthetic appearance.
   B. Probing Depth. Disease progression (a worsening of periodontitis) is indicated by 1- to 2-mm increase in probing depth.
   C. Attachment Loss
      1. Currently, the most reliable way to evaluate periodontal disease stability.
      2. Disease progression is indicated by a 2- to 3-mm increase in clinical attachment loss.
      3. Furcation Involvement. The more advanced the furcation involvement, the greater the risk of tooth loss.
      4. Tooth Mobility. The more severe the mobility experienced by a tooth, the greater the risk of tooth loss.
      5. Mucogingival involvement is assessed to determine the width of the attached gingiva.

   D. Bleeding on Probing
   1. Bleeding on probing is generally visible 10 seconds after probing.[4]
   2. Research suggests that after a few years of maintenance, a high frequency of bleeding on probing is a predictor of increased risk for progressive attachment loss.[5]
   3. Bleeding sites should be charted because these sites may need more attention during periodontal instrumentation.[4]
   E. Levels of Plaque and Calculus
   1. Plaque scores are a good indication of the patient's level of self-care compliance.
   2. Scores may reveal that the patient is in need of renewed instruction in plaque-control methods.
   3. Plaque scores should be documented to provide an objective record of the level of self-care at a particular time and to permit comparison over time.
   F. Occlusal Analysis
4. **Plaque-Control Evaluation**
   A. Reinforcement of Self-Care. Most patients will need reinforcement of their motivation for plaque control. Pointing out areas where there is less redness, reduced bleeding, or decreased plaque accumulation is a positive way to motivate patients to continue with their self-care.
   1. Patients often spend considerable time on self-care and expect to be informed about the effects of their efforts.
   2. Failure to provide this information may give a patient the impression that the dental hygienist is not interested in his or her dental health status.
   3. A disclosing solution can be used to allow the patient to see where bacterial plaque has accumulated.
   B. Plaque accumulation can be related to many factors, such as:
   1. Lack of the manual dexterity needed to carry out the self-care regimen that was recommended previously. Alternative self-care techniques should be considered.
   2. Discontinued use of one or more of the self-care methods recommended previously. Consideration should be given to making the self-care regimen less complicated (i.e., fewer aids or aids that are easier for the patient to use).
   3. Gingival recession or shrinkage may have occurred following periodontal surgery. Introduction of a new interdental aid may be indicated for plaque removal on proximal root surfaces.
   C. Microbial monitoring may be indicated for high-risk patients.
   1. Microbial monitoring may be used to determine the specific periodontal pathogens before antimicrobial or other therapy is initiated.
   2. Types of tests that may be used on certain patients include bacterial culture, immunoassay, nucleic acid probe assay, and enzyme assay.
5. **Periodontal Instrumentation**
   A. Deplaquing and removal of calculus is one of the most important steps for disease control. The goal of periodontal debridement is to disrupt the subgingival biofilm and create an environment that is biologically acceptable to the tissues of the periodontium.
   B. Root instrumentation is accepted as the most important means of disrupting the subgingival biofilm. Repeated root surface debridement over time may result in substantive loss of root substance (cementum and dentin) and increase the risk for exposure of the dentinal tubules to the oral environment and even pulp exposures.
   1. Following periodontal therapy, some patients will present for periodontal maintenance with little or no subgingival calculus deposits. In these patients firm stroke pressure with the instrument against the tooth is not necessary and should be avoided.

2. Conservation of root substance is an important goal of periodontal debridement.
   a. Ultrasonic instrumentation with a precision-thin tip has been shown to remove less root substance than hand instrumentation and offers the added benefit of the antimicrobial effect created by the vibrating ultrasonic tip.
   b. *Plastic curets (such as those used to debride dental implants) are effective for deplaquing root surfaces and minimize trauma to the hard tissues of the root for periodontally treated patients during maintenance care.*[6]

6. **Counseling**

   Counseling, such as smoking cessation counseling, should be provided regarding control of any risk factors that might be contributing to a patient's periodontal disease.

7. **Application of Fluorides**
   1. Routine application of professional fluoride treatments during periodontal maintenance care is indicated to promote remineralization, aid in the prevention of root caries, and aid in the control of dentinal hypersensitivity.
   2. Research studies suggest that high concentrations of topical fluorides may have some antimicrobial properties and may be of some benefit in decreasing plaque accumulation.[2,7–9]

PLANNING FOR ADDITIONAL TREATMENT NEEDS AND MAINTENANCE INTERVAL

1. **Recommendations for Treatment Needs and/or Referrals**
   A. At the end of the periodontal maintenance visit, the patient should be informed of his or her current periodontal health status. Any additional treatment needs are recommended at this time.
      1. These recommendations include communication or consultation with other dental and medical healthcare providers who will be providing care.
      2. Relationship between the General and Periodontal Practices
         a. Mild chronic periodontitis patients can receive total dental and periodontal maintenance in a general dental practice.
         b. Moderate chronic periodontitis patients should alternate periodontal maintenance between the general dental practice and the periodontal practice.
         c. Severe chronic periodontitis patients should receive periodontal maintenance in a periodontal practice. In addition, annual or semiannual visits should be scheduled with a general dentist who will provide restorative and other general dental care.
         d. Aggressive periodontitis patients should receive all periodontal therapy in a periodontal practice. In addition, annual or semiannual visits should be scheduled with a general dentist who will provide restorative and other general dental care.

2. **Determination of Maintenance Interval**
   A. The frequency of periodontal maintenance visits must be determined on an individual basis. Factors to consider in determining the maintenance interval between maintenance visits include the following:
      1. Severity of Disease. The more severe the disease, the more frequently the patient should be seen.

2. Adequacy of Patient Self-Care. The better the self-care, the less frequently the patient needs to be seen. Intervals should be more frequent when a patient has less than optimal self-care.

3. Host Response. Systemic or genetic factors may negatively affect the host response. For example, a patient who continues to smoke or one with poorly controlled diabetes should be seen more frequently.

B. An important general guideline for determining the frequency of maintenance care is based on the time interval for the repopulation of periodontal pathogens after periodontal debridement.

    1. Studies indicate that following periodontal debridement the subgingival pathogens return to predebridement levels in 9 to 11 weeks in most patients.[10,11]

    2. *Research evidence strongly shows that periodontal maintenance should be performed at least every 3 months or less for the removal and disruption of subgingival periodontal pathogens.*[1,12]

    3. Patients who receive frequent periodontal maintenance will experience less attachment loss and tooth loss than patients who have less frequent maintenance care.[13,14]

SECTION 3: PREVENTION OF ROOT CARIES

INTRODUCTION OF ROOT CARIES

1. Occurrence of Root Caries in Patients with Periodontitis

A. Root caries, decay on the root surfaces, is a common problem in patients with periodontitis.

B. According to the 1985–1986 United States Public Health Service (USPHS) survey of adults:

    1. About half of the adults in the United States are afflicted with root surface caries by age 50.

    2. The percentage increases to 70% by age 60, with an average prevalence of about three lesions by age 70.[15]

C. A 2004 systematic review on root caries incidence found that 23.7% of older adults *develop at least one new lesion annually.*[16]

2. Clinical Appearance

A. Root caries occurs only if the root surface is exposed to the oral environment due to loss of attachment.[17]

    1. In health, the root surface is protected by the periodontal attachment apparatus and is not exposed to the oral environment.

    2. The root may be exposed to the oral environment due to gingival recession or within a periodontal pocket.

B. New root caries usually is seen as a shallow, softened area that is yellow to light brown. As the lesion develops, it may have a leathery consistency. Older lesions appear brown to black and may be hard (**Fig. 23-2**).

C. Lesions usually begin at or slightly occlusal to the free gingival margin but can extend into the periodontal pocket. The lesion usually spreads laterally and can extend circumferentially around the root surface.[18]

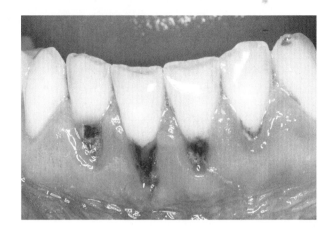

Figure 23-2. Root caries.
Root caries on the mandibular incisors of a person with periodontitis. (Courtesy of Dr. Richard J. Foster, Guilford Technical Community College, Jamestown, NC.)

3. **Etiology of Root Caries**
   A. No specific microorganisms have been proven to cause root caries.
      1. Root caries is most likely a mixed infection or a succession of bacterial populations.
      2. Mutans streptococci and *Lactobacillus* are associated with root caries.
      3. Recent studies, with few exceptions, fail to find association between *Actinomyces* and root caries.[19]
   B. Like enamel caries, root caries requires a susceptible tooth surface, dental plaque, and time to initiate and progress. However, root caries differs from enamel caries in some aspects.
      1. Root surfaces are more vulnerable to demineralization. Root surfaces demineralize at a pH of 6.2 to 6.7.[20]
      2. Mineral loss for the root surface during demineralization is up to 2.5 times greater than enamel.[21]
   C. Risk factors for the development of root caries include: attachment loss, inadequate oral hygiene, cariogenic diet, infrequent dental visits, past caries experience, inadequate salivary flow, lack of fluoride exposure, and removable partial dentures.
   D. Individuals who have coronal caries are 2 to 3.5 times more likely to develop root caries.[22]

FLUORIDE THERAPY AND THE PREVENTION OF ROOT CARIES

1. **Research on Fluoride for the Prevention of Root Caries.** Root lesions can be arrested by remineralization.
   A. Fluoridated Drinking Water. Several studies have demonstrated that the presence of fluoridated drinking water throughout the lifetime of an individual reduces the development of root surface caries.[23]
   B. Toothpaste.
      1. The use of an 1100 ppm sodium fluoride (NaF) dentifrice results in a significant decrease in root surface caries of 67%.[24]
      2. A recent clinical trial demonstrated that prescription strength fluoride toothpaste, containing 5000 ppm NaF, was effective in reversing root caries. 57% of patients using the high strength dentifrice had reversal of root caries.
   C. Mouth rinses. Fluoride mouthrinses containing 0.05% NaF have been shown to significantly reduce root caries incidence.[25]
   D. Professional Application.
      1. A large long-term clinical study showed that semiannual applications of 1.23% APF gel significantly reduced the formation of new root caries and the number of remineralized lesions was significantly increased by daily rinsing with a 0.05% NaF rinse.[26]
      2. Fluoride varnish applied every 3 months has been shown to reduce new root caries formation by over 50 percent.[27]
2. **Recommendations for Use of Fluoride in Root Caries Prevention**
   A. The prevention of periodontal disease and the associated attachment loss is the most effective way to prevent root caries. In patients with existing periodontal disease, prevention of further attachment loss will reduce the surface area susceptible to decay.
   B. Recommendations for fluoride use are summarized in Table 23-2. A variety of fluoride products can be helpful in preventing root caries (**Fig. 23-2**).
      1. **Patients with a Low Risk for Root Caries**
         a. Low risk is defined as no root caries in 3 years.
         b. Fluoridated drinking water
         c. NaF toothpaste. Patients should avoid rinsing with large volumes of water after the use of fluoride toothpaste.[28]
         d. A semi-annual application of 1.23% APF. If contraindications exist for the use of APF, apply 2.0% NaF or consider use of fluoride varnish. Apply fluoride gels or foams for a full four minutes.

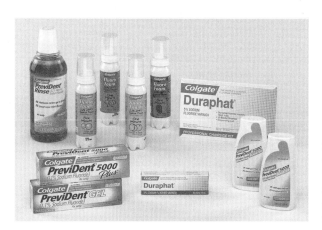

Figure 23-3. Fluoride Products. There are a variety of fluoride products for professional or home use that are helpful in the control of root caries. These include toothpastes, gels, foams, rinses, and varnishes. (Courtesy of Colgate-Palmolive Company)

2. **Patients with a Moderate Risk for Root Caries**
   a. Moderate risk is defined as less than 2 new root lesions in 3 years.
   b. Fluoridated drinking water
   c. NaF mouthrinse (225 ppm), 1.1% NaF brush on gel, or a 1.1% NaF toothpaste (5000 ppm) in addition to daily fluoride toothpaste
   d. Daily rinse or gel. Rinses or gel applications at bedtime result in fluoride retention.[29]
   e. Dietary counseling
   f. A semi-annual application of 1.23% APF.
3. **Patients with a High Risk for Root Caries**
   a. High risk is defined as more than 2 new root lesions in 3 years.
   b. Fluoridated drinking water
   c. For high risk patients, use a 1.1% NaF gel in a custom tray/brush on or a 1.1% NaF toothpaste. In addition, consider use of .12% chlorhexidine and a 5-10 gram daily consumption of xylitol in the form of gum.[18]
   d. Daily rinse or gel. Rinses or gel applications at bedtime result in fluoride retention.[29]
   e. Dietary counseling.
      1) Selection of noncariogenic foods. Avoid consumption or limit the frequency of intake of foods with high sucrose content, such as candy and sugar-containing beverages and soft drinks.
      2) Consider the use of a 5-10 gram daily consumption of xylitol in the form of gum.
   f. Meticulous daily plaque control to minimize the amount of cariogenic bacteria.
   g. Professional fluoride applications every 3 to 4 months with 1.23% acidulated phosphofluoride (APF) or 5.0% NaF varnish.

Table 23-2. Preventive Strategies for Root Caries

Root Caries Risk Level	Criterion	Strategy
Low Risk	No root caries in 3 years	Fluoridated water Fluoride toothpaste Professional application of fluoride every 6 months
Moderate Risk	Less than 2 new root lesions in 3 years	Fluoridated water Fluoride toothpaste Professional application of fluoride every 6 months Daily rinse (approximately 225 ppm) or gel (1.1% NaF) Dietary counseling
High Risk	More than 2 new root lesions in 3 years	Fluoridated water Fluoride toothpaste Professional application every 3 to 4 months Daily gel (1.1% NaF) Dietary counseling; Consider: Chlorhexidine gluconate mouth rinse

SECTION 4: OUTCOMES ASSESSMENT

At each periodontal maintenance visit, the most important determination to be made is whether the periodontal health status of the patient is stable. Inadequate periodontal maintenance and/or inadequate patient compliance may result in progression of the recurrence of the periodontitis.

PERIODONTAL DISEASE RECURRENCE

1. **Concepts of Disease Recurrence**
   A. **Recurrence** of periodontitis occurs when signs and symptoms of disease return after having subsided. The term recurrence implies that the periodontitis was brought under control during nonsurgical periodontal therapy (or nonsurgical periodontal therapy plus periodontal surgery) and that the periodontitis is once again resulting in progressive attachment loss.
   B. Recurrence of periodontitis may occur in specific sites only. For example, it would be possible for a patient treated for periodontitis to experience disease recurrence on the mesial surface of a single premolar tooth and for all other teeth in the dentition to show good disease control.
2. **Clinical Signs of Recurrence of Periodontitis.** Clinical signs of recurrence of periodontitis (Box 23-2) can include:
   A. Progressive attachment loss
   B. Pockets that bleed on probing or that exhibit exudate
   C. Pockets that get deeper over time
   D. Progressing radiographic evidence of bone loss
   E. Increasing tooth mobility
3. **Reasons for Recurrence of Periodontitis.** Periodontitis recurs in patients for a variety of reasons, and the dental team should be aware that it is not always possible to determine a specific reason for disease recurrence. The most common reasons for recurrence of periodontitis (Box 23-3) are:
   A. Inadequate plaque control by the patient
   B. Incomplete professional treatment
      1) Incomplete periodontal debridement
      2) Failure to control all local risk factors
   C. Failure to control systemic factors
   D. Inadequate control of occlusal contributing factors
   E. Improper periodontal surgical technique
   F. Attempting to treat teeth with a poor prognosis

Box 23-2

Clinical Signs of Recurrence

- Progressive attachment loss
- Pockets that bleed upon probing or exhibit exudate
- Pockets that get deeper over time
- Radiographic evidence of progressing bone loss
- Increasing tooth mobility

Box 23-3

Reasons for Recurrence

- Inadequate plaque control by the patient
- Incomplete professional treatment
- Failure to control systemic factors
- Inadequate control of occlusal contributing factors
- Improper periodontal surgical technique
- Attempting to treat teeth with a poor prognosis

PATIENT COMPLIANCE

1. **Definition**
   A. **Compliance** is defined as the extent to which a person's behavior coincides with medical or health advice.[30]
      1. A patient who does not follow recommendations for daily self-care is described as **noncompliant**.
      2. A patient who meets regularly scheduled periodontal maintenance appointments is described as **compliant**.
   B. Compliance is also called adherence and therapeutic alliance; however, compliance is the most common term used in dental literature.
   C. **Reasons for Noncompliance.** The reasons for patient noncompliance are complex, because the reasons for noncompliance can be different for each patient and for the same patient in different situations. Some common reasons that have been suggested for noncompliance include.[31]
      1. Fear of dental treatment
      2. The expense of dental treatment
      3. Low priority for the patient in the face of competing demands on the patient's time and/or financial resources
      4. Denial—some individuals want to deny that they have a problem; this may be due to a lack of information about their disease
      5. Failure to understand the implications of noncompliance
      6. Perceived indifference on the part of dental healthcare providers
2. **Strategies for Improving Compliance.** Figure 23-4 highlights some ideas for improving patient compliance.[31,32]

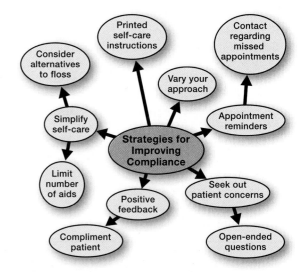

Figure 23-4. Suggestions for Improving Patient Compliance. An idea map of various strategies for improving patient compliance.

   A. Printed Self-Care Instruction. Giving patients printed self-care instructions that they can refer to at home.
      1. Place the instruction sheet in a plastic sheet protector, like those available for use in three-ring notebooks. These sheet projectors are readily available in office supply stores and are priced economically.
      2. Note the next periodontal maintenance appointment at the bottom of the instruction sheet.
      3. Have instructions translated into the patient's native language.

4. Simplifying self-care recommendations. Patients often perceive self-care instructions as being difficult to follow and as time-consuming.
    a. Plaque control instructions should be as clear and simple as possible while addressing the specific needs of the patient. The use of dental terminology should be avoided and replaced by words that are easily understood by the patient.
    b. A limited number of self-care aids should be recommended. Studies indicate that patients are less likely to comply with self-care when they are instructed to use multiple aids on a daily basis.
    c. Alternatives to traditional dental floss should be considered since compliance with flossing is poor.
5. Varying the approach to patient education and self-care instructions. Patients often complain about having to listen to the "same old lecture" from the dental hygienist at each periodontal maintenance appointment.

B. Seeking Out Patient Concerns
1. Provide opportunities for communication by asking open-ended questions such as:
    ■ "What are your concerns about this suggestion, treatment, etc.?"
    ■ "How do you think you will fit this self-care recommendation into your daily schedule?"
    ■ "How would you compare using this powered flossing device to using traditional dental floss?"
2. Accommodate the patient's needs whenever possible. A satisfied patient is more likely to comply with self-care and maintenance appointments.

C. Informing Patients
1. Counsel the patient about his or her periodontal health status.
2. Explain the benefits of having regularly scheduled periodontal maintenance visits and the risks of infrequent professional care.

D. Monitoring Appointments
1. Use a postcard or telephone call to remind the patient of upcoming appointments.
2. Contact the patient when an appointment is missed. The sooner the patient is contacted after missing an appointment, the more likely he or she is to reschedule.

E. Providing Positive Feedback to Patients
1. Areas of improvement should be pointed out to the patient, such as less plaque, fewer bleeding sites, or less inflamed tissue.
2. The patient should be complimented in front of the dentist by describing how the patient's efforts have led to improved periodontal health.
3. Positive reinforcement should be used to convey a motivational message rather than criticism.

CHAPTER SUMMARY STATEMENT

The **periodontal maintenance** phase of treatment includes all measures used by the dental team and the patient to keep periodontitis under control. The goal of this stage of treatment is to prevent the recurrence of periodontal diseases. Among those patients treated for periodontitis, the disease tends to recur, and constant vigilance is needed on the part of the dental team to keep periodontitis under control. Periodontal maintenance provides the professional assistance that most patients need for renewal of motivation, instruction in plaque control, and elimination or reduction of primary and secondary risk factors.

SECTION 5: FOCUS ON PATIENTS

CASE 1
Your dental team has just completed a reevaluation of the results of nonsurgical therapy for a patient with generalized slight chronic periodontitis. The findings of the reevaluation reveal that the periodontitis is under control and that periodontal maintenance is the next logical step. When should the first maintenance appointment be scheduled?

CASE 2
One of your dental team's chronic periodontitis patients has recently undergone periodontal surgery and now has several sites of gingival recession exposing tooth roots. Unfortunately, this patient has had a high incidence of caries over the past few years. What measures might your team take to minimize the risk of root caries in this patient?

CASE 3
A patient who has been treated for chronic periodontitis by your team has been followed for periodontal maintenance for more than 3 years. During each maintenance visit, there have been no indications of recurrence of the periodontitis. The patient calls you before her next maintenance visit to inform you that she has just been diagnosed with diabetes mellitus. She looked up diabetes on the Web and now wants to know if this will affect her periodontal condition. How should you respond to the patient's concern?

References

1. Axelsson P, Lindhe L. The significance of maintenance care in the treatment of periodontal disease. *J Clin Periodontol*. 1981;8:281–294.
2. McGuire MK. Prognosis versus actual outcome: A long-term survey of 100 treated periodontal patients under maintenance care. *J Periodontol*. 1991;62:51–58.
3. Parameters of care. American Academy of Periodontology. *J Periodontol*. 2000;71(5 Suppl):I–ii, 847–883.
4. Lang NP, Joss A, Tonetti MS. Monitoring disease during supportive periodontal treatment by bleeding on probing. *Periodontol 2000*. 1996;12:44–48.
5. Claffey N, Nylund K, Keger R, et al. Diagnostic predictability of scores of plaque, bleeding, suppuration and probing depth for probing attachment loss. 3 1/2 years of observation following initial periodontal therapy. *J Clin Periodontol*. 1990;17:108–114.
6. Bardet P, Suvan J, Lang NP. Clinical effects of root instrumentation using conventional steel or non-tooth substance removing plastic curettes during supportive periodontal therapy (SPT). *J Clin Periodontol*. 1999;26:724–742.
7. Brambilla E. Fluoride—Is it capable of fighting old and new dental diseases? An overview of existing fluoride compounds and their clinical applications. *Caries Res*. 2001;35(Suppl 1): 6–9.
8. Mazza JE, Newman MG, Sims TN. Clinical and antimicrobial effect of stannous fluoride on periodontitis. *J Clin Periodontol*. 1981;8:203–212.
9. ten Cate JM. Consensus statements on fluoride usage and associated research questions. *Caries Res*. 2001;35(Suppl):71–73.
10. Greenstein G. Periodontal response to mechanical non-surgical therapy: a review. *J Periodontol*. 1992;63:118–130.
11. Slots J. Subgingival microflora and periodontal disease. *J Clin Periodontol*. 1979;6:351–382.
12. Haffajee AD, Socransky SS, Smith C, et al. Relation of baseline microbial parameters to future periodontal attachment loss. *J Clin Periodontol*. 1991;18:744–750.

13. De Vore CH, Duckworth JE, Beck FM, et al. Bone loss following periodontal therapy in subjects without frequent periodontal maintenance. *J Periodontol*. 1986;57:354–359.

14. Wilson TG, Jr, Glover ME, Malik AK, et al. Tooth loss in maintenance patients in a private periodontal practice. *J Periodontol*. 1987;58:231–235.

15. National Institute of Dental Research (U.S.). Epidemiology and Oral Disease Prevention Program, Oral health of United States adults: the National Survey of Oral Health in US. Employed Adults and Seniors, 1985–1986: National findings. NIH publication no.87-2868. 1987, Bethesda, MD.: U.S. Dept. of Health and Human Services Public Service National Institutes of Health: p. iii, 168.

16. Griffin SO, Griffin AM, Swann JL, et al. Estimating rates of new root caries in older adults. *J Dent Res.*,2004;83:634–638.

17. Brown LJ, Brunelle JA, Kingman A. Periodontal status in the United States 1988–1991: prevalence, extent and demographic variation. *J Dent Res*. 1996;75(Special Issue):672–683.

18. Berry TG, Summitt JP, Sift EJ Jr., et al. Root caries. *Oper Dent*. 2004;29:601–607.

19. Zambon JJ, Kasprzak SA. The microbiology and histopathology of human root caries. *Am J Dent.*, 1995;8:323–328.

20. Atkinson JC, Wu AJ. Salivary gland dysfunction: Causes, symptoms, treatment. *J Am Dent Assoc*. 1994;125:409–416.

21. Øgaard B, Arends J, Rolla G. Action of fluoride on initiation of early root surface caries in vivo. *Caries Res*. 1990;24:142–144.

22. Pappas A, Koski A, Giunta J. Prevalence and intraoral distribution of coronal and root caries in middle-aged and older adults. *Caries Res*. 1992;26:459–465.

23. Brustman BA. Impact of exposure to fluoride-adequate water on root surface caries in elderly. *Gerodontics*. 1986;2:203–207.

24. Jensen ME, Kohout F. The effect of a fluoridated dentifrice on root and coronal caries in an older adult population. *J Am Dent Assoc*. 1988;117:829–832.

25. Ripa LJ, Leske GS, Forte F, et al. Effect of a 0.05% neutral NaF mouthrinse on coronal and root caries in adults. *Gerodontology*. 1987;6:131–136.

26. Wallace MC, Retief DH, Bradley EL. The 48-month increment of root caries in an Population of older adults participating in a preventive dental program. *J Public Health Dent*. 1993;53:133–137.

27. Schaeken MJM, Keltjens HMAM, van der Hoeven JS. Effect of fluoride and chlorhexidine on the microflora of dental root surfaces. *J Dent Res*. 1991;70:150–153.

28. Sjogren K, Birkhed D. Factors related to fluoride retention after use of fluoride. *Caries Res*. 1993;27:474–477.

29. Zero DT, Raubertas RF, Fu J, et al. Fluoride concentrations in plaque, whole saliva, and ductal saliva after application of home-use topical fluorides. *J Dent Res*. 1992;71:1768–1775.

30. Haynes RB, Sackett DL. *Compliance with Therapeutic Regimens*. 1976, Baltimore: Johns Hopkins University Press; 1976:xiv, 293.

31. Wilson TG, Jr. How patient compliance to suggested oral hygiene and maintenance affect periodontal therapy. *Dent Clin North Am*. 1998;42:389–403.

32. Wilson TG, Jr. Compliance: a review of the literature with possible applications to periodontics. *J Periodontol*. 1987;58:706–714.

SECTION 6: CHAPTER REVIEW QUESTIONS

1. Other terms for periodontal maintenance are supportive periodontal treatment and periodontal recall.
   A. True
   B. False

2. Which of the following is NOT an objective of periodontal maintenance?
   A. Control inflammation in the periodontium
   B. Decrease attachment levels
   C. Preserve alveolar bone levels

3. Periodontal examination during a periodontal maintenance appointment should include an evaluation of attachment loss, an evaluation of tooth mobility, as well as an evaluation of gingival recession.
   A. True
   B. False

4. Which of the following has NOT been demonstrated to reduce root caries?
   A. Fluoride varnish
   B. Sodium fluoride (NaF)
   C. Calcium tablets

5. Research evidence suggests that a proper interval for periodontal maintenance is at least
   A. Every 3 months
   B. Every 6 months
   C. Once each year

6. Compliance is defined as the
   A. Ability of a patient to use dental floss successfully
   B. Extent to which a patient's behavior coincides with medical advice
   C. Likelihood that a patient will pay for services rendered

7. Giving the patient multiple self-care aids to use each day is a proven technique for improving patient compliance.
   A. True
   B. False

Chapter

24 Maintenance of the Dental Implant Patient

 Refer to the CD packaged with this book for full color versions of the clinical photographs in this chapter.

Learning Objectives

- Define the term dental implant and describe the components of a typical dental implant.
- Define the term peri-implant tissues.
- Compare and contrast the periodontium of a natural tooth with the peri-implant tissues that surround a dental implant.
- Define the terms osseointegration and biomechanical forces as they apply to dental implants.
- Compare and contrast the terms peri-implant gingivitis and peri-implantitis.
- Discuss the special considerations for periodontal instrumentation of a dental implant.
- Describe an appropriate maintenance interval for a patient with dental implants.
- In the clinical setting, select appropriate self-care aids for a patient with dental implants.

KEY TERMS

Dental implant

Implant fixture

Transgingival abutment post

Biocompatible

Peri-implant tissues

Biologic seal

Osseointegration

Peri-implant disease

Peri-implant gingivitis

Peri-implantitis

Biomechanical forces

SECTION 1: ANATOMY OF THE DENTAL IMPLANT

A **dental implant** is a nonbiologic (artificial) device surgically inserted into the jawbone to (i) replace a missing tooth or (ii) provide support for a prosthetic denture. The dental hygienist plays an important role in patient education and professional maintenance of the dental implant. Understanding the basics of implantology and the anatomy of the peri-implant tissues is a prerequisite to understanding the maintenance of dental implants.

COMPONENTS OF THE DENTAL IMPLANT

1. **Implant Fixture**
   A. An **implant fixture** is the portion of the implant that is surgically placed into the bone (**Fig. 24-1**).
   B. The implant fixture acts as the root of the implant.
      1. The metal used for dental implants is titanium. Titanium is an ideal material for dental implants because it is a bone-loving metal that is biocompatible and because it is a poor conductor of heat and electricity.
      2. The major disadvantage of titanium is that it scratches easily.
2. **Transgingival Abutment Post**
   A. The **transgingival abutment post** is a titanium post that protrudes through the tissue into the mouth (**Fig. 24-1**).
   B. The abutment post supports the restorative prosthesis (crown or denture) (**Fig. 24-2**).
   C. The titanium abutment is extremely **biocompatible** (not rejected by the body) and allows tissue healing around the implant.
   D. Modern dental implants may be difficult to recognize since they often have the same appearance as the crowns and fixed bridges used to restore natural teeth. *For this reason, dental implants should be clearly noted in the chart so that all dental team members are alerted to the fact that this is a dental implant patient.*

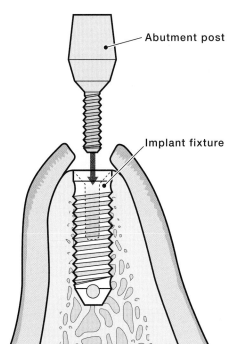

Abutment post

Implant fixture

Figure 24-1. Implant Components.
The abutment post and implant fixture of a dental implant. The implant fixture is placed into living alveolar bone. The abutment extends through living gingival tissue into the mouth. A crown or prosthesis is connected to the abutment post.

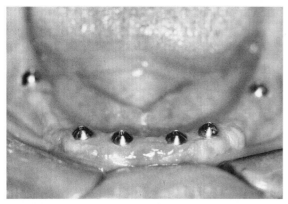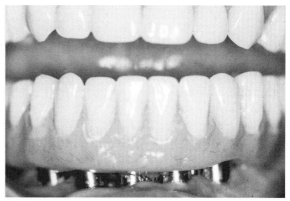

A

B

Figure 24-2. Dental Implants. A: Abutment posts on the mandibular arch. B: Abutment posts supporting a restorative prosthesis.

3. **Peri-implant Tissues.** The **peri-implant tissues** are the tissues that surround the dental implant (**Fig. 24-3**). The peri-implant tissues are similar in many ways to the periodontium of a natural tooth but there are some important differences (**Table 24-1**).

A. Implant-to-Epithelial Tissue Interface

   1. The epithelium adapts to the titanium abutment post, creating a **biologic seal**. The union of the epithelial cells to the implant surface is very similar to that of the epithelial cells to the natural tooth surface.
   2. The biologic seal functions as a barrier between the implant and the oral cavity.
   3. As in a natural tooth, a sulcus lined by sulcular epithelium surrounds the implant abutment post.

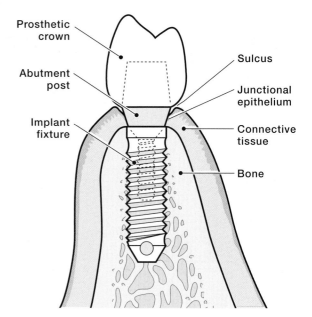

Figure 24-3. Peri-implant Tissues. The implant is surrounded by junctional epithelium, connective tissue, and alveolar bone. There are no periodontal ligament fibers between the implant fixture and the alveolar bone.

B. Implant-to-Connective Tissue Interface

   1. *The implant-to-connective tissue interface is significantly different from that of connective tissue of a natural tooth.*
   2. The implant surface lacks cementum, so the gingival fibers and the periodontal ligament cannot insert into the titanium surface as they do into the cementum of a natural tooth.

    a. On a natural tooth:
  1) The supragingival fibers brace the gingival margin against the tooth and strengthen the attachment of the junctional epithelium to the tooth
  2) The periodontal ligament suspends and maintains the tooth in its socket.
  3) The periodontal ligament fibers also serve as a physical barrier to bacterial invasion.

    b. The connective tissue is unable to accomplish any of these protective functions for the dental implant. *Therefore, periodontal pathogens can destroy bone much more rapidly along a dental implant than along a natural tooth with its protective barrier of periodontal ligament fibers.*

3. The connective tissue fiber bundles in the gingiva around an implant have been shown to be either (i) oriented parallel to the implant surface or (ii) encircling the implant abutment.[1]

4. Keratinized tissue may or may not be present around the dental implant.

C. Implant-to-Bone Interface

1. Osseointegration is the direct contact of the bone with the implant surface (with no intervening periodontal ligament). Osseointegration is a major requirement for implant success.

2. Clinically, osseointegration is regarded as successful if there is:

    a. An absence of clinical mobility

    b. An absence of gingival inflammation of peri-implant tissues

    c. No discomfort or pain when the implant is in function

    d. No increased bone loss or radiolucence around the dental implant on a radiograph

Table 24-1. Tissues Surrounding a Dental Implant

Tissues of the Periodontium	Peri-implant Tissues
Junctional epithelium	Attaches to the implant surface (biologic seal)
Connective tissue fibers	Run parallel or circular to the implant surface
Periodontal ligament	No periodontal ligament
Cementum	No cementum
Alveolar bone	In direct contact with the implant surface (osseointegration)

SECTION 2: PERI-IMPLANT DISEASE

1. **Pathologic Changes in Implant Tissues**
   A. Plaque deposits can accumulate on the surfaces of teeth, restorations, oral appliances, and also on dental implants. The continuous presence of bacterial deposits can result in inflammation of the soft tissues around the implant. When the disease process progresses further, partial or total loss of osseointegration can occur.
   B. Pathologic changes of the peri-implant tissues can be referred to as **peri-implant disease**.
      1. **Peri-implant gingivitis** is plaque-induced gingivitis (with no loss of supporting bone) that occurs in the gingival tissues surrounding a dental implant.
      2. **Peri-implantitis** is the term for chronic periodontitis in the tissues surrounding an osseointegrated dental implant, resulting in loss of alveolar bone.
         a. Peri-implantitis begins at the coronal portion of the implant, while the apical portion continues to be osseointegrated.
         b. An advanced peri-implantitis lesion can be diagnosed by the detection of bone loss around the implant fixture.
            1) The implant does not become mobile until the final stages of peri-implantitis.
            2) Implants that show mobility and signs of loss of osseointegration should be removed.

2. **Etiology of Peri-Implant Disease.** The major etiologic factors associated with peri-implant disease are bacterial infection and biomechanical factors. Smoking is an additional factor that has been implicated in implant failure.
   A. Bacterial Infection
      1. The pathogenesis of periodontal disease—in natural teeth and dental implants—requires the presence of bacterial plaque and the host inflammatory response.
      2. It appears that periodontal disease in both peri-implant tissues and periodontium in natural teeth progresses in a similar fashion. *The rate of tissue destruction, however, tends to be more rapid in peri-implant tissues than in periodontal tissues.*
      3. The same bacteria that are pathogenic to natural teeth can be detrimental to dental implants.
         a. It is theorized that the natural teeth in a partially edentulous mouth act as a reservoir of periodontal pathogens that reinfect the implants.
         b. This finding makes meticulous self-care of dental implants even more critical for the partially edentulous patient than for the fully edentulous patient.
   B. Biomechanical Factors.
      1. In a natural tooth the periodontal ligament helps absorb some of the forces placed on the tooth. These forces placed on natural teeth can arise from chewing food, supporting a dental appliance, or perhaps from habits such as bruxing.
      2. Dental implants lack the protective structure of the periodontal ligament that is found on natural teeth. For all practical purposes, the dental implant is in direct contact with the alveolar bone.
      3. Since dental implants do not have a periodontal ligament, forces placed on an implant are transmitted directly to the alveolar bone. It is critical to minimize forces placed on an implant to avoid damage to the surrounding alveolar bone.
      4. Collectively forces placed on an implant have been called **biomechanical forces** to underscore the importance of both biologic and mechanical aspects of controlling those forces to achieve long term success with implants.
      5. Biomechanical forces on implants are influenced by a variety of factors that must be assessed by the clinician. Factors that influence the biomechanical forces include: the position of the implant fixture; the number of implants supporting the prosthesis; and the force load distribution among the implants.

CONSIDERATIONS FOR IMPLANT MAINTENANCE

1. **Maintenance of Peri-Implant Tissues**
   A. One of the most important factors in the long-term success of dental implants is the maintenance of the peri-implant tissues. Maintenance therapy for dental implants is similar to a maintenance visit for a patient treated for periodontitis (**Table 24-2**).
   B. Meticulous self-care is of the utmost importance in preventing peri-implant disease.
      1. Some patients undergoing implant therapy may have had a long history of dental neglect and/or poor plaque control.
      2. The dental hygienist can assist the patient in maintaining dental implants by providing self-care education pertinent to dental implant care and home care tools that are appropriate and simple to use.
2. **Objectives of Maintenance Therapy for Dental Implants**
   A. Maintenance of Alveolar Bone Support
      1. Alveolar bone support is evaluated by use of good-quality radiographs taken with long-cone paralleling technique at specific time intervals.
      2. The bone height and density around the implants is compared with previous radiographs of the site.
   B. Control of inflammation
      1. Patient and professional plaque control is important for proper gingival health.
      2. Patient self-care must be reevaluated and, if necessary, reinforced each time the patient is seen for maintenance. The better the patient self-care, the better the possibilities of maintaining stable results.
   C. Maintenance of a healthy and functional implant
      1. Implant components should be checked for prosthesis integrity (such as loose screws, cement washout, material wear); implant, screw, or abutment fracture; unseating of attachments; solder joint wear; and proper adaptation.
      2. Any implant mobility requires immediate consultation with a dentist or specialist.
3. **Peri-Implant Radiography**
   A. Maintenance of bone levels around dental implants is an important criterion for determining treatment success. Radiographic evaluation of bone height and topography is important for the longitudinal monitoring of peri-implant stability.
      1. Vertical bone loss of less than 0.2 mm annually following the implant's first year of function is a criterion utilized to determine treatment success.
      2. Radiographs also allow for the evaluation of the fit of the prosthesis and the integrity and adaptation of the different implant components.
   B. Dental implants should be checked radiographically at least once a year and should be checked more often in patients in whom periodontal breakdown around the implant was noted at a previous visit.

Table 24-2. Assessment of Dental Implants

Characteristics of a Healthy Implant Site	Characteristics of a Disease Implant Site
Firm, pink tissue	Red, swollen tissue
No mobility	Mobility present
Radiographic evidence of bone in close contact with the implant	Radiographic evidence of radiolucency around the implant

4. **Implant Mobility**
   A. Absence of mobility is a very important clinical criterion for dental implants.
      1. Implants should not move if osseointegrated and healthy.
      2. Signs of mobility could indicate the presence of a loose abutment or the rupture of the cement seal on cemented restorations. Mobility also can result from a loosening of the internal screw that attaches the abutment post to the implant fixture. Severe mobility accompanied with discomfort also might indicate fracture of the implant itself.
      3. Implant mobility may indicate a lack of osseointegration or prosthetic failure between the components. Long-term failure between the prosthetic components (i.e., screws between the crown and implant fixture) may lead to bone loss and complete failure of the implant fixture and the dental implant.
   B. The technique for assessing mobility of a dental implant is similar to that used to assess a natural tooth. The use of instruments with plastic handles is recommended if the implant fixture itself must be touched.
   C. Radiographic evaluation is recommended when mobility is noted. Loose internal screws will appear as a gap in the implant components on a radiograph.
5. **Periodontal Instrumentation of Dental Implants**
   A. The use of traditional metal curets is contraindicated around implant components. Implant components are made of titanium, a soft metal, that can be permanently damaged (grooved, scratched) if treated with metal instruments (**Fig. 24-4**).
      1. There is an increased likelihood of plaque retention and peri-implantitis if the titanium is scratched.
      2. Metal instruments can also disturb the surface coating of the implant, reducing the biocompatibility with the peri-implant tissues.
      3. The use of ultrasonic or sonic devices with metal tips is also contraindicated with implants.

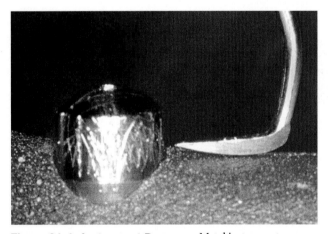

Figure 24-4. Instrument Damage. Metal instruments can scratch the surface of the implant.

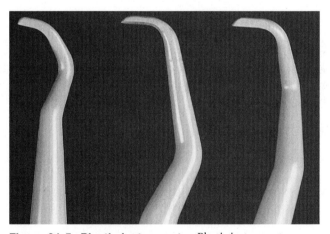

Figure 24-5. Plastic Instruments. Plastic instruments are safe for use on a dental implant.

   B. Instruments used for assessment and debridement of implant teeth should be made of a material that is softer than the implant (Box 24-1). Plastic instruments are most commonly used (**Fig. 24-5**).
      1. Plastic instruments are safe for use on all types of implants without damage to the abutment surface.
      2. A separate category of implant instruments is composed of instruments made of plastic materials that contain graphite fillers. Plastic instruments with graphite fillers can be used on the prosthetic crown covering a dental implant or on the prosthetic denture that is attached to the implant abutment. Care must be taken, however, not to use these instruments apical to the margin of the prosthetic crown.

3. Calculus is removed readily from implants because there is no interlocking or penetration of the deposit with the implant surface. Light lateral pressure with a plastic instrument is recommended.

Box 24-1

Guidelines for Debridement of Dental Implants

- The titanium surface of the abutment is easily removed; great care must be taken not to scratch the titanium abutment or disrupt the biologic seal
- Plastic instruments are recommended; metal instruments and ultrasonic or sonic devices with metal tips are contraindicated
- Instrumentation should be restricted to supragingival deposit removal
- Strokes should be short, controlled, and activated with light pressure; calculus does not adhere to titanium as tenaciously as on natural teeth
- Direction of strokes is in an oblique, vertical, or horizontal direction away from the peri-implant tissues

---

6. **Peri-Implant Probing**
   A. When a dental implant shows signs of either radiographic or clinical changes, clinical attachment levels can be used to monitor peri-implant health. No probing is necessary if the peri-implant tissue is healthy.
      1. To interpret probe readings, the clinician must have baseline data relating to the implant such as abutment type, size, prosthetic design, the baseline probed levels of attachment, and fixed reference point for probing.
      2. Probing measurements should be made from a fixed reference point on the abutment or prosthetic implant crown. Due to the length of the abutment and the connective tissue interface with the abutment post, probing depths may be deeper than the 1- to 3-mm depths that are considered normal in natural teeth.
   B. Probing should be avoided until postoperative healing is complete, approximately 3 months after abutment connection.
      1. Only a light probing technique should be used since the biological seal is weakly adherent to the abutment. Heavy probing force may be invasive since the probe may penetrate through the biological seal and could introduce bacteria into the peri-implant environment.
      2. Penetration of the plastic probe tip is dependent on the health (or inflammatory stage of the peri-implant tissues) and the thickness of the tissue around the abutment.
   C. Although peri-implant probing depth measurements may vary from patient to patient, research studies have indicated that successful implants generally allow probe penetration of approximately 3 mm.
7. **Maintenance Frequency**
   A. A 3-month maintenance interval is usually appropriate for dental implant patients.
      1. However, the clinician must determine the best interval for each specific case.
      2. Periodontal maintenance appointments should be scheduled as frequently as necessary to keep the periodontium and peri-implant tissues healthy.
   B. The following are indications for more frequent maintenance intervals.
      1. Reduced Bone Support Around Implants. Reduced bone support indicates that close monitoring of bone support is needed or the dental implant might be lost.
      2. Inflammation. A patient who has signs of inflammation around implants, even in the presence of good plaque control, needs more frequent maintenance visits.
      3. Host Response. Systemic conditions or diseases may affect the host–bacterial interaction. A shorter interval is needed for these cases.

PATIENT SELF-CARE OF DENTAL IMPLANTS

1. Care of a Fixed Prosthetic Crown
    A. Definition. A fixed prosthetic crown is a porcelain, acrylic, or composite tooth that fits over the abutment (**Fig. 24-6**).
    B. Techniques and Tools
        1. The single tooth prosthesis (crown) can present a challenge for plaque control in that the patient may quickly begin to regard it as a natural tooth.
        2. Usually the crown covering the implant abutment is larger in circumference than the abutment post. The bulky surface of the crown contacts the tissue and then dips in to meet the abutment post. Dental floss should be adapted along the margin of the crown, directed into the sulcus and around the abutment post (**Fig. 24-7**).
        3. In some cases, the restoration may be similar to that of a fixed bridge (e.g., a pontic supported by two dental implants). Tufted dental floss and a toothpick in a holder (Perio-Aid, Marquis Dental Mfg., Aurora, CO) make an effective combination of tools for deplaquing the large embrasure spaces and into the sulci of these fixed-bridge–type restorations.

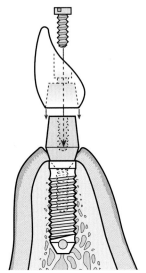

Figure 24-6. Fixed Prosthetic Crown. The crown fits over the abutment.

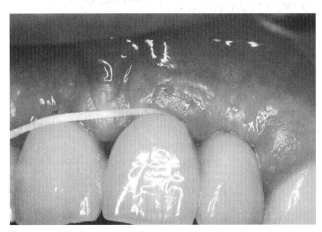

Figure 24-7. Implant Self-Care. Dental floss is used to clean a single implant with a prosthetic crown.

2. Care of a Removable Prosthesis
    A. Definition. A removable prosthesis is similar to a traditional full denture except that it is attached to the abutment posts by O-rings, magnets, or clips (**Fig. 24-8**). This type of prosthesis is also referred to as a tissue supported prosthesis or an overdenture. The patient can remove the prosthesis to clean the denture and around the abutments.
    B. Techniques and Tools
        1. A removable prosthesis is the easiest type of prosthesis for the patient to clean. The prosthesis itself is removed from the mouth for cleaning and once removed, exposes the abutment posts for cleaning.
        2. Tools for plaque removal around the abutments may include a soft bristle brush, a single-tufted manual toothbrush, and interdental brushes (**Fig. 24-9**). Tufted dental floss or implant floss can be wrapped around the abutment post for deplaquing. *Note that interdental brushes used to clean implants should be nylon-coated.* The use of a standard interdental brush (that has nylon filaments twisted into wire) should be avoided since the wire could scratch the abutment post.

3. In some cases, a metal bar joins the abutment posts and is used to attach the prosthetic denture in the mouth. Tufted dental floss or a 2 × 2 gauze square can be useful in cleaning underneath the metal bar and around the abutment posts (**Fig. 24-10**).

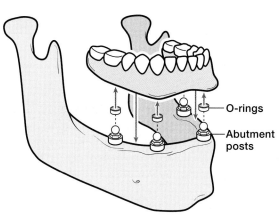

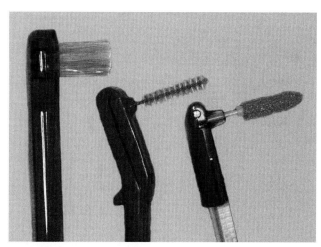

Figure 24-8. Removable Prosthesis. A removable prosthesis is similar to a traditional full denture except that it is attached to the abutment posts of dental implants by O-rings, magnets, or clips.

Figure 24-9. Oral Hygiene Aids. End-tuft and interdental brushes are helpful self-care aids for individuals with dental implants.

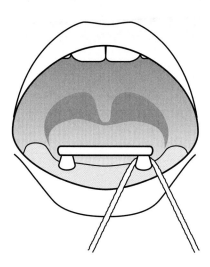

Figure 24-10. Abutments Joined by Metal Bar. Tufted dental floss is useful in cleaning the implant abutments and underneath the connecting metal bar.

CHAPTER SUMMARY STATEMENT

As dental implant therapy becomes more common, dental hygienists will care for more patients needing implant maintenance. An important role of the dental hygienist is the education of patients about the importance of meticulous self-care and frequent maintenance visits. Implant maintenance appointments should include monitoring of plaque levels, soft tissue examination, assessment of the restorative integrity, reinforcement of patient plaque-control measures, periodontal debridement of implant abutment posts/prostheses, and radiographic examination.

SECTION 4: FOCUS ON PATIENTS

CASE 1
While you are performing nonsurgical therapy on a chronic periodontitis patient, the patient tells you that he is thinking about having all of his teeth removed, since they are not healthy anyway, and just having some implants placed. He tells you that this would be easier, since he would not have to worry about the implants like he does his teeth. How should you respond?

CASE 2
You are scheduled to record the information needed to make a periodontal diagnosis on a patient new to your dental team. Radiographs have not yet been ordered for the patient. As you begin your probing, the patient informs you that she has two dental implants. Visual examination of the patient's dentition does not immediately reveal which teeth are replaced by the implants. How should you proceed?

CASE 3
At a maintenance visit for one of your team's patients you note obvious mobility of a crown supported by an implant. How should you proceed?

Reference

1. Lang NP, Karring T, British Society of Periodontology: *Proceedings of the 1st European Workshop on Periodontology*, Charter House at Ittingen, Thurgau, Switzerland, February 1–4, 1993. London: Quintessence: 1994:478.

SECTION 5: CHAPTER REVIEW QUESTIONS

1. In a dental implant, the titanium post that protrudes through the tissue into the mouth is termed:
   A. Abutment post
   B. Implant fixture
   C. Peri-implant post
   D. Biologic seal

2. The tissues that surround a dental implant are the:
   A. Periodontium
   B. Peri-implant tissues

3. The implant-to-connective tissue interface for a dental implant is similar to the connective tissue on a natural tooth.
   A. True
   B. False

4. Periodontal pathogens can destroy bone much more rapidly along a dental implant than along a natural tooth.
   A. True
   B. False

5. Chronic periodontitis in the tissues surrounding a dental implant is termed:
   A. Periodontitis
   B. Peri-implant gingivitis
   C. Peri-implantitis
   D. Osseointegration

6. Standard metal periodontal instruments are safe for use on dental implants.
   A. True
   B. False

25 Periodontal Emergencies

Refer to the CD packaged with this book for full color versions of the clinical photographs in this chapter.

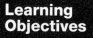

Learning Objectives

- Name and describe the three types of abscesses of the periodontium.
- Define the terms acute and circumscribed.
- List the possible causes of abscesses of the periodontium.
- Compare and contrast the abscess of the periodontium and the endodontic abscess.
- Outline the typical treatment steps for a gingival abscess and a periodontal abscess.
- Describe the clinical situation that can result in a pericoronal abscess.
- Outline the typical treatment for a pericoronal abscess (pericoronitis).
- List the two types of necrotizing periodontal diseases.
- Describe the characteristics of necrotizing ulcerative gingivitis.
- Outline the typical treatment steps for necrotizing ulcerative gingivitis.
- Describe the symptoms of primary herpetic gingivostomatitis.

KEY TERMS

Abscess of the periodontium
Acute
Circumscribed
Localized
Pus
Endodontic abscess
Gingival abscess
Periodontal abscess
Pericoronal abscess

Operculum
Necrotizing ulcerative gingivitis
Necrotizing ulcerative periodontitis
Necrosis
Ulceration
Punched out papillae
Pseudomembrane
Primary herpetic gingivostomatitis

SECTION 1: ABSCESS OF THE PERIODONTIUM

There are several periodontal conditions that can bring patients to the dental office for emergency care. It is imperative that all members of the dental team be alert for these conditions because their recognition and early intervention can limit the permanent damage to the periodontium. This chapter outlines the more common periodontal emergency conditions and briefly describes the treatment that may be recommended and performed by the dentist or the dental hygienist. Some of these conditions can be encountered in their early stages by the dental hygienist during routine treatment and recall appointments.

The emergency conditions described in this chapter are examples of *acute periodontal conditions*.

- Acute conditions are commonly characterized by a rapid onset and rapid course
- Acute conditions are frequently accompanied by pain and discomfort
- Acute conditions may not be related to the presence of preexisting gingivitis or periodontitis

OVERVIEW OF ABSCESS OF THE PERIODONTIUM

There are three types of abscesses of the periodontium: (i) the gingival abscess, (ii) the periodontal abscess, and (iii) the pericoronal abscess.

1. **Abscess of the periodontium** is usually described as an acute, circumscribed collection of pus in the periodontium (**Fig. 25-1**). In its earliest stages, the abscess of the periodontium can be discovered by the dental hygienist during oral inspection at a routine treatment visit. When an abscess of any type is suspected, the condition should immediately be brought to the attention of the dentist for early treatment.
   A. Definitions
      1. **Acute** means that the condition has a rapid onset, has a rapid course and that it can be accompanied by pain or discomfort.
      2. The term **circumscribed** means that the abscess is **localized** (confined to a small area). Note that other types of oral infections can be spread throughout soft tissue and do not necessarily result in a localized collection of pus.
      3. **Pus** is a collection of dead white blood cells that result from the body defense mechanisms involved in fighting the infection.
   B. Types of Abscesses of the Periodontium
      1. Gingival abscess
      2. Periodontal abscess
      3. Pericoronal abscess

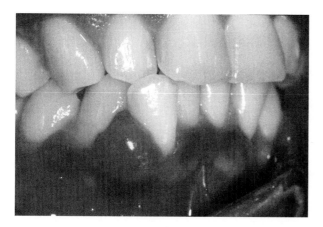

Figure 25-1. Abscess of the Periodontium. Note the localized swelling between the mandibular right canine and first premolar. Palpation of the swelling would reveal what feels like a fluid-filled sack.

2. Signs and Symptoms of Abscess of the Periodontium (Box 25-1)

   A. Symptoms. Typical patient complaints are pain and localized swelling. Pain resulting from an abscess of the periodontium is usually described by the patient as constant and easy to localize (the patient can point to the exact spot that hurts).

   B. Signs

      1. Localized swelling. Oral examination will usually reveal the presence of a localized, circumscribed swelling of the soft tissue.

      2. Alveolar Bone Loss. The radiographs of a tooth with an abscess of the periodontium frequently reveal alveolar bone loss in the area of the abscess (**Fig. 25-2**).

         a. Alveolar bone loss resulting from an abscess of the periodontium can occur extremely rapidly when compared with the rate of alveolar bone loss usually associated with periodontitis.

         b. Although a dental radiograph of an abscess of the periodontium may reveal alveolar bone loss, it is not possible to tell what part of the missing bone resulted from the abscess and what part of the missing bone was caused by chronic periodontitis that was present before the abscess formed.

      3. Pus Drainage. When there is delay in treating an abscess of the periodontium, the collection of pus can break through the surface tissues, thus establishing a path of drainage on its own (**Fig. 25-3**). This course of events is similar to other abscesses in other parts of the body. For example, if a pimple is allowed to develop without any treatment, it will eventually come to a head and drain.

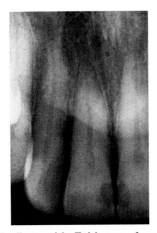

Figure 25-2. Radiographic Evidence of an Abscess of the Periodontium. This radiograph shows bone loss around the right central. Radiographic findings must always be correlated with the clinical findings to confirm the diagnosis.

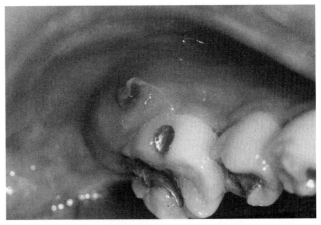

Figure 25-3. Path of Drainage. The abscess of the periodontium shown here has broken through the surface tissues, establishing a path of drainage on its own.

Box 25-1

Signs and Symptoms of an Abscess of the Periodontium

- Patients usually describe the pain as localized and constant
- Localized swelling in the soft tissue
- Radiographic evidence of alveolar bone loss that does not involve the tooth apex
- Tooth has a vital pulp

3. **Causes of Abscess of the Periodontium.** Theories about the origin of the abscess of the periodontium vary, but most investigators attribute formation of this type of abscess to one of the following:

   A. Blockage of the orifice (or opening) of an existing periodontal pocket. Most periodontal pockets have readily accessible openings that give easy access to a periodontal probe. Some authors have theorized that in certain instances the opening of a periodontal pocket can become restricted in size because of temporary improvement of the surface tissue tone. This improvement of tissue tone can result in trapping bacteria and fluids in a pocket, leading to an abscess of the periodontium.

   B. Forcing a foreign object into the supporting tissues of a tooth.

      1. A variety of foreign objects have been implicated in the formation of some abscesses of the periodontium. For example, an abscess could result when a patient accidentally punctures the gingiva with a toothpick, forcing bacteria into the tissue.

      2. Another common event that can result in an abscess of the periodontium is accidentally forcing some food product like a husk from a kernel of popcorn or a peanut skin into a periodontal pocket.

   C. Incomplete calculus removal in a periodontal pocket. Incomplete calculus removal also has been implicated in the formation of some abscesses of the periodontium.

      1. When this occurs, it is usually in a site with a deep probing depth where the calculus deposits are removed only in the most coronal aspects of the pocket near the gingival margin, but calculus deposits deeper in the pocket are not removed because of difficulty of access.

      2. It is theorized that removal of the more coronal deposits allows the gingival margin to heal somewhat and to tighten around the tooth, like a drawstring of a pouch, preventing drainage of bacterial toxins and other waste products from the pocket. Bacteria remaining in the deeper aspects of the periodontal pocket can result in the formation of an abscess.

4. **Abscess of the Periodontium versus Endodontic Abscess**

   A. Differentiation of Types of Abscess. Abscesses affecting the tissues around a tooth can result for two separate sources: (i) the periodontium itself or (ii) the pulpal tissues of the tooth. It is helpful for the dental hygienist to be familiar with the characteristics of these two types of abscesses, since abscess of the periodontium and the endodontic abscess sometimes appear to have somewhat similar clinical characteristics. **Table 25-1** shows the characteristics of both the abscess of the periodontium and the endodontic abscess.

   B. Abscess of the Periodontium—an abscess that results from an infection of the periodontium.

   C. Endodontic Abscess

      1. An **endodontic abscess** is an abscess that results from an infection of the tooth pulp.

      2. An endodontic abscess can be caused by death of the tooth pulp from trauma or from deep dental decay. A dead pulp is termed a nonvital pulp.

      3. Management of a patient with an endodontic abscess usually requires root canal treatment and will not be discussed in this chapter.

Table 25-1. Differentiation of the Types of Abscess

Clinical Characteristic	Abscess of the Periodontium	Endodontic Abscess
Vitality test results	Vital pulp	Usually nonvital pulp
Radiographic appearance	Bone loss present but does not involve the apex of the tooth	Bone loss frequently seen around the apex of the tooth
Symptoms	Localized, constant pain	Difficult to localize, intermittent pain

GINGIVAL AND PERIODONTAL ABSCESSES

1. **Gingival and Periodontal Abscesses.** Two of the three types of abscesses of the periodontium are the gingival abscess and the periodontal abscess.
   A. **Gingival Abscess.** One variation of the abscess of the periodontium occurs in a periodontally healthy mouth when some foreign object is forced into a healthy gingival sulcus. An abscess of the periodontium that is limited to the gingival margin area can follow this event. Some authors refer to this abscess as a gingival abscess to emphasize that it is limited in extent only to the marginal gingiva (**Fig. 25-4**).
   B. **Periodontal Abscess.** Another variation of the abscess of the periodontium—the periodontal abscess—usually occurs in a site with preexisting periodontal disease including preexisting periodontal pockets. *The periodontal abscess usually affects the deeper structures of the periodontium and is not limited to the gingival margin area only as is the gingival abscess.*

2. **Treatment of the Gingival and Periodontal Abscess**
   A. Treatment of the gingival abscess and the periodntontal abscess is similar and requires (i) establishment of a path of drainage for the pus and (ii) thorough periodontal debridement of the tooth surfaces in the area of the abscess (Box 25-2). Treatment of a painful dental emergency also always involves control of the discomfort.
   B. Steps commonly followed in treatment are outlined below.
      1. During treatment it is usually necessary to anesthetize the tooth to be treated, since manipulation of the tissues involved by an abscess can be quite uncomfortable.
      2. Drainage of the abscess can be established either through the pocket itself or by performing periodontal surgery (as discussed in Chapter 21). When drainage is established through the pocket, it can be done by puncturing the soft tissue wall of the pocket with the toe of a sterile curet.
      3. Thorough periodontal instrumentation of the tooth surfaces in the site of the abscess is important in bringing this type of abscess under control.
      4. Some adjustment of the tooth occlusion is usually also indicated since inflammation resulting from the abscess can force a tooth to extrude slightly from its socket, leading to trauma from occlusion.
      5. In more advanced cases of abscesses antibiotics may be needed, as with any other serious oral infection.
      6. Some clinicians recommend warm saltwater (saline) rinses to help keep the abscess draining until completely healed.
      7. Following emergency treatment of a patient with an abscess of the periodontium, the dental team should appoint the patient for a thorough periodontal assessment, since the abscess of the periodontium frequently occurs in a patient with existing untreated periodontal disease.

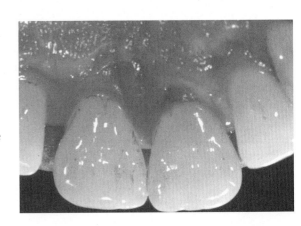

Figure 25-4. An Abscess of the Periodontium Limited to Gingival Tissues or Gingival Abscess. A gingival abscess of the maxillary central incisor. Note that the swelling accompanying this abscess is near the free gingival margin and that the gingival tissue at adjacent sites appears healthy.

Box 25-2

Typical Treatment Steps for an Abscess of the Periodontium

1. Anesthetize the involved tooth
2. Establish a path for drainage of the collection of pus
3. Periodontal instrumentation of the tooth surfaces in the area of the abscess
4. Flush the site with sterile saline
5. Adjust the tooth occlusion if needed
6. Instruct the patient to rest, drink fluids, and rinse with warm saline
7. Reappoint the patient for comprehensive clinical assessment

PERICORONAL ABSCESS

1. **Pericoronal Abscess.** The third type of abscess of the periodontium is the pericoronal abscess (also referred to as **pericoronitis**). The **pericoronal abscess** is an infection in the soft tissue surrounding the crown of a partially erupted tooth. This type of abscess is seen in teeth where some of the soft tissues surrounding the teeth actually cover part of the occlusal surface of the teeth.
   A. Description
      1. *Pericoronal abscess (or pericoronitis) is most frequently seen around mandibular third molar teeth.* Since a third molar tooth frequently does not have space to erupt fully, the tooth can have a flap of tissue covering part of the occlusal surface.
      2. The flap of gingival tissue that covers a portion of the crown of a partially erupted tooth can become infected, and it is this type of infection under this flap of tissue that is referred to as a pericoronal abscess.
      3. This flap of tissue is called an **operculum**, and some authors refer to pericoronitis as operculitis.
   B. Signs and Symptoms of Pericoronal Abscess (Box 25-3)
      1. Pain. Pain is common with this infection. Figure 25-5 shows a patient with pericoronitis under a soft tissue flap on a third molar tooth.
      2. Soft Tissue Swelling and Redness. In patients with pericoronitis, the soft tissue flap or operculum can exhibit redness (erythema) and swelling (edema).
      3. Damage to Tissue Covering the Partially Erupted Tooth. As pericoronitis progresses and the tissue swelling increases, the opposing tooth can frequently be seen to impinge (press) on the swollen tissue, creating additional tissue damage and additional patient discomfort.
      4. Limited Mouth Opening. In advanced cases of pericoronitis, limited mouth opening (called trismus) can be seen.
      5. Fever and Swollen Lymph Nodes. Elevated body temperature (fever) and swollen lymph nodes (lymphadenopathy) also can be seen in advanced cases of pericoronitis.

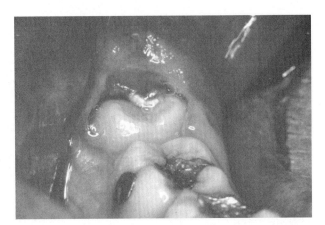

Figure 25-5. Pericoronitis.
A patient with pericoronitis under a soft tissue flap on a third molar. The tissues of the flap are red and swollen. Manipulation of the flap causes discomfort for the patient.

2. **Treatment of Pericoronitis** (Box 25-4)
   A. Treatment of a patient with pericoronitis involves (i) drainage of the pus (ii) irrigation of the undersurface of the flap of tissue with warm saline and (iii) relief of pain.
   B. Because of discomfort in the site of the pericoronitis, patients frequently discontinue plaque control in the area. Patients should be instructed to resume cleaning the site with gentle plaque control techniques.
   C. As with any other oral infection, advanced cases may require the use of antibiotics.
   D. Occasionally the dentist will find it necessary to remove the opposing tooth— usually a malposed maxillary third molar tooth—as part of the emergency visit. This would eliminate additional trauma to the mandibular tissues and facilitate resolution of the infection.
   E. Following resolution of the pericoronitis, the dentist may recommend extraction of the third molar that was the source of the pericoronal abscess. In some cases it is possible to remove the flap of tissue with periodontal surgery to prevent recurrence of the abscess rather than remove the tooth.
   F. Pericoronitis tends to recur if definitive treatment (extraction of the partially erupted tooth or surgical removal of the operculum) is not provided.

Box 25-3

Signs and Symptoms of Pericoronitis

- Pain around a partially erupted tooth
- Soft tissue swelling and redness around a partially erupted tooth
- In advanced cases, limited mouth opening, fever, and swollen lymph nodes

Box 25-4

Typical Treatment Steps for Pericoronitis

1. Administer local anesthesia if needed to control discomfort caused by tissue manipulation
2. Using sterile saline irrigate the undersurface of the operculum thoroughly
3. Remove any debris or plaque that has accumulated in the site
4. Instruct the patient to rinse frequently with warm saline, get plenty of rest, and drink fluids
5. Extract the opposing third molar when severe tissue trauma is part of the clinical picture
6. Reschedule the patient for further clinical assessment and further treatment, as indicated

SECTION 2: NECROTIZING PERIODONTAL DISEASES

Necrotizing periodontal diseases include necrotizing ulcerative gingivitis (NUG) and necrotizing ulcerative periodontitis (NUP). Both of these diseases are acute infections of the periodontium that can bring patients to the dental office for emergency treatment.

- NUG is an acute infection of the gingival tissues only.
- NUP is an acute infection that mimics NUG but can also affect the deeper structures of the periodontium such as the alveolar bone.
- Both conditions have been reported to occur in patients with compromised immune systems who therefore have limited host defense mechanisms.

NECROTIZING ULCERATIVE GINGIVITIS

1. **NUG** is an acute infection of the periodontium that is limited to gingival tissues. Other names for this condition are Vincent's infection and trench mouth. As the name implies, patients with NUG exhibit necrosis and ulceration of the gingiva.
   A. Necrosis of the epithelium. **Necrosis** refers to cell death, in this instance referring to the death of the cells comprising the gingival epithelium.
   B. Ulceration of the gingival tissue. **Ulceration** is the loss of the epithelium normally covering underlying connective tissue. Ulceration results from death of the epithelial cells and subsequent loss of the epithelial covering of the underlying gingival connective tissue.

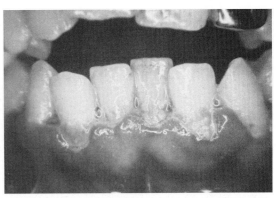

Figure 25-6. Necrotizing Ulcerative Gingivitis. Note that the necrotic areas have extended from the papillae onto the facial surfaces of the teeth. The necrotic areas of the gingiva are covered with gray–white layer called the pseudomembrane.

2. **Appearance, Signs, and Symptoms of NUG**
   A. Description
      1. Punched out papillae. The typical clinical appearance of NUG is necrotic papillae that are usually called **punched out papillae** to underscore their craterlike appearance.
      2. Pseudomembrane formation. The necrotic areas of gingiva are covered with a gray–white layer referred to as a **pseudomembrane (Fig. 25-6)**.
         a. The pseudomembrane consists of dead cells, bacteria, and oral debris. Underlying this pseudomembrane is raw connective tissue.
         b. Patients with NUG usually exhibit bleeding with the slightest manipulation of the gingival tissues. This bleeding results from breakage of some of the tiny blood vessels in the connective tissues that are normally protected by the epithelium.
   B. Signs and Symptoms of NUG (Box 25-5)
      1. Pain. Patients with NUG usually seek emergency care for oral pain since the ulceration associated with the infection results in exposure of connective tissue, which can be quite painful.
      2. Swollen lymph nodes. Patients with NUG can display swollen lymph nodes (lymphadenopathy), a vague feeling of discomfort (malaise), and elevated temperature.
      3. Halitosis. Because of the necrosis or death of cells involved with this disease there is usually noticeable halitosis or bad breath. Some authors have described this halitosis as fetid breath.
   C. Patient Characteristics
      1. History of smoking. NUG frequently occurs in smokers.
      2. History of poor nutrition. NUG frequently occurs in patients with poor nutrition.
      3. Recent history of stress. NUG has been reported to occur in patients experiencing severe stress, such as college students at the time of examinations.
      4. Human immunodeficiency virus (HIV)-positive status. NUG has also been reported to occur in some patients with HIV infection. HIV is the virus that causes acquired immunodeficiency syndrome (AIDS).
3. **Treatment of NUG** (Box 25-6)
   A. Treatment of the patient with NUG involves gentle debridement (removal) of the pseudomembrane, periodontal instrumentation of the tooth surfaces, and reinstitution of gentle personal plaque control (**Fig. 25-7**).
   B. In more advanced cases, antibiotics may be needed as in any other severe oral infection.
   C. It is helpful to instruct patients to rest, drink fluids, and avoid spicy foods.

Box 25-5

Signs, Symptoms, and Patient Characteristics in Necrotizing Ulcerative Gingivitis

- Oral pain
- Gingival bleeding with even slight manipulation of the gingival tissues
- Necrotic or punched out gingival papillae
- Presence of pseudomembrane on affected sites
- Swollen lymph nodes (lymphadenopathy)
- Vague feeling of discomfort (malaise)
- Elevated body temperature
- Extreme halitosis
- History of smoking, poor nutrition, and stress

Box 25-6

Typical Treatment Steps for a Patient with Necrotizing Ulcerative Gingivitis

1. **At the first appointment.**
   - The pseudomembrane should be removed carefully.
   - *Supragingival* periodontal instrumentation is performed. Instrumentation is limited because of the discomfort elicited by tissue manipulation.
   - The patient is instructed regarding a gentle self-care regimen.
2. **One to 2 days later.**
   - *Subgingival* periodontal instrumentation usually can be begun at this appointment.
   - Further instruction in self-care should be included at this visit.
3. **Three to five days after initial visit.**
   - Subgingival instrumentation usually can be completed.
4. **Following the resolution of the infection.** The patient should be appointed for a comprehensive clinical assessment to identify any underlying chronic periodontal disease.

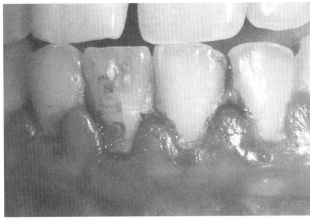
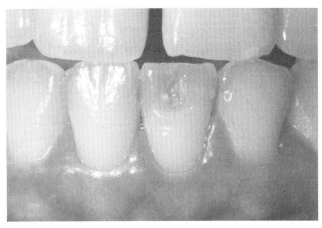

A   B

Figure 25-7. Necrotizing Ulcerative Gingivitis: Before and After Treatment.
A: Necrotizing ulcerative gingivitis before treatment. **B:** The same patient after treatment. (Courtesy
of Dr. Don Rolfs, Periodontal Foundations, Wachatee, WA.)

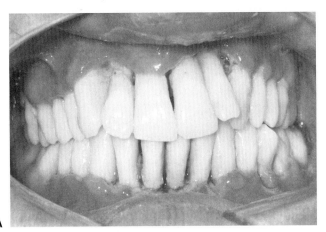
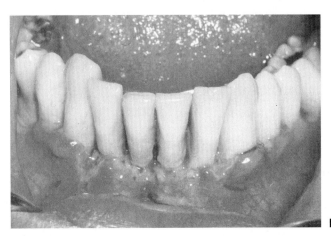

A   B

Figure 25-8. Necrotizing Ulcerative Periodontitis. **A:** A patient with necrotizing ulcerative
periodontitis. **B:** Close-up of the mandibular arch. (Courtesy of Dr. Don Rolfs, Periodontal
Foundations, Wachatee, WA.)

NECROTIZING ULCERATIVE PERIODONTITIS

1. **NUP**
   A. Symptoms of necrotizing ulcerative periodontitis are similar to those of NUG but
      this condition also affects the deeper structures of the periodontium such as the
      alveolar bone **(Fig. 25-8)**.
   B. One unusual finding in NUP is that it can be accompanied by the formation of
      bone sequestra (dead pieces of alveolar bone).

2. **Treatment of NUP**
   A. The treatment of patients with NUP is complex and usually requires medical
      consultation since the patients that develop this condition usually have serious
      underlying medical compromising conditions that must be managed
      simultaneously with dental therapy.
   B. *When patients with NUP are encountered in a general dental office, immediate
      referral to a periodontist is indicated.*

SECTION 3: PRIMARY HERPETIC GINGIVOSTOMATITIS

PRIMARY HERPETIC GINGIVOSTOMATITIS

Primary herpetic gingivostomatitis is actually a medical condition resulting from a viral infection. It is listed here as a periodontal emergency condition since patients with this condition frequently first seek care in a dental office because of the nature of the oral symptoms as described below.

1. **Description. Primary herpetic gingivostomatitis** is a painful oral condition that results from initial infection with the herpes simplex virus (HSV).
   A. There are two types of herpes simplex virus, oral herpes virus (HSVI) and genital herpes virus (HSVII). Primary herpetic gingivostomatitis is usually caused by initial infection with HSVI, but can also be caused by initial infection with HSVII.
   B. In some patients, the initial infection with these viruses produces no noticeable clinical signs and can go undetected clinically. In other patients, however, the symptoms resulting from this initial infection can be quite severe, and it is these severe symptoms that are known as primary herpetic gingivostomatitis.
   C. *Primary herpetic gingivostomatitis is contagious and requires careful attention to prevent its spread.*
   D. The initial infection with HSVI usually occurs in children or in young adults, but it can occur at any age.
   E. Once a patient is infected with this virus, the infection can recur periodically throughout the life of the patient in the form of herpes labialis (fever blisters and cold sores).

2. **Signs and Symptoms of Primary Herpetic Gingivostomatitis** (Box 25-7)
   A. Oral Pain. Discomfort results in difficulty in eating and drinking.
   B. Swollen, Red, Bleeding Gingiva. In primary herpetic gingivostomatitis the gingiva is swollen, fiery red, and bleeds easily.
   C. Painful Oral Ulcers. Careful inspection of the gingival tissue can reveal small clusters of blisters (vesicles) on the tissues that burst, leaving numerous, painful oral ulcers (**Fig. 25-9**). The ulcers are surrounded by a red halo.
      1. These ulcers can occur on lips, palate, and tongue as well as the gingival tissue.
      2. Pain caused by these ulcers can be such a major problem that eating and drinking can be impaired. Restricting fluids can lead to dehydration, and dehydration in a child can be a serious medical emergency.
   D. In the more severe clinical manifestation, this infection is associated with symptoms such as pain, elevated temperature, a vague feeling of discomfort (malaise), headache, and swollen lymph nodes (lymphadenopathy).

3. **Treatment of Primary Herpetic Gingivostomatitis** (Box 25-8)
   A. Primary herpetic gingivostomatitis usually regresses spontaneously (goes away without treatment) in approximately 12 to 20 days, and treatment is mainly supportive. Controlling discomfort and ensuring fluid intake are the main focus for supportive treatment.
   B. In some patients, treatment will include antiviral medications, medications to reduce fever (antipyretics), and systemic medications to control pain (analgesics).
   C. Topical oral anesthetics can be used to control oral discomfort temporarily to allow the patient to eat or to drink fluids. Examples of topical anesthetics that can be used are (i) 2% lidocaine viscous and (ii) Orabase with benzocaine.
   D. The dental hygienist should keep in mind that primary herpetic gingivostomatitis is contagious, and any plan for periodontal debridement of the teeth should be postponed until the initial infection regresses.

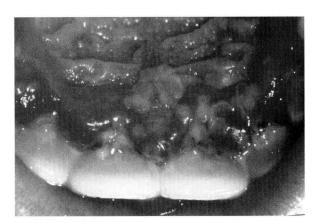

Figure 25-9. Primary Herpetic Gingivostomatitis. Note the numerous ulcerations of the gingival tissue that have resulted from the formation of vesicles that have broken.

Box 25-7

Signs and Symptoms of Primary Herpetic Gingivostomatitis

- Oral pain with difficulty in eating and drinking
- Elevated body temperature
- Malaise (vague feeling of discomfort)
- Headache
- Swollen lymph nodes
- Edematous gingival tissues (swollen gingival tissue)
- Fiery red gingival tissues
- Vesicles (blisters) and ulceration of the gingival tissue and sometimes lips, tongue, and palate; ulcerations surrounded by red halo
- Bleeding from gingival tissue

Box 25-8

Typical Treatment Steps for Primary Herpetic Gingivostomatitis

1. Keep in mind that this disease is highly contagious.
2. Primary herpetic gingivostomatitis regresses spontaneously in about 12 to 20 days.
3. Control oral discomfort. Topical oral anesthetics can be used for temporary relief of oral discomfort so that the patient can eat and drink fluids.
4. Recommend frequent fluid intake to avoid dehydration.
5. Refer the patient to a physician if systemic symptoms are severe or if the patient is unable to tolerate fluid intake.

CHAPTER SUMMARY STATEMENT

This chapter discussed some periodontal conditions that can bring patients to the office for an emergency visit. All members of the dental team should be on alert for these conditions; the dental hygienist may encounter some of these conditions in their earliest stages during routine treatment visits.

SECTION 4: FOCUS ON PATIENTS

CASE 1

During a routine patient visit for periodontal maintenance, you note that there is swelling in the interdental papilla between the patient's two central incisors. The swelling is quite localized to the area between the incisors. As you manipulate the tissues, you note pus coming from the sulcus of one of the central incisors. You also note some mobility of one of the incisor teeth. When questioned, the patient informs you that she is aware that these tissues are swollen and that she has been flossing more in hope that the swelling would go down. In view of these clinical findings how should you proceed at this maintenance visit?

CASE 2

A concerned parent, who is one of your maintenance patients, calls you to tell you that her 4-year-old daughter has something wrong with her gums. She reports that her daughter's gums appear swollen and that there appears to be some raw, red areas on the gums. Her child has been complaining of pain in her mouth and has an elevated temperature. How should you respond to the parent's concerns?

CASE 3

A patient with necrotizing ulcerative gingivitis (NUG) is referred to you by the dentist for calculus removal. Your examination of the patient reveals ulceration of most interdental papillae with the typical punched out papillae often seen with this disease. The necrotic tissue pseudomembrane is present covering the ulcerations, and heavy calculus deposits are evident. The patient is quite uncomfortable. How should you proceed with the calculus removal?

SUGGESTED READINGS

Parameter on acute periodontal diseases. American Academy of Periodontology. *J Periodontol.* 2000;71(5 Suppl):863–866.

Antonelli JR. Acute dental pain, Part 1: Diagnosis and emergency treatment. *Compendium.* 1990;11:492, 494–496, 498–500.

Antonelli JR. Acute dental pain, Part II: Diagnosis and emergency treatment. *Compendium.* 1990;11: 526, 528, 530–533.

Barr CB, Robbins MR. Clinical and radiographic presentations of HIV-1 necrotizing ulcerative periodontitis. *Spec Care Dentist.* 1996;16:237–241.

Batista BL, Jr, Novaes AB Jr, Calvano LM, et al. Necrotizing ulcerative periodontitis associated with severe congenital immunodeficiency in a prepubescent subject: Clinical findings and response to intravenous immunoglobulin treatment. *J Clin Periodontol.* 1999;26:499–504.

Blakey GH, White RP Jr, Offenbacher S, et al. Clinical/biological outcomes of treatment for pericoronitis. *J Oral Maxillofac Surg.* 1996;54:1150–1160.

Christie SN, McCaughey C, Marly JJ, et al. Recrudescent herpes simplex infection mimicking primary herpetic gingivostomatitis. *J Oral Pathol Med.* 1998;27:8–10.

Cuenin MF, Scheidt MJ, O'Neal RB, et al. An in vivo study of dentin sensitivity: The relation of dentin sensitivity and the patency of dentin tubules. *J Periodontol.* 1991;62:668–673.

Fliss DM, Tovi F, Zirkin HJ. Necrotizing soft-tissue infections of dental origin. *J Oral Maxillofac Surg.* 1990;48:1104–1108.

Glick M, Muzyka BC, Salkin CM, et al. Necrotizing ulcerative periodontitis: A marker for immune deterioration and a predictor for the diagnosis of AIDS. *J Periodontol.,* 1994;65:393–397.

Gowdey G, Alijanian A. Necrotizing ulcerative periodontitis in an HIV patient. *J Calif Dent Assoc.* 1995;23:57–59.

Homing GM, Cohen ME. Necrotizing ulcerative gingivitis, periodontitis, and stomatitis: Clinical staging and predisposing factors. *J Periodontol.* 1995;66:990–998.

Lewis MA, MacFarlane TW, McGowan DA. A microbiological and clinical review of the acute dentoalveolar abscess. *Br J Oral Maxillofac Surg.* 1990;28:359–366.

McLeod DE, Lainson PA, Spivey JD. Tooth loss due to periodontal abscess: A retrospective study. *J Periodontol.* 1997;68:963–966.

Novak MJ. Necrotizing ulcerative periodontitis. *Ann Periodontol.* 1999;4:74–78.

Peltroche-Llacsahuanga H, Reichhart E, Schmitt W, et al. Investigation of infectious organisms causing pericoronitis of the mandibular third molar. *J Oral Maxillofac Surg.* 2000;58:611–616.

Rajasuo A, Jousimies-Somer H, Savolainen S, et al. Bacteriologic findings in tonsillitis and pericoronitis. *Clin Infect Dis.* 1996;23:51–60.

Topoll HH, Lange DE, Muller RF. Multiple periodontal abscesses after systemic antibiotic therapy. *J Clin Periodontol.* 1990;17:268–272.

Wade DN, Kerns DG. Acute necrotizing ulcerative gingivitis-periodontitis: A literature review. *Mil Med.* 1998;163:337–342.

Wyss C, Dewhirst FE, Gmur R, et al. Treponema parvum sp. nov., a small, glucoronic or galacturonic acid- dependent oral spirochaete from lesions of human periodontitis and acute necrotizing ulcerative gingivitis. *Int J Syst Evol Microbiol.* 2001;51(Pt 3):955–962.

SECTION 5: CHAPTER REVIEW QUESTIONS

1. The three types of abscesses of the periodontium are:
   A. The apical abscess, the periodontal abscess, and the gingival abscess
   B. The pericoronal abscess, the periodontal abscess, and the gingival abscess
   C. The coronal abscess, the periradicular abscess, and the gingival abscess

2. One possible cause of the abscess of the periodontium is blockage of the orifice (or opening) of an existing periodontal pocket.
   A. True
   B. False

3. The endodontic abscess originates in the periodontium, while the abscess of the periodontium originates from pulp of the tooth.
   A. True
   B. False

4. Pericoronitis results from which of the following conditions?
   A. Ingesting too much sugar
   B. Short tooth roots
   C. Tissue over a tooth crown

5. During treatment of a periodontal abscess, drainage of the pus is a critical step.
   A. True
   B. False

6. The acronym NUG stands for which of the following?
   A. Never underestimate gingiva
   B. Necrotizing ulcerative gingivitis
   C. Not usually generalized

7. Treatment of NUG includes which of the following steps?
   A. Rinses with caustic chemicals
   B. Instructions to rest and drink fluids
   C. Placement of a periodontal dressing

Chapter

26 Documentation and Insurance Reporting of Periodontal Care

Learning Objectives

- Understand the foundations of tort law and how it applies to the profession of dentistry.
- Define the term liability as it applies to provision of periodontal care.
- Identify situations in the dental office that trigger liability for dental hygienists.
- Define the terms intentional torts and negligence and give examples of each.
- In the clinical setting, thoroughly document all periodontal treatment including treatment options, cancellations, patient noncompliance, refusal of treatment, and follow-up telephone calls.
- Define the terms insurance codes and insurance form and explain their use in periodontal care.

KEY TERMS

Liability
Malpractice
Tort

Intentional torts
Negligence
Insurance codes

Insurance forms

It is important for every dental hygienist to practice to the highest established standards of care, not only to ensure the safety of the patient receiving treatment but also to avoid costly malpractice litigation. Potential liability is a reality for every health care provider. *While patients can sue a dentist or dental hygienist for many reasons, the success of such a suit often depends on the quality of the chart notes. The dental hygienist has a moral and ethical obligation to deliver high-quality care and maintain thorough chart notes for each patient visit to protect the practice against liability.*

CONCEPTS OF MALPRACTICE AND TORT LAW

1. In the context of health care, **liability** is a health care provider's obligation or responsibility to provide services to another person (the patient). The health care provider's liability entails the possibility of being sued if the person receiving the services feels as if he has been treated improperly or negligently.
2. **Malpractice** is the improper or negligent treatment by a health care provider that results in injury or damage to the patient.
3. **Tort.** The legal basis for most lawsuits in dental and dental hygiene practice is founded on tort law. A tort is a civil wrong where a person has breached a duty to another. A **tort** is the law that permits an injured person to recover compensation from the person who caused the injury.
   A. **Intentional torts** are actions designed to injure another person or that person's property. There are many specific types of intentional torts, including the following:
      1. Battery is the unlawful and unwanted touching or striking of one person by another, with the intention of bringing about a harmful or offensive contact. Forceful discipline of unruly children in the dental chair could be construed as battery.
      2. Assault is an unlawful threat or attempt to do bodily injury to another. A doctor who treats a minor patient without proper parental or guardian informed consent could be charged with assault or battery.
      3. Infliction of emotional distress. An example is talking in a loud or harsh voice to an unruly child.
      4. Fraud is deception carried out for the purpose of achieving personal gain while causing injury to another party.
      5. Misrepresentation occurs when a health care provider deliberately deceives a patient about possible outcomes.
      6. Defamation is communication to third parties of false statements about a person that injure the reputation of or deter others from associating with that person. For example, a dental hygienist learns that another hygienist has been making disparaging comments about the quality of care that he or she provides. The hygienist being disparaged could sue for defamation.
      7. Trespass is to infringe on the privacy, time, or attention of another. An example is discussing a patient's personal information with someone without the patient's permission.
      8. Defamation by computer. E-mail correspondence and other written documents are discoverable in court, so disparaging remarks in e-mail communications should be avoided.

B. **Negligence** is a failure to exercise reasonable care to avoid injuring others. It is the failure to do something that a reasonable person would do under the same circumstances, or the doing of something a reasonable person would not do. Negligence is characterized by carelessness, inattentiveness, and neglectfulness rather than by a positive intent to cause injury.

1. Negligence is different from an intentional tort in that negligence *does not require* the intent to commit a wrongful action; instead, the wrongful action itself is sufficient to constitute negligence.

2. Examples of negligence include: accidentally spilling a chemical on a patient, not updating the patient's health history resulting in the patient's health being jeopardized, and incorrect treatment of periodontal disease. *Professional liability insurance typically covers only unintentional torts or negligence.*

AREAS OF POTENTIAL LIABILITY

In judging whether a professional has been negligent, the courts use a standard called the *reasonable prudent person or professional*. This means the court compares what a reasonably prudent person or professional would have done in a similar situation. Thus, providing periodontal care that meets or exceeds the standard of care is extremely important for dental hygienists. Failure to include a procedure or step in treatment because the dental hygienist claims to be unaware of the current standard will not hold up in court.

Box 26-1

Top Ten Areas of Potential Liability for Dental Hygienists

1. Failure to ask and document whether the patient has taken his or her premedication.
2. Failure to detect and document oral cancer.
3. Failure to update the patient's medical history.
4. Failure to detect and thoroughly document the presence of periodontal disease.
5. Injuring a patient.
6. Failure to document treatment thoroughly in the patient chart or computerized record.
7. Failure to protect patient privacy or divulging confidential patient information.
8. Failure to inform the patient about treatment options and the consequences of non-treatment.
9. Practicing outside the legal scope of practice. All dental hygienists should be well informed about the state practice act and follow the rules and regulations explicitly.
10. Failure to provide care that meets the established standards of care.

DOCUMENTATION OF PERIODONTAL CARE

The dental chart is a legal document. It is the first line of defense in a malpractice suit. *When a patient decides to file a lawsuit, the dental chart becomes the single most important piece of information relative to the suit. Faulty records can be the most important reason for the loss of a lawsuit.* All periodontal assessment, educational, and treatment services should be documented in the patient chart or computerized record. Marsha Freeman's, (http://www.marshafreeman.com), recommendations for thorough documentation are summarized in Box 26-2.

Box 26-2

Adequate Chart Notes

- Today's date
- Reason for today's appointment
- Thorough documentation of medical and dental history
- Patient's chief complaint in his or her own words
- Symptoms reported by the patient
- Clinician's findings from the clinical periodontal assessment
- Treatment options and recommendations
- Discussion with patient and his or her treatment choices
- All assessment, educational, and treatment services
- Items given to patient, such as educational materials or oral hygiene aids
- Date or interval of next appointment
- Initials of the individual making the chart entry

SECTION 2: PRINCIPLES FOR THOROUGH DOCUMENTATION

Jeffery J. Tonner, J.D. recommends several principles that every dental professional should follow when documenting periodontal treatment in the patient chart or computerized record.

1. **General Guidelines for Chart Entries**
   A. All entries should be complete and accurate using accepted dental terminology and abbreviations. Chart Entry 1 is an example of a complete chart entry.

Date	Treatment Rendered	Fee
1/10/07	Reason for visit: 3-month periodontal maintenance. Medical history	
	update: pat. now taking 1 aspirin per day per his physician's	
	recommendation. Chief complaint: none. Oral cancer examination:	
	normal. Periodontal probing: changes noted in charting. Plaque:	
	light, calculus: light, bleeding areas noted on periodontal chart.	
	Periodontal maintenance: periodontal instrumentation of all four	
	quadrants; ultrasonic and hand instrumentation. Plaque removal	
	by patient using brush and interdental brush. Patient tolerated	
	all procedures well. Patient education: reviewed use of tufted	
	dental floss around distal surfaces of molars. Tray fluoride	
	application 1.23% APF gel. four bitewing radiographs. Next	
	maintenance visit in 3 months. (DG)	

Chart Entry 1. Complete Chart Entry. This chart entry is an example of a thorough chart entry that documents all the events of the patient's appointment.

   B. It is helpful to organize the services documented in sequential order so that no information is omitted.
   C. If handwritten, entries should be legible and in ink.
   D. The recorder should initial the entry. Since many different people write in the patient chart, it is important that each entry be initialed. If there are multiple dentists in the practice, the dentist that examines the hygienist's patient should be identified also.
   E. Thorough chart entries provide valuable information for the next clinician that treats this patient.
   F. The patient should be thoroughly interviewed regarding his or her medical status at each visit. Patients do not usually volunteer information when they are taking a new medicine or if there has been a change in their medical history. The medical status should be thoroughly documented at each visit.
2. **Treatment Options.** The health care provider should document all treatment options presented to the patient.
3. **Appointment Schedule and Chart Entries.**
   A. Chart entries should be consistent with the appointment schedule.
      1. With most dental software and computer scheduling, the patient's name must be on the schedule in order to make a chart entry.
      2. However, with manual appointment books, entries can be erased and changed.
   B. In the event of a lawsuit, doubt may be cast on the reliability of the office's records if the treatment dates in the chart do not match the appointment book entries.
   C. If the patient is being seen as an emergency patient that should be recorded in the chart.
4. **Cancellations and Missed Appointments.** All cancellations and missed appointments should be written in the patient chart. Infrequent periodontal maintenance appointments can lead to a recurrence and progression of periodontal disease. Chart Entry 2 and Chart Entry 3 provide examples of how to document missed and cancelled appointments.

Date	Treatment Rendered	Fee
1/10/07	Patient missed maintenance appointment because of illness. (DG)	

Chart Entry 2. Missed Appointment. This chart entry is an example of documentation of a missed appointment due to illness.

Date	Treatment Rendered	Fee
1/10/07	Telephoned patient to confirm her 3-month maintenance appt.	
	Patient canceled and said that she would call to reschedule later.	
	I reminded patient of the importance of regular maintenance. (DG)	

Chart Entry 3. Canceled Maintenance Appointment. This chart entry provides an example of the documentation for a canceled periodontal maintenance appointment.

5. **Patient Noncompliance and Refusal of Treatment**
   A. Patient noncompliance with recommendations, such as (i) inadequate self-care, (ii) continued smoking, (iii) failure to regulate diabetes, or (iv) failure to follow specific instructions, can lead to disease progression. Noncompliance should be noted in the chart (Chart Entry 4).
   B. Instances when a patient opts not to have recommended treatment or declines a referral to a specialist should be documented. Furthermore, when a patient is referred to a specialist, it is recommended that a copy of the referral letter be kept in the patient chart (Chart Entry 5). Chart Entry 5 provides an example of documentation of inadequate self-care.
6. **Follow-up Telephone Calls.** Patients appreciate a follow-up telephone call from the dentist or hygienist following a long or difficult treatment procedure. For hygienists, a good rule of thumb is to call any patient who required anesthesia for periodontal instrumentation. Follow-up telephone calls should be documented (Chart Entry 6).

Date	Treatment Rendered	Fee
1/10/07	Discussed options for smoking cessation. Patient stated that "he	
	is not interested in quitting smoking." (DG)	

Chart Entry 4. Patient Noncompliance. This chart entry provides an example of the documentation for patient noncompliance with recommendations.

Date	Treatment Rendered	Fee
1/10/07	Patient reports brushing twice daily but "does not have time to	
	use an interdental brush." Showed patient signs of periodontal	
	inflammation in the interdental areas. Explained benefits of	
	interdental plaque control and several alternatives for interdental	
	self-care. Patient decided that he was not interested and stated	
	that "he only wants to brush." (DG)	

Chart Entry 5. Inadequate Self-Care. This chart entry is an example of documentation of inadequate self-care by a patient.

Date	Treatment Rendered	Fee
1/10/07	Telephoned patient at home this evening to check on her. Patient	
	reports that she "is doing well". Reminded her to use warm salt	
	water rinse before bedtime. (DG)	

Chart Entry 6. Follow-up Telephone Call. This chart entry is an example of documentation of a follow-up telephone call after a long or difficult treatment procedure.

SECTION 3: PITFALLS IN DOCUMENTATION

Jeffery J. Tonner, J.D. outlines four common pitfalls in documentation.

1. **Making Entries in Haste.** Chart Entry 7 is an example of an *inadequate* chart entry. For example, in her haste to stay on schedule, the dental hygienist simply forgets to record that she did a periodontal charting and evaluation. Later, if the patient develops periodontal disease, he or she may accuse the doctor of failure to diagnose. The dentist or hygienist may state to a jury that a periodontal evaluation is done on every patient. *In the eyes of a jury, however, if a procedure is not written in the chart, it was not done.*

2. **Skipping Lines between Entries or Writing in Margins**
   A. Keeping in the lines or skipping lines.
      1. Chart entries should be written with small enough strokes to be contained within the space provided.
      2. No lines should be skipped on a treatment record form. All lines should be used so that there is no opportunity for anyone to add information *after* a lawsuit is initiated.
   B. Writing in margins or below the last line. All entries should be written on the lines, and no entries should be written in the margins or below the last line on the page. Doing so can cause juries to wonder if the entry was made at a later date.

3. **Altering Chart Entries.** *The single most common cause of punitive damages in a dental malpractice suit is altering the chart.*
   A. Correction fluid should never be used to correct an entry. If an error is made, a single line should be drawn through the incorrect entry so that it can still be read, the word *error* written above it, and the correct entry made on the next available line. The revised entry should be initialed.
   B. Additional information should never be added to an entry from a previous appointment. Juries perceive such added entries to be fraudulent and deceptive.
   C. Forensic ink dating analysis allows an expert to determine the date that ink was used on a particular document. Therefore, it is foolhardy to add things at a later date to a patient chart in an attempt to avoid or win a lawsuit.

4. **Not Clearly Indicating Patient Comments.** Quotation marks should be used to indicate patient comments. This is especially important when making follow-up telephone calls after a difficult or invasive procedure. A sample chart entry is shown in Chart Entry 8.

Date	Treatment Rendered	Fee
1/10/07	Px, Ex	

Chart Entry 7. Incomplete Chart Entry. Although this hygienist may have been quite thorough in delivering care, the chart does not reflect that.

Date	Treatment Rendered	Fee
1/10/07	Patient reports "my gums feel so much better now." Tissue and	
	texture much improved from three weeks ago. (DG)	

Chart Entry 8. Patient Comments. This chart entry is an example of how to include a patient's comments at a periodontal maintenance visit.

SECTION 4: INSURANCE CODES FOR PERIODONTAL TREATMENT

INSURANCE CODING

1. **Insurance codes** are numeric codes used by insurance companies and the government to classify different dental procedures. For example, periodontal maintenance procedures are designated by the insurance code D4910.
2. Insurance coding was developed to speed and simplify the reporting of dental treatments to third parties such as insurance companies and the government.
3. The most important use of codes is for insurance billing purposes. Insurance codes are entered on **insurance forms** (**Fig. 26-1**). Dental treatment is listed under the appropriate procedure number.
4. In the United States, insurance codes are published in the *American Dental Association Current Dental Terminology 2005.* These codes are very specific and should be reviewed carefully before specific dental treatment is coded.
5. Another important resource for accurate insurance coding is the *2005 Current Procedural Terminology For Periodontics and Insurance Reporting Manual, 10th Edition (CPT-10)* published by the American Academy of Periodontology. This manual includes a glossary of terms and procedures and provides a guide for reporting periodontal services to third-party agencies.

INSURANCE CODES FOR PERIODONTAL SERVICES

1. **Evolution of Dental Terminology**
   A. Members of the dental team should be aware that there is a continuous evolution of terminology used in dentistry and medicine; these evolutionary changes occur as a natural result of scientific advances and improved understanding of disease pathogenesis. Terminology related to nonsurgical therapy is currently undergoing one such a change.
   B. Traditionally in the dental literature, two terms have been used to describe the therapies employed to remove deposits from tooth surfaces. These terms are *dental prophylaxis* and *scaling and root planing.*
   C. Recently in the dental hygiene literature, increasing numbers of authors are recommending that the term periodontal debridement be used to replace the older terms dental prophylaxis and scaling and root planing. Periodontal debridement is defined as the removal or disruption of bacterial plaque, its byproducts, and plaque-retentive calculus deposits from coronal surfaces, root surfaces, and within the pocket space and tissue wall, as indicated, for periodontal healing and repair.
2. **Insurance Reporting of Periodontal Debridement Codes.** The ADA Current Dental Terminology 2005 has no insurance code designation for "periodontal debridement." So, at this time, insurance forms continue to use the terms prophylaxis and scaling and root planing to designate debridement treatment procedures. *Dental team members will have to use the currently accepted insurance codes when filling out insurance forms and in communications with insurance companies or other third-party payers.*
   A. Examination Codes
      1. **D0120**—Periodic Oral Evaluation. An evaluation performed on a patient of record to determine any changes in the patient's dental and medical health status since a previous comprehensive or periodic evaluation. This includes periodontal screening and may require interpretation of information acquired through additional diagnostic procedures.
      2. **D0180**—Comprehensive Periodontal Evaluation—New or Established Patient. This code is used for patients showing signs or symptoms of periodontal disease and for patients with risk factors such as smoking or diabetes.

Dental Claim Form

05/29/2001, 16:17:35

| 1. [ ] Dentist's pre-treatment estimate [X] Dentist's statement of actual services Provider ID # | 2. [ ] Medicaid Claim [ ] EPSDT Prior Authorization # Patient ID # 873 | 3. **Carrier name and address** Blue Cross and Blue Shield of Maryland State of Md Operations Center P.O. Box 9885 Baltimore MD 21284-9885 |

PATIENT COVERAGE

| 4. Patient name first   m.i.   last | 5. Relationship to employee [X] self [ ] child [ ] spouse [ ] other___ | 6. Sex m f X | 7. Patient birthdate MM DD YYYY | 8. If full time student school city |
| Bill   Bogus | | | | |

| 9. Employee/subscriber name and mailing address Bill Bogus 123 Main St Baltimore MD 12345 | 10. Employee/subscriber soc.sec. or ID number | 11. Employee/subscriber birthdate | 12. Employer (company) name and address | 13. Group number |

INFORMATION

| 14. Is pat. covered by another dental plan? yes   no X If yes, complete 15-a. Is patient covered by a medical plan? yes   no X | 15-a. Name and address of carrier(s) | 15-b. Group no.(s) | 16. Name and address of other employer(s) |

| 17-a. Employee/subscriber name (if different from patient's) | 17-b. Employee/subscriber dental plan I.D. number | 17-c. Employee/subscriber birthdate MM DD YYYY | 18. Relationship to patient [ ] self [ ] child [ ] spouse [ ] other___ |

19. I have reviewed the following treatment plan and fees. I agree to be responsible for all charges for dental services and materials not paid by my dental benefit plan, unless the treating dentist or dental practice has a contractual agreement with my plan prohibiting all or a portion of such charges. To the extent permitted under applicable law, I authorize release of any information relating to this claim.

> Signature on File   5 29 2001
Signed (Patient* -- see reverse)   Date

20. I hereby authorize the payment of the dental benefits otherwise payable to me directly to the below named dental entity.

> Signature on File   5 29 2001
Signed (Employee/subscriber)   Date

BILLING DENTIST

21. Name of Billing Dentist or Dental Entity U Of Md Medical System Dentistry & Maxillofacial Srg	30. Is treatment result of occupational illness or injury? No X Yes If yes, enter brief description and dates
22. Address where payment should be remitted 22 South Green St Rm NGE08	31. Is treatment result of auto accident? X
23. City, State, Zip Baltimore MD 21201	32. Other accident? X
24. Dentist Soc. Sec. or T.I.N. (see reverse**) 52-1362793	25. Dentist license no.	26. Dentist phone no. 410-328-3264	33. If prosthesis, is this initial placement?	(If no, reason for replacement)	34. Date of prior placement
27. First visit date current series	28. Place of treatment Office X Hosp. ECF Other	29. Radiographs or models enclosed? No Yes X How many?	35. Is treatment for orthodontics? X If services already commenced enter:	Date appliances placed	Mos. treatment remaining

FACIAL

RIGHT LINGUAL LEFT

FACIAL

37. Examination and treatment plan -- List in order from tooth no.1 through tooth no.32 -- Using charting system shown

Tooth # or letter	Surface	Description of service (includes x-rays, prophylaxis, materials used, etc.)	Date service performed Mo.	Day	Year	Procedure Number	Fee		For Administrative Use Only
		Int Radgrph Complete	5	29	2001	D0210	0	00	
		Topical Floride Treatment - Ad	5	29	2001	D1205	0	00	
		Prophylaxis - Adult	5	29	2001	D1110	0	00	
		Periodic Examination	5	29	2001	D0120	0	00	

38. Remarks for unusual services

39. I hereby certify that the procedures as indicated by date have been completed and that the fees submitted are the actual fees I have charged and intend to collect for those procedures. Dr. Ryan M Bailey	41. Total Fee Charged 0 00
> Signed (Treating Dentist) License Number 5 29 2001 Date	42. Payment by other plan
40. Address where treatment was performed 22 S. Greene Street City State Zip	Max. allowable
	Deductible
	Carrier %
	Carrier pays
	Patient pays

Figure 26-1. Dental Insurance Claim Form. An example of a dental insurance claim form.

B. Currently Accepted Insurance Codes Pertaining to Periodontal Instrumentation
   1. **D1110**—adult prophylaxis (four quadrants). A dental prophylaxis includes scaling and polishing procedures to remove coronal plaque, calculus, and stains. *This code is usually used for healthy patients and patients with gingivitis.* Scaling on this type of patient usually can be completed in a single appointment.
   2. **D4341**—Periodontal Scaling and Root Planing—Four or More Teeth Per Quadrant. This procedure involves instrumentation of the crown and root surfaces to remove plaque and calculus from these surfaces. *It is indicated for patients with periodontal disease and is therapeutic, not preventive in nature.* This procedure may be used as a definitive treatment in some stages of periodontal disease and/or as a part of presurgical procedures in others.
   3. **D4342**—Periodontal Scaling and Root Planing—One to three teeth per Quadrant. This code is essentially the same as the D4341 code, the difference being the number of teeth present in a quadrant.
   4. **D4910**—Periodontal Maintenance. *This procedure is instituted following periodontal therapy and continues at varying intervals for the life of the dentition or implant replacements.* It includes the removal of the bacterial plaque and calculus from supragingival and subgingival regions, site specific scaling and root planing where indicated, and polishing of the teeth.
   5. **D4381**—Localized Delivery of Antimicrobial Agents via a Controlled Release Vehicle. Synthetic fibers or other approved delivery devices containing controlled-release chemotherapeutic agents are inserted into a periodontal pocket.
C. Codes for Radiographs. The most common dental radiographs are:
   1. **D0210**—a complete intraoral radiographic series including bitewings
   2. **D0220**—an intraoral periapical (first film)
   3. **D0230**—an intraoral periapical film (each additional film)
   4. **D0240**—an intraoral occlusal film
   5. **D0250**—an extraoral first film, such as a cephalometric film
   6. **D0260**—an extraoral film (each additional film)
   7. **D0270**—a single bitewing film
   8. **D0272**—two bitewing films
   9. **D0274**—four bitewing films
   10. **D0330**—a panoramic film
   11. **D0277**—vertical bitewings: 7 to 8 films
   12. **D0350**—oral/facial images. The oral/facial image code includes traditional photographs or digital images obtained by intraoral cameras.
D. Codes for Topical Fluoride
   1. **D1204**—topical fluoride treatment–adult (prophylaxis not included)
   2. **D1205**—topical fluoride treatment–adult (including prophylaxis). This code is used to report combined procedures of a prophylaxis and fluoride treatment.
E. Counseling
   1. **D1310**—nutritional counseling for control of dental disease. Counseling on food selection and dietary habits as a part of treatment and control of periodontal disease and caries.
   2. **D1320**—tobacco cessation counseling for control and prevention of oral disease.
   3. **D1330**—oral hygiene (self-care) instructions. Examples include tooth brushing technique, flossing, and the use of special oral hygiene aids.

CHAPTER SUMMARY STATEMENT

In judging whether a professional has been negligent, the courts use a standard called the *reasonable prudent person or professional.* Thus, providing and documenting periodontal care that meets or exceeds the standard of care is extremely important for dental hygienists.

The dental chart is a legal document. All periodontal assessment, educational, and treatment services should be documented in the patient chart or computerized record. When a patient decides to file a lawsuit, the dental chart becomes the single most important piece of information relative to the suit.

Insurance coding was developed to speed and simplify the reporting of dental treatments to third parties such as insurance companies and the government. These codes are very specific and should be reviewed carefully before specific dental treatment is coded.

SECTION 5: FOCUS ON PATIENTS

CASE 1
During a social gathering one evening, a dental hygienist tells her friend about human immunodeficiency virus (HIV)-positive patient she had treated that day. As the news traveled down the grapevine and the patient learned that the hygienist had revealed his HIV status, he sued her. What specific charge could he bring against the hygienist? Would she be covered under the dentist/employer's malpractice coverage or her own personal malpractice coverage?

CASE 2
The dental hygienist performed an oral cancer screening on every patient, but she never wrote it in her progress notes. When a patient found out he had oral cancer, he sued his dentist and the dental hygienist. The patient had been seen for a prophylaxis and restorative care 6 months before his diagnosis of oral cancer, and the basis for his suit was that he felt the hygienist and dentist had been negligent in failing to detect the lesion. How could this suit have been avoided?

CASE 3
During the informed consent process, the patient is informed of (i) his diagnosis; (ii) purpose, description, benefits, and risks of the proposed treatment; (iii) alternative treatment options; (iv) prognosis of no treatment, and (v) costs. The patient asks questions and demonstrates that he understands all information presented during the discussion. Then the patient refuses any treatment. What, if anything, should the dental hygienist do?

SUGGESTED READINGS

Baxter C. A review of dental negligence. *Woman Dentist J.*, September, 2004.

Montero D, Buffa D, Kranes M. Late night hospital drama keeps tragic Bronx boy on life support. *New York Times* [online edition] April 23, 2005.

O'Hagan M. Appeals Court rules against dentist. *Seattle Times* June 16, 2005.

Schofield JC, Gutmann ME, DeWald JP, Campbell PR. Disciplinary actions associated with the administration of local anesthetics against dentists and dental hygienists. *J Denl Hyg., 2005;*9:8.

Tonner J. *Malpractice: What They Don't Teach You in Dental School.* Tulsa, OK: PennWell Publishing, 1996.

Tonner J. Are your dental charts working against you? *DentalTown Magazine.* November 2003.

Walker P. *Dentistry and North Carolina Law* (self-published). PO Box 16157, Chapel Hill, NC, 27516; 2005.

Wilder R. Understanding your legal liability. *Dimens Dent Hyg.* February 2005.

SECTION 6: CHAPTER REVIEW QUESTIONS

1. Which of these terms is defined as the health care provider's obligation to provide services to another person?
   A. Liability
   B. Tort
   C. Intentional tort
   D. Negligence

2. Which term is defined as the failure to do something that a reasonable person would do under the same circumstances?
   A. Liability
   B. Tort
   C. Intentional tort
   D. Negligence

3. Yelling at a child in a loud voice is an example of:
   A. Liability
   B. Tort
   C. Intentional tort
   D. Negligence

4. A dental chart or computerized record is considered a legal document.
   A. True
   B. False

5. Patient comments should **NOT** be documented in a chart or computerized record.
   A. True
   B. False

6. Three days after treating a patient, the hygienist realizes that she forgot to document a treatment procedure in a patient's chart. Since hers was last entry in the chart, it is acceptable for her to just add the procedure to her previous entry. No one will ever know that she added this information 3 days later.
   A. True
   B. False

7. If an error is made, the hygienist should erase the error or cover it with correction fluid.
   A. True
   B. False

8. The hygienist just completed periodontal instrumentation on a new patient with chronic periodontitis. Which of the ADA insurance codes should he or she enter on the insurance form?
   A. D1110—adult prophylaxis
   B. D4341—periodontal scaling and root planing
   C. D4910—periodontal maintenance procedures

9. Which code would be entered on an insurance form for periodontal instrumentation completed during a 3-month periodontal maintenance appointment?
   A. D1110—adult prophylaxis
   B. D4341—periodontal scaling and root planing
   C. D4910—periodontal maintenance procedures

Chapter

27 Future Directions for Management of Periodontal Patients

Learning Objective

■ Discuss ways in which the management of periodontal patients may evolve in the future.

KEY TERMS

Digital radiographic techniques
Computed tomographic techniques
Host modulation therapies

There are not many absolutes in periodontics, but there is undoubtedly one–the simple fact that management of periodontal patients will continue to evolve and change over time.

- Periodontal journals are filled with new and exciting ideas, and these ideas can give us some small insight into what the future of periodontics may hold for both clinicians and patients.
- Dental hygienists should expect many changes to take place in recommendations for successful management of patients with periodontal diseases as we continue to study these diseases.
- This chapter offers an overview of a few of the possibilities for directions in the management of periodontal patients by dental hygienists.

SECTION 1: DIAGNOSTIC TECHNOLOGY FOR PERIODONTAL DISEASES

PROBING DEPTHS AND ATTACHMENT LEVELS

1. The diagnosis and monitoring of patients with periodontal diseases has been based on traditional clinical assessment methods for many years. One of these traditional clinical assessments is the use of manual periodontal probes to measure probing depths and attachment levels.
2. Probing depths can generally be recorded rapidly, and probing depths provide a reasonable assessment of periodontal problems in a patient's dentition.
3. On the other hand, attachment levels are much more difficult to measure and record, yet they provide a more accurate assessment of the precise amount of damage to the periodontium than the probing depths.
4. Computer-linked controlled-force electronic periodontal probes are already available to clinicians.
   A. These computer-linked probes can make it possible to measure both probing depths and attachment levels quickly with automatic data entry features.
   B. At present, most of these computer-linked periodontal probes have a tendency to underestimate measurements of probing depths and attachment levels in patients with subgingival calculus deposits.
   C. This technology of computer-linked periodontal probes will improve. As this technology improves, the use of these computer-linked probes in dental offices will undoubtedly become widespread, making it much easier to record attachment levels.
   D. Since the dental hygienist spends a good deal of time collecting information about patients' periodontal status, improvements in this technology will impact the practice of dental hygiene.

DIGITAL RADIOGRAPHS

1. Another traditional clinical assessment has been the study of dental radiographs. Advances in diagnostic technology also include advances in radiograph techniques.
2. **Digital (filmless) radiographic techniques** have been developed to the stage where they are already being used by many clinicians.
   A. Digital radiographic techniques allow members of the dental team to collect radiographic information using special sensors instead of printing the information on a film.

B. These digital images are then stored on a computer and can be viewed on a computer screen or even printed when needed.

C. Modern technology for viewing these images on computer screens has substantial advantages over the traditional use of radiographic film.

D. Software for viewing these digitized images can eliminate distortion as is seen with traditional film, can allow for easy magnification of details, and can provide precise measurements.

E. The same software can also allow for enhancing aspects of a digitized image, providing members of the dental team with more details of the actual status of a tooth or of the periodontium.

F. These digital images can also be shared with other health care providers quite readily—as might be indicated during a referral or during a consultation with a specialist.

COMPUTED TOMOGRAPHIC TECHNIQUES

1. Another interesting area of technology related to radiographic techniques is the use of **computed tomographic techniques**. Computed tomographic techniques can provide clinicians with the ability to study minute details and precise dimensions of the jaws on a computer screen in a three-dimensional mode.

A. These details can be so precise that they can include a three-dimensional radiographic image of a slice made through the jaws at any specific location.

B. Computed tomographic techniques are currently in use by many clinicians in the planning for the placement of dental implants.

C. As these computed tomographic techniques become more accessible to the general dentist, treatment planning for many conditions, including periodontal diseases, will improve.

2. Digital radiographic techniques and computed tomographic techniques are only two examples of enhanced diagnostic technology in the area of radiography. As this radiographic imaging technology improves, the improvements will undoubtedly come into widespread use by members of the dental team. This enhanced radiographic technology will provide a greater ease in assessing clinical parameters such as measuring alveolar bone loss or documenting healing of a site affected by periodontitis following thorough therapy by the dental hygienist or the dentist.

SECTION 2: THE PERIODONTAL DISEASE/SYSTEMIC DISEASE CONNECTION

Dental and medical researchers have been interested in study of the connection between periodontitis and certain systemic diseases for some time. Research into this critical topic is ongoing and continues to offer insights into this connection.

SYSTEMIC DISEASES WITH A CONNECTION TO PERIODONTAL DISEASE

Some examples of systemic diseases or conditions that have a connection to periodontitis are listed below. Review of the dental literature will reveal many studies about how these systemic conditions are related to periodontal diseases, but all of these areas require further scientific study.
- Smoking
- Diabetes mellitus
- Osteoporosis
- Lung abscesses
- Bacterial endocarditis
- Low birth weights for newborns

DIABETES MELLITUS

1. One specific example of an important periodontitis/systemic disease connection is the disease diabetes mellitus.
   A. It is clear that additional research into this connection may indeed impact the practice of dental hygiene.
   B. Research has clearly demonstrated that patients with poorly controlled diabetes have an increased risk for periodontitis.
   C. Since periodontitis is a type of infection, and since diabetes can lower the body's resistance to infections in general, it is not surprising that there is a connection between poorly controlled diabetes and periodontitis in some patients.
   D. In addition, research suggests that periodontal infection (and periodontal therapy) have the potential for altering the body's control of blood sugar levels.
   E. It has even been suggested that thorough treatment of periodontitis in a diabetic patient may make it easier for the patient's physician to control the diabetes.
2. There are many, many research questions that need to be answered related to this periodontitis/diabetes connection, but a few of those questions that can have a direct impact on the practice of dental hygiene are outlined below.
   A. Are the measures used to prevent or control periodontitis in the patient without diabetes adequate for the patient with diabetes mellitus?
   B. Since wound healing appears altered in patients with diabetes, are there adjustments clinicians need to make in dental hygiene therapy to maximize the potential for healing in these patients?
   C. What precise periodontal maintenance protocols are the most effective for patients with diabetes?
   D. When the dental hygienist treats a patient with diabetes, what communication protocols can be most effective in insuring that the patient's physician is aware of the patient's periodontal status so that adjustments in the therapy for diabetes can be made where needed?

3. In examining the periodontitis/diabetes connection there is another line of inquiry that will affect dental hygiene practice also.

   A. In medicine there have been dramatic improvements in the treatment regimens for patients with diabetes, and these regimens now frequently include intensive treatment with oral agents and with insulin.

   B. Unfortunately, some of these medical treatments have increased the risk for medical emergencies (such as hypoglycemia) during dental office treatment in the patient with diabetes.

   C. This medical trend in intensive therapies for patients with diabetes will continue.

   D. As more intensive therapies are used by physicians to manage patients with diabetes, the dental hygienist of the future will need to have more knowledge about these therapies, about how to manage these patients in a dental setting, and about how to respond when a medical emergency arises.

SECTION 3: PROTOCOLS FOR MAINTAINING DENTAL IMPLANTS

1. For dental patients today, dental implants are a viable option as one alternative for replacing most missing teeth, and dental implants available today have a remarkable success rate. Even though dental implantology has been intensively studied for several decades, there are still many unanswered questions related to this field, and research will continue.

2. Much additional investigation is needed in the area of dental implantology, but some examples of questions related to dental implantology and dental hygiene that are in need of further study are listed below.

   A. What self-care measures can best prevent peri-implant infections?

   B. What are the best protocols for effective maintenance of implants?

   C. Should we use the same techniques for minimizing the bacterial challenge to an implant that we apply to a natural tooth?

3. Answering these questions with appropriate scientific investigation is quite likely to have a substantial impact on clinical care delivered by the dental hygienist.

SECTION 4: THE USE OF LASERS IN PERIODONTAL CARE

1. Lasers have been widely used in many fields of medicine since the early 1960s. Lasers produce a narrow beam of light with a single wavelength that can produce intense energy.
   A. In dentistry these intense light beams can be passed down narrow tubing and can be focused on a small area of tissue within the mouth.
   B. Some laser beams are so intense that they can actually be used to remove oral soft tissue or to cut tissues in the mouth.
   C. There are different types of lasers that have been studied for use in dentistry, and each type has a different effect on enamel, dentin, pulp, and bone.
2. Lasers have been suggested for use in dentistry for a variety of applications, and some of these devices even have Food and Drug Administration (FDA) safety clearance for some intraoral soft tissue removal procedures.
   A. However, there is more study needed to clarify how these devices can be used appropriately in subgingival applications.
   B. Some preliminary investigations have suggested a possible use for these devices as part of periodontal therapies such as root debridement.
   C. Investigations into these issues are ongoing.
3. The routine use of lasers in treating patients with chronic periodontitis does not appear to be supported by the scientific studies available at this time.
   A. Additional research will clarify appropriate uses for these devices in periodontal patients and may impact some of the therapy provided for patients with periodontitis.
   B. If further study of these devices shows that periodontal patients can benefit from their use, they may one day be a routine part of the care of patients with periodontitis and perhaps even a part of the practice of dental hygiene.

SECTION 5: THE USE OF GENETIC TECHNOLOGY IN PERIODONTAL CARE

1. Clinicians have known for a long time that there are many factors that can increase the risk of developing periodontitis in their patients.
   A. One factor that is known to increase the risk of developing periodontitis is failure to control bacterial plaque growth on the teeth, thereby increasing the bacterial challenge to the periodontium.
   B. Scientific studies also seem to indicate that certain genetic factors determine how an individual patient's host defenses actually react to an increased bacterial challenge.
   C. Based upon the current research literature available, it now appears that a key factor in determining whether a patient actually develops periodontitis in response to the bacterial challenge appears to be how the body reacts to the bacterial challenge.
   D. One major determinant of how the body reacts to the bacterial challenge is genetics (or inherited characteristics).
2. Much more study into the genetic factors that increase the risk for periodontitis is needed, but it is already possible to use some types of genetic information to guide clinical decision-making in a small group of selected patients.
   A. Genetic testing can identify patients carrying gene mutations for several rare syndromes that are often accompanied by a form of periodontal disease.

    B. In addition to identifying patients with rare syndromes, there is already a commercially available genetic susceptibility test for severe chronic periodontitis.

    C. In this test specific gene polymorphisms (forms) that have been associated with the development of periodontitis can be detected.

    D. Ongoing scientific investigations will undoubtedly clarify how such genetic testing can be used in periodontitis patient management.

3. As more and more scientific information about identifying genetic control of host defenses becomes available, it is quite likely that this information can impact how we manage patients with periodontal diseases and impact the practice of dental hygiene.

SECTION 6: LOCAL DELIVERY MECHANISMS IN PERIODONTAL CARE

1. Research has demonstrated that using local delivery mechanisms for antimicrobial chemicals in periodontal patients has a small but measurable impact upon clinical parameters such as attachment levels. This topic has been already been discussed in other chapters of this book.

2. There are several areas of research investigation that are needed related to these local delivery mechanisms:

    A. Can local delivery mechanisms be designed that have a greater clinical impact than those currently available for clinical use?

    B. What specific treatment protocols should be followed to produce the most benefit for individual patients?

    C. Are there additional antimicrobial agents that can be delivered safely using the local delivery concept?

    D. Can other therapy provided by the dental hygienist be enhanced by using some of these local delivery mechanisms?

3. Research into the use of local delivery mechanisms for antimicrobial agents continues. It is entirely possible that as this modality improves in clinical effectiveness, using local delivery mechanisms may become more and more useful in the care of the periodontal patient by the dental hygienist.

SECTION 7: HOST DEFENSES IN PERIODONTAL PATIENTS

1. As already discussed in this book, research has demonstrated that host defenses can play a significant role in the actual development of attachment loss and alveolar bone loss in periodontitis patients.
   A. A variety of **host modulation therapies** have been investigated that might be used as adjunctive (supplemental) treatment in periodontitis patients.
   B. Host modulation therapies usually involve using medications that can alter biochemical pathways in a manner that will (i) slow attachment loss, (ii) slow alveolar bone loss, or (iii) decrease inflammation in periodontal patients.
2. As discussed in Chapter 22, investigations into possible host modulation therapies have already resulted in one commercially available medication that can be used as adjunctive treatment in patients with chronic periodontitis.
   A. This medication is a low dose of doxycycline that can be used to lower levels of collagenase, an enzyme involved in the destruction of collagen.
   B. Collagen is one of the components of many of the structures that make up the periodontium, and lowering the levels of collagenase can slow the progress of periodontitis.
   C. Investigations are ongoing into a number of other possible host modulation therapies that include studies into (i) modulation of cytokines (chemicals involved in periodontitis that can result in increased periodontal disease progression), (ii) reduction of prostaglandins (chemicals that enhance inflammation in the gingiva and in the periodontium), and (iii) slowing alveolar bone loss with chemical agents called bisphosphonates.
3. As further scientific investigations improve our understanding of host modulation therapies in the management of periodontitis patients, there are likely to be a variety of therapeutic options for members of the dental team to use in patient management.

SECTION 8: PERIODONTAL DISEASE RISK ASSESSMENT

1. Recently there has been increased interest in identifying clinical tools that can be used to quantify a patient's risk for developing periodontitis.
   A. Traditionally clinicians have assessed the risk of developing periodontitis subjectively, but studies have shown that subjective risk assessment is variable even among clinicians who are experts.
   B. Periodontal disease risk assessment tools would be quite useful to members of the dental team if they provided an objective method of risk assessment that could accurately predict which patients are most likely to develop periodontitis.
   C. Using these tools to identify the patients with the highest risk for developing periodontitis would allow members of the dental team to provide more aggressive treatment for those patients.
   D. In addition, these tools might identify which patients should be referred to a specialist early in their treatment and which patients might not need such early and aggressive referrals.
2. Studies have already been published that document that some of these risk assessment tools are predictors of loss of alveolar bone loss and loss of periodontally affected teeth. It is likely that some of these tools for quantifying a patient's risk will be in more widespread use in dental offices in the near future. These risk assessment tools would be useful to the dental hygienist and the dentist in planning therapy or preventive measures for patients and in identifying patients in need of immediate referral.

CHAPTER SUMMARY STATEMENT

Dental hygienists should expect many changes to take place in recommendations for successful management of patients with periodontal diseases as we continue to study these diseases. This chapter presented a brief overview of a few of the possibilities for directions in the management of periodontal patients by dental hygienists.

SUGGESTED READINGS

American Academy of Periodontology. Consensus report. Discussion section I, *Proceedings of the World Workshop in Clinical Periodontics*. Chicago: American Academy of Periodontology; 1989:I-23–I-32.

Armitage GC. Clinical evaluation of periodontal diseases. *Periodontol 2000.* 1995;7:39–53.

Armitage GC. Development of a classification system for periodontal diseases and conditions. *Ann Periodontol.* 1999;4:1–6.

Barnett ML, Press KP, Friedman D, et al. The prevalence of periodontitis and dental caries in a Down's syndrome population. *J Periodonto.l* 1986;57:288–293.

Becker W, Becker B, Newman M, et al. Clinical and microbiologic findings that may contribute to dental implant failure, *Int J Oral Maxillofac Implants.* 1990;5:31–38.

Benn DK. A review of the reliability of radiographic measurements in estimating alveolar bone changes. *J Clin Periodontol.* 1990;17:14–21.

Cobb CM. Lasers in periodontics: A review of the literature. *J Periodontol.* 2006;77:545–564.

Eickholz P, Kim TS, Benn DK, et al. Validity of radiographic measurement of interproximal bone loss, *Oral Surg Oral Med Oral Pathol Oral Radiol Endod.* 1998;85:99–106.

Eickholz P, Hausmann E. Accuracy of radiographic assessment of interproximal bone loss in intrabony defects using linear measurements. *Eur J Oral Sci.* 2000;108:70–73.

Golub LM, Lee H-M, Ryan ME. Tetracyclines inhibit connective tissue breakdown by multiple non-antimicrobial mechanisms. *Adv Dent Res.* 1998;12:12–26.

Goodson JM. Clinical measurements of periodontitis. *J Clin Periodontol.* 1986;13:446–455.

Goodson JM, Haffajee AD, Socransky SS. The relationship between attachment level loss and alveolar bone loss. *J Clin Periodontol.* 1984;11:348–359.

Hausmann E. A contemporary perspective on techniques for the clinical assessment of alveolar bone. *J Periodontol.* 1990;61:149–156.

Jeffcoat MK. Osteoporosis: A possible modifying factor in oral bone loss. *Ann Periodontol.* 1998;3:312–321.

Jeffcoat MK, Reddy MS. Digital subtraction radiography for longitudinal assessment of peri-implant bone change: Method and validation. *Adv Dent Res.* 1993;7:196–201.

Jeffcoat MK, Wang IC, Reddy MS. Radiographic diagnosis in periodontics. *Periodontol 2000.* 1995;7:54–68.

Kircos LT, Misch CE. Diagnostic and imaging techniques. In Misch CE, ed. *Contemporary Implant Dentistry.* St. Louis:Mosby; 1999:73–87.

Lindhe J, Ranney R, Lamster I, et al. Consensus report: chronic periodontitis. *Ann Periodontol.* 1999;4:38.

Loe H. Periodontal disease. The sixth complication of diabetes mellitus, *Diabetes Care.* 1993;16(Suppl 1):329–334.

Mealey BL. Diabetes mellitus. In Rose LF, Genco RJ, Mealey BL, Cohen DW, eds. *Periodontal Medicine*, Toronto:BC Decker Publishers; 2000:121–151.

Mealey BL. Periodontal implications: Medically compromised patients. *Ann Periodontol.*1996;1:256–321.

Minsk L, Polson AM, Weisgold A et al. Outcome failures of endosseous implants from a clinical training center. *Compend Contin Educ Dent.* 1996;17:848–859.

Mullally BH, Linden GJ. Comparative reproducibility of proximal probing depth using electronic pressure-controlled and hand probing. *J Clin Periodontol.* 1994;21:284–288.

Offenbacher S. Periodontal diseases: Pathogenesis. *Ann Periodontol.* 1996;1:821–878.

Page RC, Martin J, Krall EA, et al. Longitudinal validation of a risk calculator for periodontal disease. *J Clin Periodontol.* 2003;30:819–827.

Persson GR, Mancl LA, Martin J, et al. Assessing periodontal disease risk. *J Am Dent Assoc.* 2003;134:575–582.

Rees TD, Biggs NL, Collings CK. Radiographic interpretation of periodontal osseous lesions. *Oral Surg Oral Med Oral Pathol.* 1971;32:141–153.

Ritchey TR, Orban BJ. Three-dimensional roentgenographic interpretation in periodontal diagnosis. *J Periodontol.* 1960;31:275–282.

Rosenfeld AL, Mecall RA. Using computerized tomography to develop realistic treatment objectives for the implant team. In Nevins M, Mellonig JT, Fiorellini JP, eds. *ImplantTherapy: Clinical Approaches and Evidence of Success.* Chicago: Quintessence.; 1998.

Smith RA, Berger R, Dodson TB. Risk factors associated with dental implants in healthy and medically compromised patients. *Int J Oral Maxillofac Implants.* 1992;7:367–372.

Taylor GW. Bidirectional interrelationships between diabetes and periodontal diseases: An epidemiological perspective. *Ann Periodontol.* 2001;6:99–112.

Tupta-Veselicky L, Famili P, Ceravolo FJ, et al. A clinical study of an electronic constant force periodontal probe. *J Periodontol.* 1994;65:616–622.

Wang S-F, Leknes KN, Zimmerman GJ, et al. Reproducibility of periodontal probing using a conventional manual and automated force-controlled electronic probe. *J Periodontol.* 1995;66:38–46.

28 Periodontal Resources in Dental Literature and on the Internet

SECTION 1	GUIDELINES FOR READING DENTAL LITERATURE
	Selecting and Reading a Research Study
	Definitions Relevant to Dental Literature
SECTION 2	PROCEDURE FOR SEARCHING THE INTERNET
SECTION 3	PERIODONTAL RESOURCES ON THE INTERNET
	General Suggestions for Using the Internet

Learning Objectives

- Demonstrate the ability to gather relevant information from the Internet.
- Given a topic in periodontics, research it in the dental literature using both print and online resources.

KEY TERMS

MEDLINE
PubMed
LONESOME DOC

SECTION 1: GUIDELINES FOR READING DENTAL LITERATURE

For a dental health care professional, keeping current on the standards of health care delivery, disease prevention, and treatment is a requirement. The practicing dental hygienist should stay current with the latest standards of treatment and techniques. One of the best methods for staying current is to read the dental literature either in the form of printed journals or electronically, using Internet services such as MEDLINE.

MEDLINE is the English-language database for biomedical information. MEDLINE can be accessed free of charge through several gateways. One example is **PubMed**, a gateway hosted by the National Library of Medicine (NLM) at **http://www.nlm.nih.gov** By using **LONESOME DOC**, the dental hygienist can have a printed version of any journal article listed on MEDLINE mailed or faxed to the dental office for a small fee.

SELECTING AND READING A RESEARCH STUDY

One of the most useful types of journal articles is the primary research study. This Chapter contains a summary of the typical format of a research study; terminology used in dental literature, and suggested questions for critiquing a primary research study (Box 28-1).

1. **Sources.** As discussed in Chapter 15, there are many sources of information, however, these sources can vary greatly in the quality and reliability of information presented. Time is limited and no one individual can read everything that is published in the field of dental hygiene. It is of primary importance for the dental hygienist to be able to locate the best sources of information.
   A. Scientific Journals
      1. Often published by a professional group (American Dental Hygienists' Association or American Academy of Periodontology) or scientific publishers.
      2. Peer-reviewed by a panel of experts who review research articles for study design, statistics, and conclusions.
      3. Supported with references.
      4. The best source for randomized clinical trials and learning about new research findings.
   B. Practice or Trade Magazines
      1. Can be commercial in nature. Some magazines may look like journals, but in reality are produced by a company as advertisements for its products.
      2. May or may not be peer-reviewed.
      3. May or may not be supported with references.
      4. Can vary widely in quality. Some magazines are appropriate sources of information for the general public but not as a source of evidence-based information needed by a dental healthcare professional.
2. **Format of a Research Study**
   A. Title. The title indicates the topic of the research study.
   B. Abstract
      1. Located at the beginning of the article and containing a brief description of the article.
      2. Includes a summary of the (i) focus of the study, (ii) experimental strategy, and (iii) findings.
      3. Reading the abstract can be a good means of selecting an article of interest.
      4. It is important for the reader to be aware that the abstract does not always present the study or its results in an accurate manner. The reader must study the entire article and draw his or her own conclusions about the study and its relevance to dental hygiene practice.

Box 28-1

Suggested Questions for Critiquing a Primary Research Study

Title, Authors, Funding

1. What is the title of the article? Who published the article? What is the date of the publication?
2. Is the journal peer-reviewed?
3. What are the authors' qualifications?
4. What are the funding sources for the research? Did a company with economic interests in the outcome of this study provide funding?

Abstract

1. Does the abstract contain the necessary elements (purpose, sample, methods, results, and conclusion)? What necessary elements, if any, are missing from the abstract?

Question/Purpose/Hypothesis

1. What research question is being asked?
2. How are the variables described? What is the dependent and independent variable? Are there extraneous variables?
3. Does the question (topic) apply to your patients?

Research Methods

1. What type of study is this (*in vivo* or *in vitro*)?
2. What population was sampled? How were subjects selected and was the sample selection appropriate? How many groups were studied and compared (control group, experimental group)?
3. Was the assignment of patients to treatment randomized? Were patients, examiners, and therapists blinded to treatment?
4. What research question was asked (was the right question asked)? What are the outcomes being measured and are they appropriate?
5. Briefly describe the research methods. Were scorers/examiners calibrated for reliability?
6. How long was the research study? Was the study long enough for the outcome to become apparent?

Results

1. What data analysis method was used?
2. Were tables, graphs, or charts clear (helpful)?
3. Were the results clearly explained in terms of the original research question? Were the findings currently relevant or obsolete (out of date)?

Discussion

1. Were the results clearly interpreted? Does the author fully explain any flaws in the study design and their effect upon the results?
2. Briefly summarize the results and interpretations *as presented by the author(s)*.
3. Explain the results, as *you* would interpret them. Compare your explanation of the results with those of the author(s).
4. Do the results conflict or substantiate (agree with) the results from other studies on the same subject? If the results are different, how do they differ?

Conclusion

1. Briefly state the author(s) conclusions.
2. Are the conclusions appropriate? Is there an evidence-base to support the authors' interpretation and recommendations? Does the conclusion fall in line with the results?
3. Compare your thoughts about the study's importance with those of the author(s). Do you agree with the authors' conclusions?
4. Can you apply the finding to patient treatment? If yes, explain how.

    C. Introduction
1. Presents a background of past research on the topic (a literature review).
2. Provides an introduction to the study and defines the purpose and major questions to be addressed in the study.

    D. Methods. This section provides information about how the research was conducted including the:
1. Population studied (animal or human subjects)
2. Design (parallel, cross-over, split-mouth)
3. Number of subjects studied (did the study involve 2 subjects or 200?)
4. Length of time the study was conducted (did the study last 2 weeks or 5 years?)
5. Techniques used to gather information in the study
6. Outcomes measured

    E. Results. This section presents a statistical analysis and the findings of the research study. This section should present the findings in an objective manner without interpreting them.

    F. Discussion. This section contains the author's interpretation and explanation of the results of the research study. This section often includes a description of the strengths and weaknesses of the study as well as suggestions for future research.

    G. Conclusion. In this section, the author summarizes the importance of the research findings.

    H. References
1. References should be current (most of the references should have been published within the past 5 years).
2. References provide an opportunity for the dental hygienist to read additional articles to learn more about the topic.

DEFINITIONS RELEVANT TO DENTAL LITERATURE

1. A randomized clinical trial is a study in which a group of subjects that is receiving an experimental treatment is compared to a control group that is receiving a placebo or an alternative treatment.

2. Randomization is the unbiased assignment of subjects or objects in a research study to a control or experimental group on a random basis.

3. Blinding is the assignment of a subject to a study group without the subject and/or the investigator knowing the assignment. For example, Mr. Jones is a subject in an investigation of a new blood pressure medication. Half the subjects will receive the blood pressure medication and the other half will receive a placebo, but the investigator will not know whether Mr. Jones is receiving the placebo or the blood pressure medication.

4. Control groups consist of subjects who did not receive the active treatment. They may have received a placebo, alternate therapy, or no therapy at all.

5. A placebo is an inactive or harmless substance, such as distilled water or sugar, used in experimental clinical trials to compare the effects of the inactive substance with those of the experimental drug or treatment.

6. Validity is the degree to which a measurement is appropriate for the question being addressed or that it measures what it is intended to measure. The measure used must be appropriate for the question being answered. The measure must have been shown to be accurate in measuring the observed outcome.

7. Reliability is the extent to which a test measurement or device produces the same results with different investigators, observers, or administration of the test over time. If several tests produce the same result, the measurement is considered reliable. Reliability is demonstrated by well-trained, calibrated examiners that can produce consistent results on the same person using the same instrument.

8. Statistical significance tells whether the observed outcome from one therapy is statistically different from a comparative therapy. Statistical significance may also tell if the observed outcome of one therapy is statistically different from observations at baseline of the same therapy.

9. Clinical relevance tells whether the finding is important enough to affect a treatment decision (to cause the clinician to incorporate it in a patient's treatment). The Results section describes the findings from a statistical perspective. Very small changes are often statistically significant, but this does not necessarily mean that the treatment being investigated is *superior* to another treatment.

10. *In vivo* research is conducted on a living organism.

11. *In vitro* research is not conducted on a living organism.

SECTION 2: PROCEDURE FOR SEARCHING THE INTERNET

Table 28-1. Procedure for Searching the Internet

Equipment: Computer with Web browser software, a modem to connect to the Internet, and an active Internet connection

Steps	Purpose
1. Connect the computer to the Internet and open your Internet browser. Some of the most popular browsers are Internet Explorer, Safari, and Netscape.	An Internet connection is necessary to search the Internet. An Internet browser is a software program used for searching and viewing various kinds of Internet resources such as information on a Website.
2. Locate a search engine. Most browsers have a built-in search engine. Popular search engines include Google, Lycos, AltaVista, Yahoo, and Excite.	Search engines help you sift through all those pages to find the information that you need.
3. Look at the search engine's Web page. Near the top of the page you will see a white box with the word SEARCH next to it. Click the search box and type a word or phrase that describes what you are looking for. Next, (i) press the GO button next to the search box on the Web pages or (ii) hit the Return key on your keyboard. The words that you type in the search box are called "key words." For best results, it is important to choose the key words carefully. Use one to three words that are as specific as possible.	Key words tell the search engine what to look for.
4. View the results of your search. If you did not find what you are looking for, check your spelling and retype or choose new key words and try the search again.	If the key words are misspelled or not specific enough, the search engine will not find the information that you are looking for.
5. From the search results page, select an appropriate site and double click the address written in blue to open the Website.	This allows you to view the information on the Website.
6. If the Website information is helpful; either download the information or bookmark the page. If you need additional information, return to the results page or conduct another search.	Downloading the information or bookmarking the Website gives you access to it in the future.
7. Try to complete the search process within 10 or 15 minutes.	The ability to search the Internet effectively is a vital information-accessing tool for dental health care providers.

From Nield-Gehrig JS. *Patient Assessment Tutorials A Step-by-Step Guide for the Dental Hygienist*, Lippincott Williams & Wilkins, 2006.

SECTION 3: PERIODONTAL RESOURCES ON THE INTERNET

GENERAL SUGGESTIONS FOR USING THE INTERNET

1. Be careful to type the Website address exactly as written.
   A. Most Website addresses will begin with "http://www" but there are some exceptions. Some addresses may not include "www" and others may include "www1" in the address.
   B. Some addresses end in "html" and others in "htm." It makes all the difference in the world if you type "http:// www.umn.edu/perio/tobacco/tobhome.html" instead of "http://www1.umn.edu/perio/tobacco/ tobhome.html."
2. The Website addresses listed here were current at the time of publication.
   A. Website addresses change frequently, however, since the Internet is such a dynamic resource.
   B. If the listed Website address is no longer valid, try using an Internet search engine (such as Excite, Lycos, or LookSmart) to locate the new Website for the organization. Simply type the organization's name (such as "American Medical Association") into the search box and click on search. The search engine will find the new Website address for you.

SEARCH ENGINES FOR JOURNAL ARTICLES

- MEDLINE (PubMed) Literature Search Facility
  http://www.ncbi.nlm.nih.gov/pubmed
  Provides free access to more than 11 million MEDLINE journal citations dating back to the mid-1960s.
- NHS Centre for Reviews
  http://www.york.ac.uk/inst/crd/darehp.htm
  To access online abstracts, click on "Search DARE."

EVIDENCE-BASED DENTISTRY/MEDICINE— ELECTRONIC SEARCHING

- Centre for Evidence-Based Dentistry
  http://www.cebd.org
  Resources include evidence-based tools, evidence-based dentistry journal, and evidence-based links.
- Centre for Evidence-Based Medicine
  http://www.cebm.utoronto.ca
  Provides information that can be used to learn about and develop resources that can be used to practice and teach evidence-based medicine.

LINKS TO PERIODONTAL JOURNALS

- *Journal of Periodontology*
  http://www.perio.org/journal/journal.html
  Use search engine to search the journal archives. Free abstracts are available online. Full-text articles are available by subscription only.

- Blackwell Synergy Dental Journals
  **http://www.blackwell-synergy.com/servlet/useragent?func=showHome&type
  =journals&action=0&open=427#C427**
  Free online abstracts and full-text articles for selected journal issues for the following
  journals:
  Journal of Periodontal Research
  Oral Microbiology and Immunology
  Periodontology 2000
  Journal of Clinical Periodontology
  The Periodontology and Oral Implantology Journal
- Tuith online
  http://www.Dundee.ac.uk/tuith
  Online Journal of the Scottish Dental Practice Research Network. Includes online full-
  text articles from current and previous journal issues.
- International Academy of Periodontology
  http://www.perioiap.org/publications.htm
  Review abstracts from previous issues of the *Journal of the International Academy of
  Periodontology*

ONLINE ARTICLES AND ABSTRACTS

- International Academy of Periodontology
  http://www.perioiap.org/publications.htm
  Online abstracts from the *Journal of the International Academy of Periodontology*. Select
  "review abstracts" to access the abstracts.
- National Institute of Dental & Craniofacial Research
  http://www.nidr.nih.gov
  Online access to full text publications of the NIDCR under the topic of "disease and
  conditions" including "diabetes and periodontal disease."
- European Periodontology
  http://www.od.mah.se/depts/par/peri52.html
  Online lectures presented at the Academy of Periodontology in 1995. Some topics are
  outdated, but others are helpful.
- International Academy of Periodontology
  http://www.perioiap.org/publications.htm
  Online abstracts from the *Journal of the International Academy of Periodontology*. Select
  "review abstracts" to access the abstracts.

ONLINE LECTURES AND COURSES

- Basic Periodontology: Centre for Oral Health Sciences, Malmo University,
  http://cert.od.mah.se/vip/basic.periodontology/main.html
  An online mini-textbook with such topics as: gingivitis, periodontitis, pathogenesis,
  attachment loss, subgingival colonization, subgingival bacteria, periodontal pathology,
  nonsurgical treatment, healing, surgery, gingivectomy, and periodontal flap
  procedures.
- European Periodontology
  http://www.od.mah.se/depts/par/peri52.html
  Online lectures presented at the Academy of Periodontology in 1995. Some topics are
  outdated, but others are helpful.

- International Academy of Periodontology
  http://www.perioiap.org/publications.htm
  Online abstracts from the *Journal of the International Academy of Periodontology*. Select "review abstracts" to access the abstracts.
- National Institute of Dental & Craniofacial Research (NIDCR)
  http://www.nidr.nih.gov
  Online access to full-text publications of the NIDCR under the topic of "disease and conditions" including "diabetes and periodontal disease."
- UCLA Periodontics Information Site
  http://www.dent.ucla.edu/pic/index.html
  Free online periodontology courses.
- Virtual Periodontology
  http://www.od.mah.se/depts/par/virtual.html
  Glossary of periodontal terms and a large selection of online mini-courses in periodontics.
- Histology of the Periodontium
  http://www.dental.pitt.edu/informatics/periohistology/en/gutoc.htm
  An online course presented by University of Pennsylvania and Temple University, hosted by the University of Pittsburgh.
- Periodontal Immunology by Dr. Ken Miyasaki
  http://www.dent.ucla.edu/pic/members/immunology
- HIV—AIDS in Dental Care
  HIVdent
  A case-based self-study module for dental health care personnel
  http://www.hivdent.org/Dental%20HIV.pdf

MULTIMEDIA ON PERIODONTAL DISEASE

- The National Library of Medicine Multimedia Index
  http://locatorplus.gov
  Select LOCATORplus. Enter periodontal disease in the search box and select *audiovisuals and computer files* in the Quick Limit box. Click search.

NEWS ARCHIVES RELATING TO PERIODONTAL DISEASE

- MEDLINE Plus News By Health Topic
  http://www.nlm.nih.gov/medlineplus/alphanews_a.html
  Read health-related news articles from Reuters Health Information (articles display for 30 days) and HealthDay (articles display for 90 days), plus the most recent press announcements from major medical organizations.

BOOKS ON PERIODONTAL DISEASE

- The National Library of Medicine Book Index
  http://locatorplus.gov
  Select LOCATORplus. Enter periodontal disease in the search box and select *books only* in the Quick Limit box. Click search.

PROFESSIONAL SOCIETIES AND GOVERNMENTAL AGENCIES

These organizations have a broad range of information for dental professionals and patient education.

- American Academy of Periodontology (AAP)
  http://www.perio.org
  Clinical and scientific papers and information for patients. AAP offers a wide range of excellent clinical publications.
- British Society of Periodontology
  http://www.bsperio.org
  Online journal abstracts; patient information; links to other Websites.
- National Institute of Dental & Craniofacial Research
  http://www.nidr.nih.gov
  Online access to full-text publications of the NIDCR under the topic of "disease and conditions" including "diabetes and periodontal disease."
- British Society of Periodontology
  http://www.bsperio.org.uk/patients/
  Information for patients on periodontal disease and treatment.

DIRECTORY OF HEALTH HOTLINES AND ASSOCIATIONS

- National Library of Medicine
  Directory of Health Organizations
  http://sis.nlm.nih.gov/dirline.html
  This site is a comprehensive source of information on associations and health hotlines.

BROCHURES ON PERIODONTAL DISEASE FOR PATIENT EDUCATION

- American Academy of Periodontics
  http://www.perio.org/consumer/request.htm
  Samples of oral health/periodontal disease patient education brochures produced by the American Academy of Periodontics.

PATIENT INFORMATION/ EDUCATION: ORAL HEALTH/ PERIODONTAL DISEASE

- American Academy of Periodontology
  http://www.perio.org
  Patient resources such as "find a periodontist," "what are periodontal diseases?," "protecting your oral health," and "periodontal procedures."
- American Dental Association
  http://www.ada.org/public/index.asp
- American Dental Hygienists' Association
  http://www.adha.org/oralhealth/index.html
- British Dental Association
  http://www.BDA-dentistry.org.uk
- Proctor and Gamble Dental Resource Net
  http://www.dentalcare.com

- The Combined Health Information Database
  http://chid.nih.gov
  Enter "periodontal disease" in the simple search box and click on search.
- Simple Steps to Better Dental Health
  http://www.simplestepsdental.com/SS/ihtSS/r.WSIHW000/st.31819/t.31819/pr.3.html
  A wealth of patient education topics including: how to prevent problems, dental conditions, treatments, periodontal disease, dry mouth, bad breath, tobacco, gum surgery,
  implants, scaling and root planing, emergencies, and diseases.
- The Wisdom Tooth, School of DH, University of Manitoba
  http://www.umanitoba.ca/outreach/wisdomtooth/index.html
  Patient education topics including stages of gingivitis and periodontits, periodontal
  disease and kissing, smoking and oral health, diabetes and oral health, bad breath, dry
  mouth, and pregnancy gingivitis.

ORAL AND SYSTEMIC HEALTH INFORMATION FOR PATIENTS

- Patient UK
  http://www.patient.co.uk
  A directory of health- and disease-related Websites for patients.
- National Electronic Library for Health
  http://www.nhsdirect.nhs.uk
  Gateway to health information for patients. Search under "gum disease."

PORPHYROMONAS GINGIVALIS

- Porphyromonas gingivalis Genome Project
  http://www.pgingivalis.org
  Information and photo gallery on the periodontal pathogen, *Porphyromonas gingivalis*.

ENDOCARDITIS/ANTIBIOTIC PREMEDICATION

- American Heart Association
  http://www.americanheart.org/presenter.jhtml?identifier=11086
  Endocarditis: guidelines for antibiotic premedication.

FACTS AND STATISTICS

- National Center for Health Statistics
  http://www.cdc.gov/nchs/fastats/dental.htm
  Statistics: FASTATS: Oral health.
- World Health Organization (WHO)
  http://www.whocollab.od.mah.se
  Global information on dental diseases, including periodontal conditions.

INFORMATION ON SYSTEMIC RISK FACTORS FOR REFERENCE AND PATIENT EDUCATION

- American Diabetes Association
  http://www.diabetes.org

- American Heart Association
  http://www.americanheart.org
- American Lung Association
  http://www.lungusa.org
- American Medical Association
  http://www.ama-assn.org
- National Institute of Dental & Craniofacial Research
  http://www.nidr.nih.gov
  Enter "periodontal" in the search box to obtain a list of articles on the link between systemic disease and periodontal disease.
- HIV Dent
  http://www.hivdent.org
  Extensive information on the dental care of human immunodeficiency virus (HIV)-positive patients.
- National Oral Health Information Clearing House
  http://www.nohic.nidcr.nih.gov/publinks.html
  Online full-text special care publications.
- Catalog link
  http://www.dentaldidactics.com
  Contains topics such as "Alzheimer's disease" and "cardiovascular risks of periodontitis."

AIDS/HIV AND PERIODONTAL DISEASE

- HIVdent
  http://www.hivdent.org/main.htm
  An excellent source of information on HIV/acquired immunodeficiency syndrome (AIDS).
- HIVdent
  HIV—AIDS in Dental Care
  http://www.hivdent.org/Dental%20HIV.pdf
  A case-based self-study module for dental health care personnel.
- HIVdent
  5th World Workshop on Oral Health and Disease in HIV/ AIDS
  http://www.hivdent.org/oralm/5thWorldWorkshopOnOralHealthAndDisease InAIDS/5WWOHDA-MAIN.htm
- HIVdent
  Oral Manifestations & Dental Care Issues for HIV
  http://www.hivdent.org/oralm/oralm.htm

PERIODONTAL QUIZ FOR PATIENTS

- Periodontal Quiz
  http://www.barfielddds.com/perioquiz.htm
  A brief, eight-question quiz on periodontal health.

GINGIVITIS, PERIODONTITIS, GUM DISEASE FOR PATIENTS

- MEDLINE Plus
  http://www.nlm.nih.gov/medlineplus/gumdisease.html
  Gum disease.
- US Food and Drug Administration.
  http://www.fda.gov/fdac/features/2002/302_gums.html
  Fighting gum disease: how to keep your teeth.
- Mayo Foundation for Medical Education and Research
  http://mayoclinic.com/health/trench-mouth/DS00363
  Gingivitis.
- The Gum Disease
  http://www.gumsbleeding.com/
  Full color photographs and information about gum disease sponsored by a group of Ohio dentists.
- American Academy of Periodontology
  http://www.perio.org/consumer/2a.html
  Periodontal disease.
- Mayo Foundation for Medical Education and Research
  http://mayoclinic.com/health/periodontitis/DS00369
  Periodontitis—a great overview for patients.

RESOURCES FOR PATIENT EDUCATION IN SPANISH

- Tratamiento Gingivitis Y Periodontitis
  http://www.periodontitis.net/
  Información para pacientes sobre la periodontitis y la gingivitis.

FACTS AND FALLACIES ABOUT PERIODONTAL DISEASE

- American Academy of Periodontology
  http://www.perio.org/consumer/f1.html
  Facts and fallacies about periodontal disease.

WOMEN AND PERIODONTAL DISEASE

- American Academy of Periodontology
  http://www.perio.org/consumer/women.htm
  Women: Protecting your teeth throughout life.

TEENAGERS AND PERIODONTAL DISEASE

- Nemours Foundation
  http://kidshealth.org/teen/diseases_conditions/mouth/gum_disease.html
  Teenagers: gum disease.

TREATING PERIODONTAL DISEASE

- American Dental Association
  www.ada.org/prof/resources/ pubs/jada/patient/patient_23.pd
  Treatment of periodontal diseases.

TOOTH PROBLEMS: SELF-CARE FLOW CHARTS

- American Academy of Family Physicians
  http://familydoctor.org/511.xml
  Tooth problems: self-care flow charts.

BODY–MOUTH CONNECTION

- American Academy of Periodontology
  http://www.perio.org/consumer/mbc.top2.htm
  The body–mouth connection.

DIABETES AND PERIODONTAL DISEASE

- National Diabetes Information Clearinghouse
  http://diabetes.niddk.nih.gov/dm/pubs/complications_teeth/index.htm
  Prevent diabetes problems: keep your teeth and gums healthy.
- About Senior Health
  http://seniorhealth.about.com/cs/oralconditions/a/diabetic_gum.htm
  Diabetes and oral health.

NECROTIZING ULCERATIVE GINGIVITIS

- Mayo Foundation for Medical Education and Research
  http://mayoclinic.com/health/trench-mouth/DS00457
  Trench mouth (necrotizing ulcerative gingivitis).

PERICORONITIS

- Pericoronitis
  http://www.simplestepsdental.com/SS/ihtSS/r.WSIHW000/st.32219/t.29748/pr.3.html
  Simple steps to better dental health.

NUTRITION INFORMATION

- U.S. Dept. of Agriculture
  http://www.mypyramid.gov/
  Information, images, and patient information on the Food Guide Pyramid for proper nutrition.
- Dietary Guidelines for Americans 2005
  http://www.healthierus.gov/dietaryguidelines/
- The US Department of Agriculture's web site for nutrition information
  http://www.nutrition.gov/
- International Bibliographic Information on Dietary Supplements (IBIDS) Database
  http://ods.od.nih.gov/Health_Information/IBIDS.aspx
  Click on IBIDS. Enter periodontal disease in the search box. The search engine allows you to retrieve up to 100 fully explained references.

TOBACCO USE AND PERIODONTAL DISEASE

■ American Academy of Periodontology
http://www.perio.org/consumer/smoking.htm
Tobacco use and periodontal disease.

SMOKING CESSATION RESOURCES

■ Smoking Cessation Leadership Center
http://smokingcessationleadership.ucsf.edu
The Smoking Cessation Leadership Center (SCLC) is a national program office of the Robert Wood Johnson Foundation that aims to increase smoking cessation rates and increase the number of health professionals who help smokers quit. Click on *Health Profession Resources* for a downloadable toolkit including print-and-post flyers for the dental office and downloadable PowerPoint slide presentations.

■ **National Cancer Institute Quitline**.
http://www.nci.nih.gov/cancertopics/tobacco
The quitline is toll free at **1-877-44U-QUIT** (1-877-448-7848). Information specialists are available to answer smoking-related questions in English or Spanish, Monday through Friday, 9:00 AM to 4:30 PM local time.

■ The **U.S. Department of Health and Human Services** has a national quitline number, **1-800-QUIT-NOW** (1-800-784-8669). This toll free number is a single access link to the national network of tobacco cessation quitlines. Callers are automatically routed to a state-sponsored quitline, if one exists in their area. If there is no state-run quitline, the call goes to the National Cancer Institute (NCI) quitline.

■ American Cancer Society quitline: **1-800-277-2345**

■ American Lung Association quitline: **1-800-586-4872**

■ Smoke Free
http://www.smokefree.gov/usmap.html#
On this Website, click on a state to find smoking cessation resources in that state.

■ American Cancer Society Resources for Health Professionals
http://www.cancer.org/docroot/PED/PED_10_6.asp?sitearea=PED
American Cancer Society website with resources of health professionals. Smoking cessations resources include free brochures to keep smokers motivated, patient education materials, and a link to find a quitline in your area.

■ American Dental Hygienists' Association
http://www.askadviserefer.org
Website for the **American Dental Hygienists' Association's** smoking cessation initiative. The site has resources including links to fact sheets, presentations, and quitline resource lists.

■ American Dental Association
http://www.ada.org/prof/resources/topics/cancer.asp
The **American Dental Association's** Website provides oral cancer information for dental health care providers.

■ University of Manitoba, Division of Periodontology
http://www1.umn.edu/perio/tobacco/tobperio.html
Tobacco and periodontal disease.

Chapter

29 Patient Cases: Radiographic Analysis

CASE 1

CASE 2

CASE 3

CASE 4

CASE 5

CASE 6

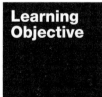
Learning Objective

■ Apply concepts from the chapters in this book to complete a radiographic analysis of Cases 1 to 6.

Directions:
■ Practice your skills in radiographic analysis by doing a radiographic analysis for each patient case in this chapter.
■ Using sheets of notebook paper, recreate the Radiographic Analysis Worksheet shown on the facing page. Complete a radiographic analysis for each case.

Radiographic Analysis Worksheet

Case:

Diagnostic Acceptability

Does this series of radiographs or panoramic radiograph exhibit minimum diagnostic acceptability? Answer: Explanation:

Diagnostic Evaluation of Radiographs

Radiographically visible anatomy:

Caries:

Calculus:

Restorative procedures:

Missing teeth:

Variations and deviations from normal:

Alveolar bone height assessment:

Figure 29-1. Sample Radiographic Analysis Worksheet.

SECTION 1: CASE 1

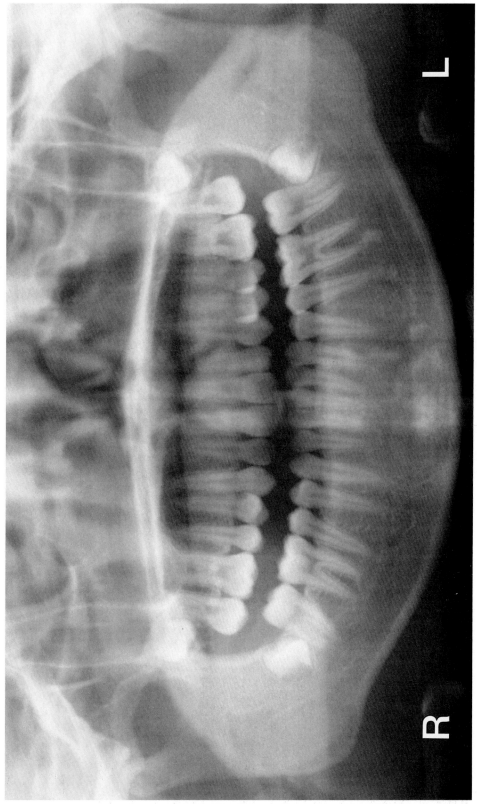

Figure 29-2. Panoramic Radiograph for Case 1.

SECTION 2: CASE 2

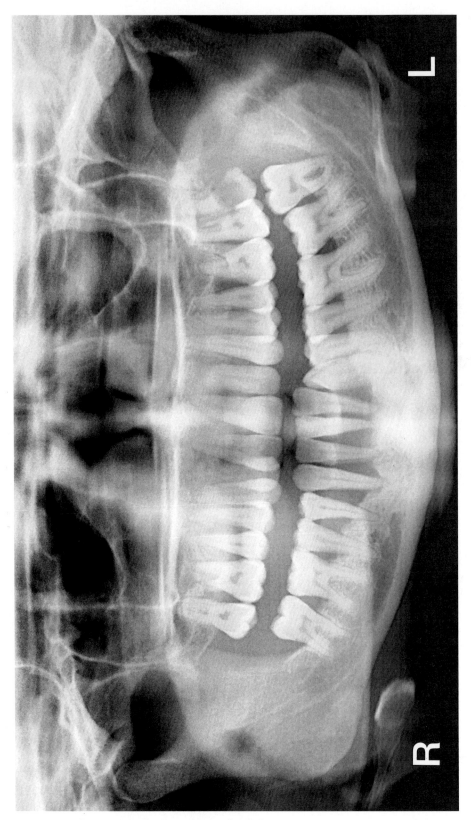

Figure 29-3. Panoramic Radiograph for Case 2.

SECTION 3: CASE 3

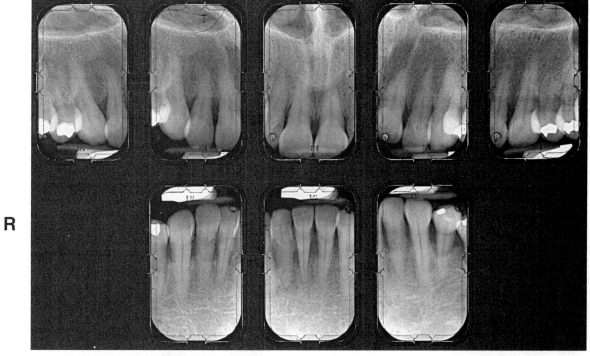

R   L

Figure 29-4A. Anterior Radiographs for Case 3.

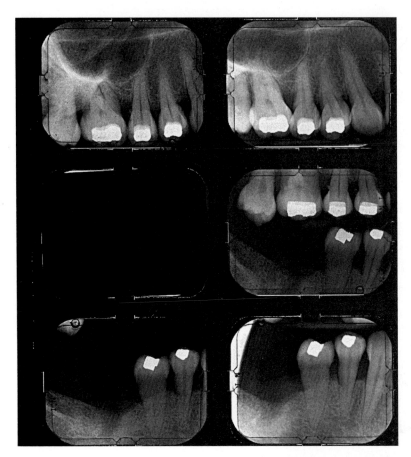

Figure 29-4B. Right Posterior Radiographs for Case 3.

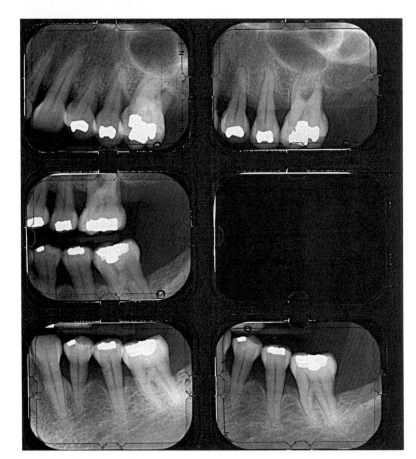

Figure 29-4C. Left Posterior Radiographs for Case 3.

SECTION 4: CASE 4

R

L

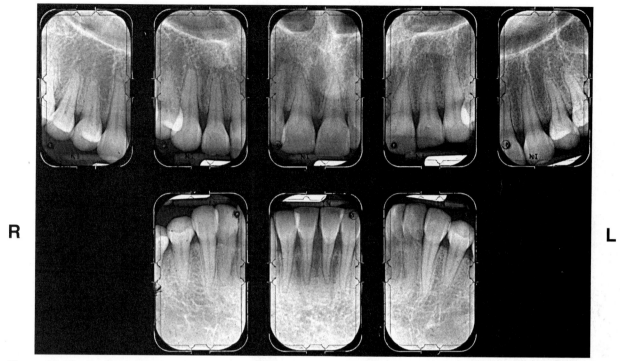

Figure 29-5A. Radiographs for Case 4.

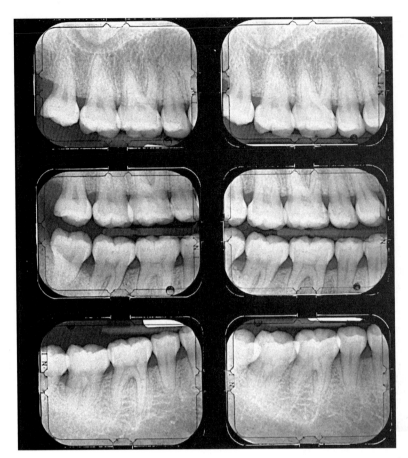

Figure 29-5B. Right Posterior Radiographs for Case 4.

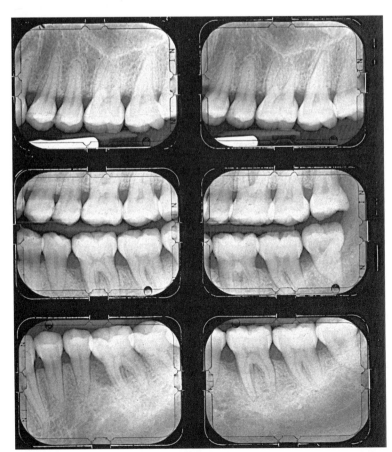

Figure 29-5C. Left Posterior Radiographs for Case 4.

SECTION 5: CASE 5

R

L

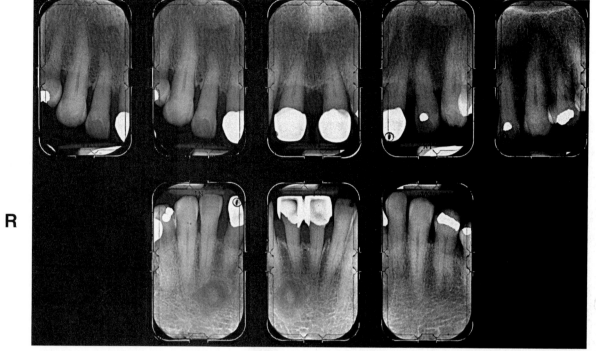

Figure 29-6A. Radiographs for Case 5.

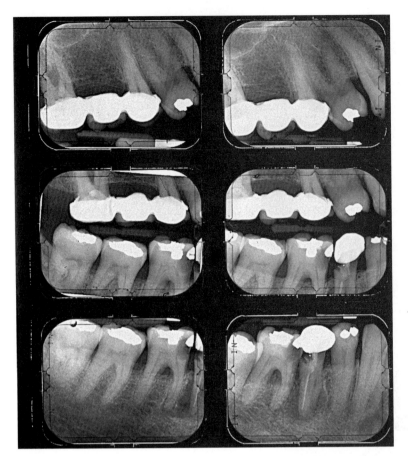

Figure 29-6B. Right Posterior Radiographs for Case 5.

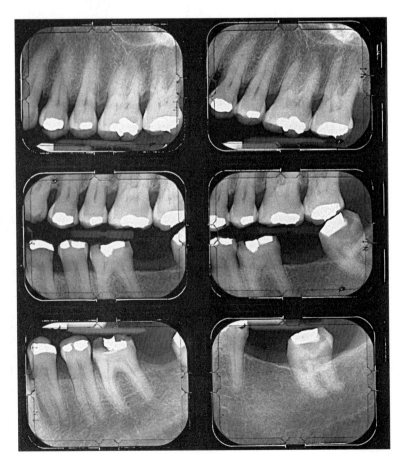

Figure 29-6C. Left Posterior Radiographs for Case 5.

SECTION 6: CASE 6

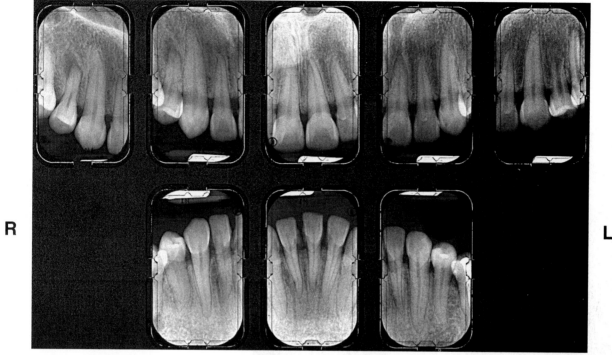

R

L

Figure 29-7A. Radiographs for Case 6.

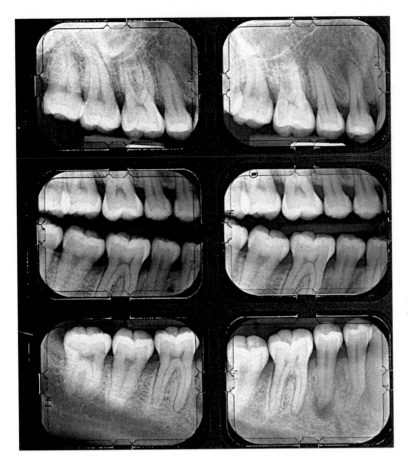

Figure 29-7B. Right Posterior Radiographs for Case 6.

Figure 29-7C. Left Posterior Radiographs for Case 6.

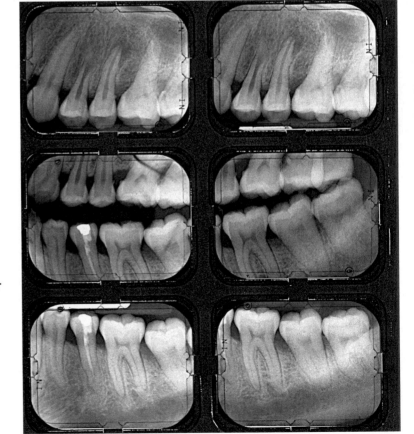

30 Comprehensive Patient Cases

FICTITIOUS PATIENT CASE 1

FICTITIOUS PATIENT CASE 2

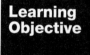

■ Apply concepts from the chapters in this book to fictitious patient case 1 and 2.

Directions:
■ Apply your knowledge and skills by answering the decision-making questions for fictitious patient case 1 and 2.

MR. KARN: DECISION-MAKING BASED UPON EXAMINATION FINDINGS

1. How will the medications Mr. Karn is taking affect the planning and delivery of any needed dental treatment?

2. What does Mr. Karn's health history reveal about his medical status that will be important for the dental team to consider during treatment?

3. Based upon the clinical photographs, can you identify any etiologic factors for either gingivitis or periodontitis?

4. What might be the cause of the gingival recession on the palatal surface of the maxillary left first molar tooth?

5. How would you describe the appearance of Mr. Karn's gingival tissues on the lingual surface of the mandibular right quadrant?

6. The mandibular left first molar has a class II furcation involvement on the facial surface. How would the presence of this furcation involvement affect any periodontal treatment?

7. What local contributing factors that can affect the progress of periodontitis are evident on the radiographs?

8. Are there any sites visible on the radiographs where there is evidence of alveolar bone loss?

9. What specific features on these radiographs indicate alveolar bone loss?

10. How would you characterize Mr. Karn's periodontal condition? Do you think that he has gingivitis, periodontitis, neither, or both? What clinical features did you use to reach your conclusion?

11. Write a plan for non-surgical periodontal therapy for Mr. Karn. Include all of the procedures to be performed by both the dental hygienist and the dentist. For each procedure indicate who should perform this procedure—dental hygienist or dentist.

12. What information should your team give Mr. Karn about his periodontal condition?

13. What should Mr. Karn be told about the possible need for periodontal surgery later in the treatment?

14. What should Mr. Karn be told about the possibility of an implant to replace his maxillary right first molar tooth?

15. What should Mr. Karn be told about the need for continuing treatment such as periodontal maintenance?

PATIENT PROFILE

Mr. Karn is a 47-year-old high school teacher who has recently moved to your city. He has made an appointment with your dental team because he wants an implant to replace his missing upper right molar tooth.

At his first visit he informs you that he has been too busy lately to get a dental check-up and that he has not seen a dentist for several years. Mr. Karn states that he brushes twice daily when he has time and that he does not floss regularly even though he knows that he should. He also uses an over-the-counter mouth rinse occasionally.

HEALTH HISTORY

At the time of his first visit Mr. Karn's blood pressure is 130/80 and his pulse is 62 beats per minute. A review of Mr. Karn's health history reveals that he takes two medications: (i) Zocor for elevated cholesterol levels and (ii) Nifedipine for hypertension. Mr. Karn also states that he smokes between one-half and one pack of cigarettes each day.

PERIODONTAL CHART

CASE #1

Maxilla

	1	2	3	4	5	6	7	8	9	10	11	12	13	14	15	16	Maxilla
Mobility (I, II, III)						I	I						I			I	
Bleeding/Purulence (+)	+	+		+	+	+	+			+	+	+	+	+	+	+	
Attachment Level (CEJ to BP)																	
Probing Depth (FGM to BP)	646	635		325	536	525	435	433	334	425	435	536	626	638	846	746	

Facial

Palatal

	1	2	3	4	5	6	7	8	9	10	11	12	13	14	15	16	
Bleeding/Purulence (+)	+	+		+	+	+	+	+	+	+	+	+	+	+	+	+	
Attachment Level (CEJ to BP)																	
Probing Depth (FGM to BP)	636	525		335	526	536	425	443	324	424	525	535	626	627	827	736	
Plaque (F/P)																	
Supragingival Calculus		✓		✓	✓				✓	✓				✓	✓	✓	
Subgingival Calculus	✓	✓		✓	✓	✓	✓	✓	✓	✓	✓	✓	✓	✓	✓	✓	
PSR Code			4					3					4				

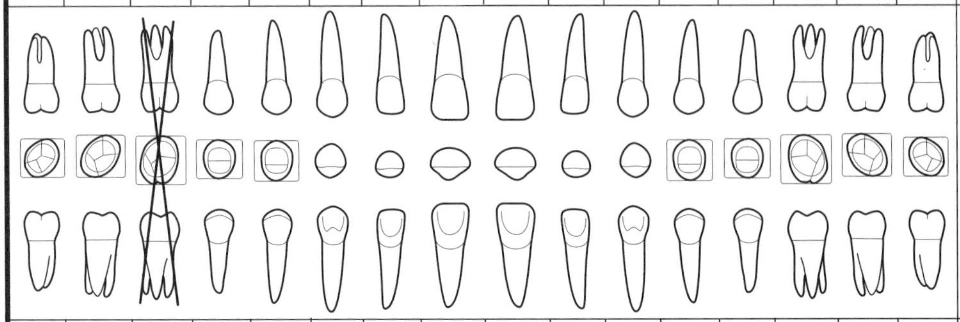

Right   Left

Mandible

	32	31	30	29	28	27	26	25	24	23	22	21	20	19	18	17	Mandible
Mobility (I, II, III)			I			I	I										
Bleeding/Purulence (+)	+		+	+	+	+		+		+	+	+		+	+		
Attachment Level (CEJ to BP)																	
Probing Depth (FGM to BP)	546	736	626	635	535	534	324	423	323	324	324	434	435	536	746	635	

Lingual

Facial

	32	31	30	29	28	27	26	25	24	23	22	21	20	19	18	17	
Bleeding/Purulence (+)	+	+	+	+	+		+	+	+		+		+		+	+	
Attachment Level (CEJ to BP)																	
Probing Depth (FGM to BP)	546	736	625	535	635	534	324	423	323	324	324	434	435	526	736	625	
Plaque (L/F)																	
Supragingival Calculus						✓	✓	✓	✓	✓			✓	✓			
Subgingival Calculus	✓	✓	✓	✓	✓	✓	✓	✓	✓	✓	✓	✓	✓	✓	✓	✓	
PSR Code			4					3					4				

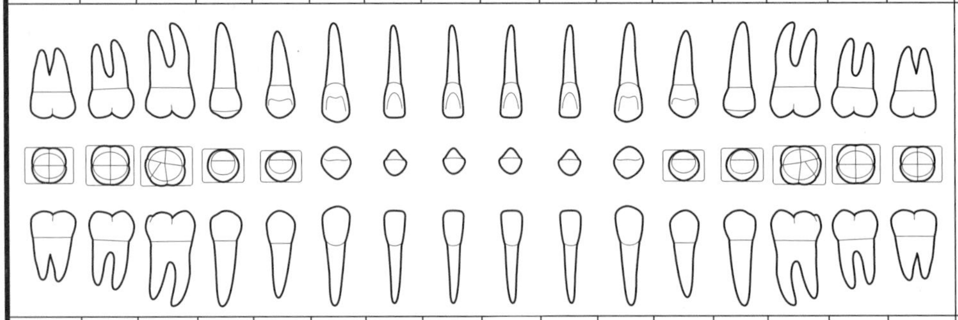

Figure 30-1. Mr. Karn's Periodontal Chart.

CLINICAL PHOTOGRAPHS

 Refer to the CD packaged with this book for full color versions of these photographs.

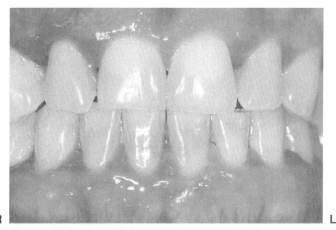

Figure 30-2. Anterior Teeth.

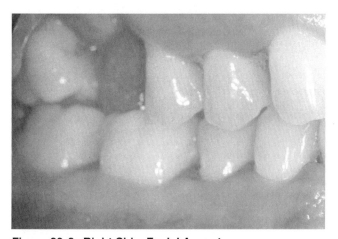

Figure 30-3. Right Side: Facial Aspect.

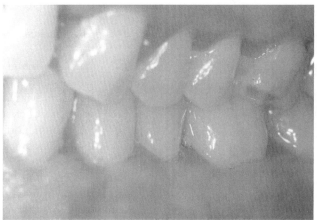

Figure 30-4. Left Side: Facial Aspect.

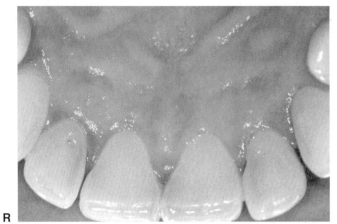

R   L

Figure 30-5. Maxillary Anteriors: Lingual Aspect.

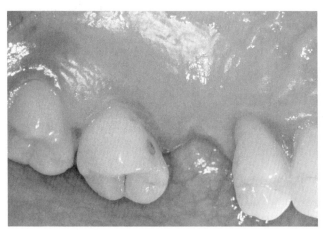

Figure 30-6. Maxillary Right Lingual.

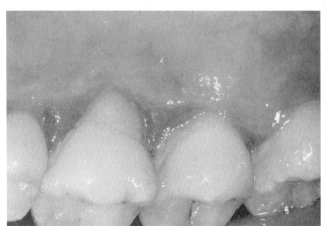

Figure 30-7. Maxillary Left Lingual.

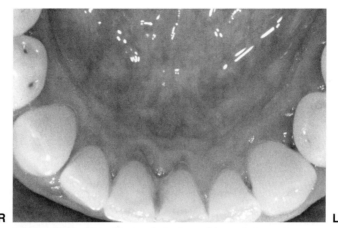

Figure 30-8. Mandibular Anteriors: Lingual Aspect.

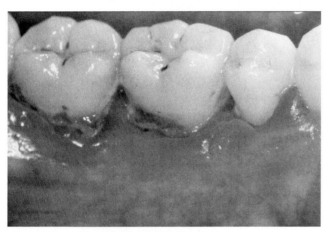

Figure 30-9. Mandibular Right Lingual.

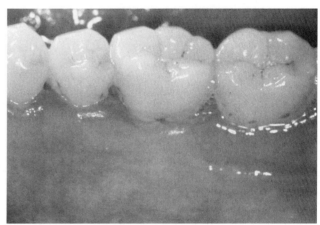

Figure 30-10. Mandibular Left Lingual.

RADIOGRAPHIC SERIES

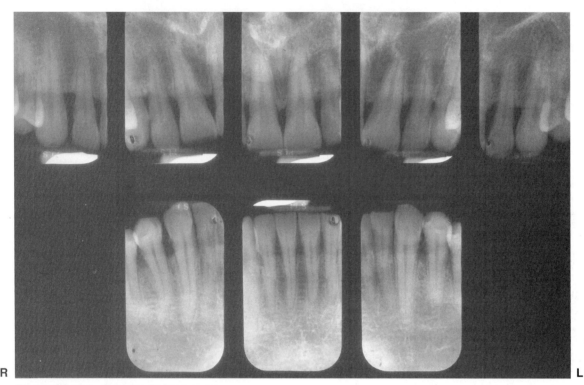

R   L

Figure 30-11A. Anterior Radiographs.

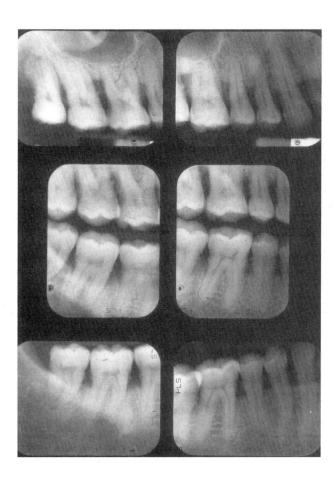

Figure 30-11B. Right Posterior Radiographs.

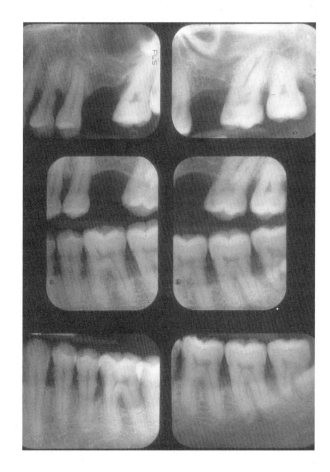

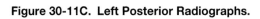

Figure 30-11C. Left Posterior Radiographs.

MR. WILTON: DECISION-MAKING BASED UPON EXAMINATION FINDINGS

1. What do Mr. Wilton's vital signs and health history reveal about his medical status that will be important for the dental team to consider during treatment?

2. What special precautions should your dental team take during a periodontal evaluation to ensure Mr. Wilton's welfare?

3. What actions should your dental team take to deal with the apparent elevation in Mr. Wilton's blood pressure?

4. Are there any etiologic factors for either gingivitis or periodontitis evident on the clinical photographs?

5. How would you describe the appearance of gingival tissues around Mr. Wilton's mandibular anterior teeth?

6. In response to your questions, Mr. Wilton informs you that the spaces between his front teeth were not there a few years ago. What do you think may be causing these spaces between his teeth to appear?

7. What do the probing depths tell you about the possible need for periodontal therapy in addition to initial periodontal therapy?

8. Were appropriate radiographs taken of Mr. Wilton? If the radiographs are appropriate, why? If not, which radiographs should have been ordered for Mr. Wilton?

9. What local contributing factors are evident on the radiographs?

10. What do the radiographs reveal about the level of bone support for the maxillary anterior teeth?

11. How would you characterize Mr. Wilton's periodontal condition? Do you think that he has gingivitis, periodontitis, neither, or both? What clinical and radiographic findings did you use to reach your conclusion?

12. Write a plan for initial periodontal therapy for Mr. Wilton. Include all of the procedures to be performed by both the dental hygienist and the dentist. For each procedure indicate who should perform this procedure—dental hygienist or dentist.

13. What information should your team give Mr. Wilton about his periodontal condition?

14. What information should your team give Mr. Wilton about his wife's concern about his bad breath?

15. What information should your team give Mr. Wilton about his concern related to the spaces between his maxillary incisor teeth?

16. What should your team tell Mr. Wilton if he refuses your team's recommendations for periodontal therapy?

PATIENT PROFILE

Mr. Wilton is a 52-year-old manager of a local gardening store who is here for his initial visit in the dental office. During his initial interview, Mr. Wilton informs you that he made this appointment at his wife's insistence. He states that his wife wants to know if there is anything that can be done about his bad breath.

HEALTH HISTORY

At the time of his initial visit, Mr. Wilton's blood pressure is 164/100 and his pulse rate is 68 per minute. Mr. Wilton informs you that he is not taking any medications at present but that he had high blood pressure once and did take a medication for that a few years ago. He tells you that he was feeling just fine so he stopped taking the medication. Mr. Wilton also informs you that he has a mitral valve prolapse.

PERIODONTAL CHART

CASE #2

	1	2	3	4	5	6	7	8	9	10	11	12	13	14	15	16	**Maxilla**
Mobility (I, II, III)			I				I	I	II	I		I					
Bleeding/Purulence (+)	+	+			+		+	+	+		+	+	+		+	+	
Attachment Level (CEJ to BP)																	
Probing Depth (FGM to BP)	635	634		338	535	537	626	625	537	625	536	725	524		435	535	

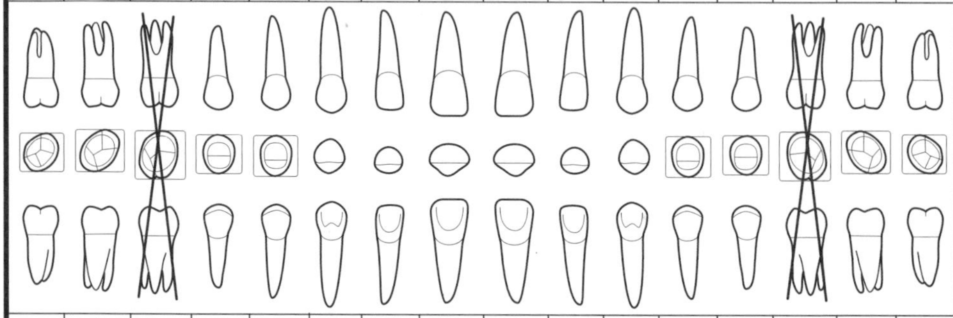

Facial / Palatal

	1	2	3	4	5	6	7	8	9	10	11	12	13	14	15	16	
Bleeding/Purulence (+)	+	+		+	+	+		+	+		+	+	+		+		
Attachment Level (CEJ to BP)																	
Probing Depth (FGM to BP)	535	634		438	534	636	536	535	635	535	536	726	534		426	535	
Plaque (F/P)																	
Supragingival Calculus		✓			✓	✓	✓	✓	✓	✓		✓		✓	✓		
Subgingival Calculus	✓	✓		✓	✓	✓	✓	✓	✓	✓	✓	✓	✓		✓	✓	
PSR Code			4					4					4				

Right — *Left*

	32	31	30	29	28	27	26	25	24	23	22	21	20	19	18	17	**Mandible**
Mobility (I, II, III)			I			II	II	II	II								
Bleeding/Purulence (+)		+	+	+		+	+	+	+	+	+	+	+	+		+	
Attachment Level (CEJ to BP)																	
Probing Depth (FGM to BP)		535	536	545	524	535	635	545	536	637	635	524	535	635	636	635	

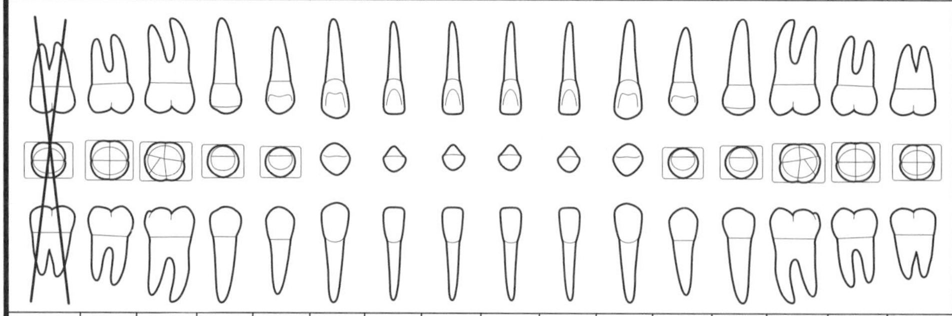

Lingual / Facial

	32	31	30	29	28	27	26	25	24	23	22	21	20	19	18	17	
Bleeding/Purulence (+)		+	+		+	+	+	+	+	+	+	+		+	+	+	
Attachment Level (CEJ to BP)																	
Probing Depth (FGM to BP)		535	526	535	424	535	624	535	525	536	524	525	425	525	526	625	
Plaque (L/F)																	
Supragingival Calculus						✓	✓	✓	✓	✓	✓					✓	
Subgingival Calculus		✓	✓	✓	✓	✓	✓	✓	✓	✓	✓	✓	✓	✓	✓	✓	
PSR Code			4					4					4				

Figure 30-12. Mr. Wilson's Periodontal Chart.

CLINICAL PHOTOGRAPHS

Refer to the CD packaged with this book for full color versions of these photographs.

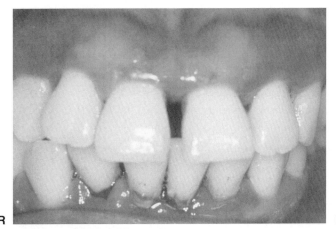

R   L

Figure 30-13. Anterior Teeth.

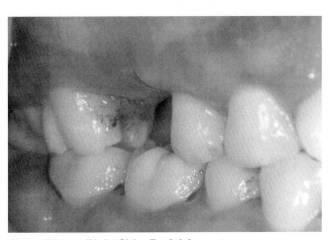

Figure 30-14. Right Side: Facial Aspect.

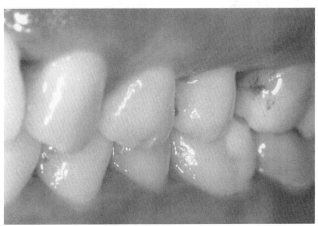

Figure 30-15. Left Side: Facial Aspect.

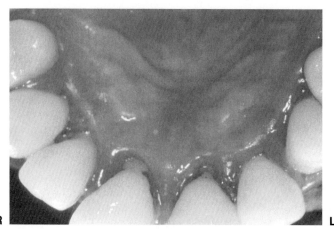

Figure 30-16. Maxillary Anteriors: Lingual Aspect.

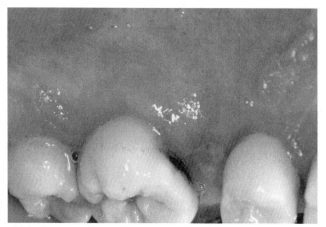

Figure 30-17. Maxillary Right Lingual.

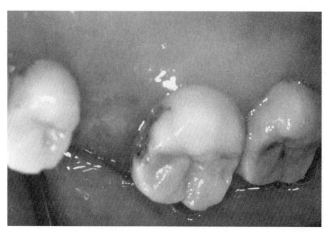

Figure 30-18. Maxillary Left Lingual.

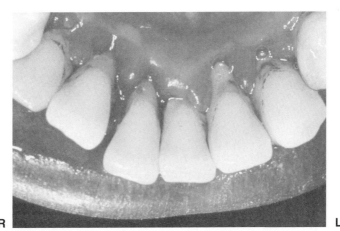

Figure 30-19. Mandibular Anteriors: Lingual Aspect.

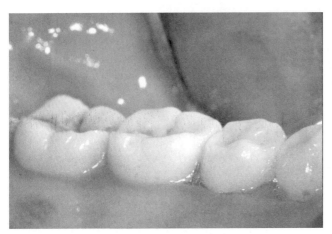

Figure 30-20. Mandibular Right Lingual.

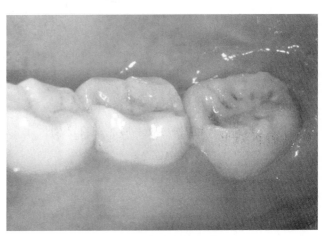

Figure 30-21. Mandibular Left Lingual.

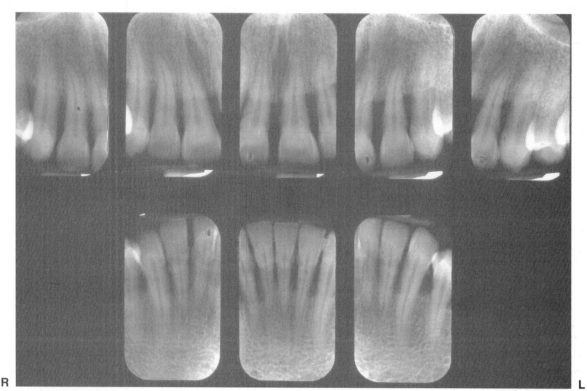

R   L

Figure 30-22A. Anterior Radiographs.

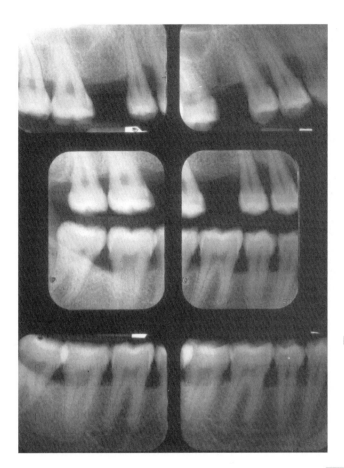

Figure 30-22B. Right Posterior Radiographs.

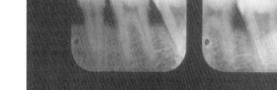

Figure 30-22C. Left Posterior Radiographs.

A Answer Key for Chapter Review Questions

Chapter 1

1. a.
2. b.
3. b.
4. b.
5. a.
6. c.
7. d.
8. a.
9. b.

Chapter 2

1. c.
2. b.
3. a.
4. d.
5. b.
6. a.
7. a.
8. c.
9. a.
10. b.
11. c.
12. a.
13. c.
14. d.
15. b.
16. Base of the sulcus, crest of the alveolar bone.
17. Tooth, bony socket
18. a.
19. a.

Chapter 3

1. a.
2. c.
3. b.
4. e.
5. a.
6. e.
7. b.
8. a.

Chapter 4

1. c.
2. b.
3. b.
4. d.
5. a.

Chapter 5

1. b.
2. d
3. c
4. b
5. c
6. d
7. a
8. a

Chapter 6

1. a.
2. b.

3. a.
4. c.
5. d.
6. d.
7. b.
8. d.

Chapter 7

1. a.
2. b.
3. b.
4. d.
5. c.
6. d.

Chapter 8

1. a.
2. a.
3. a.
4. b.
5. c.
6. a.
7. b.
8. a.
9. a.
10. b
11. c.

Chapter 9

1. c.
2. b.

3. d.
4. b.
5. c.
6. d.
7. a.

Chapter 10

1. a.
2. c.
3. a.
4. a.
5. b.
6. c.
7. a.
8. b.
9. d.

Chapter 11

1. b.
2. a.
3. c.
4. b.
5. b.
6. c.
7. a.
8. b.

Chapter 12

1. c.
2. d.
3. c.
4. a.
5. c.
6. c.
7. b.
8. a.
9. b.

Chapter 13

1. b.
2. c.
3. a.
4. d.
5. a.
6. c.
7. a.
8. b.

Chapter 14

1. a.
2. c.

3. b.
4. a.
5. d.
6. d.
7. d.
8. c.

Chapter 15

1. Evidence: research, particularly that involving clinical trials, clinical expertise meaning growth and wisdom gained from everyday experience, patient values, which are the preferences of the patient for a therapy

2. Asking good questions; utilization of the PICO process
Finding/locating good evidence; accessing a search engine
Appraising the evidence; review of the study design such as checking for randomization or blinding
Applying the evidence; develop a learning philosophy or accessing/using clinical practice guidelines
Evaluating your performance; asking yourself how sure you are that your current practice protocols are based on scientific evidence.

3. Patient: For a pediatric patient at high risk for dental caries
Intervention: would a fluoride varnish
Comparison: or a topical fluoride application
Outcome: better reduce the incidence of new decay in the next 6 months

3. A systematic review because it combines the results of several studies, particularly randomized clinical trials to uncover the most efficacious treatments.

4. I would use search engines first to find relevant articles. From what I find on the search engine I would then choose articles from peer-reviewed sources.

5. I would look for things like balancing, equal treatment of the groups, monitoring of subject behavior during the study and accountability of dropouts.

6. Systematically developed statements to assist practitioners and patients in arriving at decisions on appropriate health care for specific clinical circumstances. Professional associations are primary source for these guidelines.

7. Practitioners may not be aware of current evidence, or they may know it but don't have the skills or organizational support to apply the evidence. The practice and community may also negatively influence implementation of evidence.

8. What you do right in practice, what you might want to stop doing and/or what you should change.

9. Yes, there is a Code of Ethics for dental hygienists and it can be found by contacting the American Dental Hygienists' Association.

Chapter 16

1. c.
2. b.
3. c.
4. b.
5. c.
6. a.
7. b.
8. a.

Chapter 17

1. b.
2. b.
3. a.
4. a.
5. a.
6. a.
7. c.
8. b.

Chapter 18

1. d.
2. b.
3. b.
4. a.

5. b.
6. d.
7. a.
8. b.

Chapter 19

1. b.
2. a.
3. b.
4. b.
5. a.
6. d.
7. c.
8. a.

Chapter 20

1. a.
2. d.
3. a.
4. b.
5. a.

Chapter 21

1. a.
2. a.
3. b.
4. a.
5. a.

6. a.
7. a.
8. b.
9. b.
10. a.

Chapter 22

1. a.
2. b.
3. b.
4. a.
5. a.
6. c.
7. b.

Chapter 23

1. a.
2. b.
3. a.
4. c.
5. a.
6. b.
7. b.

Chapter 24

1. a.
2. b.
3. b.

4. a.
5. c.
6. b.

Chapter 25

1. b.
2. a.
3. b.
4. c.
5. a.
6. b.
7. b.

Chapter 26

1. a.
2. d.
3. c.
4. a.
5. b.
6. b.
7. b.
8. b.
9. c.

Glossary

A

Abscess of the periodontium—a localized infection involving the periodontium. (Compare with endodontic abscess).

Abutment—a tooth, root, or implant used to support or anchor a fixed or a removable prosthesis.

Actinobacillus actinomycetemcomitans—a gram-negative bacterium that has been identified as an etiologic agent of periodontitis.

Active disease site—a disease site that shows continued apical migration of the junctional epithelium over time.

Acute—a condition that is of rapid onset and can be accompanied by pain.

Acute inflammation—an inflammatory response that begins suddenly and is of short duration (2 weeks or less).

Aerobic bacteria—bacteria that require oxygen to live.

Aggressive periodontitis—a bacterial infection resulting in inflammation within the supporting tissues of the teeth characterized by a rapid destruction of the periodontal ligament, rapid loss of supporting bone, high risk for tooth loss, and a poor response to periodontal therapy. The severity of the tissue destruction seen in aggressive periodontitis is often inconsistent with the relatively small amounts of bacterial plaque exhibited by the patient.

Alveolar bone—the bony projection that surrounds and supports the roots of the teeth.

Alveolar bone proper—the thin layer of bone that lines each alveolus.

Alveolar crest—the most coronal portion of the alveolar process. In health, the alveolar crest is located 1 to 2 mm apical (below) the cementoenamel junctions of the teeth.

Alveolar mucosa—the apical boundary, or lower edge, of the gingiva; it can be distinguished easily from the gingiva by its dark red color and smooth, shiny surface.

Alveolus—the bony socket; a cavity in the alveolar bone that houses the root of a tooth (alveolus, singular; alveoli, plural).

American Dental Association Current Dental Terminology—a standardized system to record dental procedures for purposes of insurance billing.

Anaerobic bacteria—bacteria that cannot live in the presence of oxygen.

Anastomose—the joining together of blood vessels to create a complex system of vessels.

Antibody—a protein molecule produced and secreted by B lymphocytes in response to a microorganism. All antibodies have the same overall structure and are known collectively as **immunoglobulins**.

Anticoagulant drugs—substances that prevent or delay coagulation of the blood.

Antigen—any substance that is recognized by the immune system as being foreign, such as bacteria and viruses.

Apical—toward the tip of the root.

Apically positioned flap—a periodontal surgical procedure in which a flap is sutured at a position that is more apical to its original position.

Asynchronous multiple bursts theory—a theory of disease progression that suggests that multiple bursts of periodontal disease activity occur over short periods followed by an indefinite period of remission.

Attached gingiva—the part of the gingiva that is tightly connected to the cementum on the cervical third of the root and to the periosteum (connective tissue cover) of the alveolar bone.

Attachment apparatus—the components that hold a tooth in the mouth: periodontal ligament, cementum, and alveolar bone.

Attachment loss—the migration of the attachment apparatus apical to the level of the cementoenamel junction due to the destruction of the fibers and bone that support the teeth.

Autograft—when bone is grafted from one area of the patient's jaw to another.

Automatic defibrillator—a device that delivers an electric shock at a preset voltage that is used for restoring the normal cardiac rhythm.

Avascular—lacking a blood supply.

B

B cell—see B lymphocyte.

B lymphocyte—a white blood cell that differentiates and becomes an antibody-producing cell.

Bacteremia—the presence of bacteria in the bloodstream.

Bacterial blooms—periods when specific species or groups of species grow at rapidly accelerated rates within the dental plaque biofilm.

Bacterial endocarditis—a bacterial infection caused by bacteria that adhere to the lining of the heart chambers and the heart valves.

Bacterial enzymes—cytotoxic agents that are harmful or destructive to host cells.

Bacterial plaque—a biofilm that adheres tenaciously to tooth surfaces, restorations, and prosthetic appliances. Also see biofilm.

Bacterium (plural, bacteria)—a microorganism composed of a single cell that only can be seen through a microscope. Many bacteria cause disease.

Bacteroides forsythus—a gram-negative bacterium that has been identified as an etiologic agent of periodontitis.

Basal cells—the deepest (innermost) layer of epithelial cells; these cells are not flat but are somewhat cube-shaped and are attached to the basal lamina.

Basal lamina—a thin, tough sheet that separates the epithelial cells from the underlying connective tissue. Also see external basal lamina and internal basal lamina.

Baseline data—clinical data gathered at the beginning of treatment to which data gathered at subsequent appointments are compared.

Bifurcation—the anatomic crotch area where the roots of a two-rooted tooth divide.

Biofilm—a well-organized community of bacteria that adheres to surfaces and is embedded in an extracellular slime layer. Biofilms form rapidly on any wet surface and usually consist of many species of bacteria as well as other organisms and debris.

Biologic equilibrium—a state of balance in the internal environment of the body.

Biologic seal—adaptation of the epithelium to the titanium abutment post of a dental implant. The biologic seal also is known as the perimucosal seal.

Biologic width—the distance from the base of the sulcus or pocket to the alveolar bone (approximately 2 mm).

Bipolar pacemaker—a device surgically placed in the chest of a patient to regulate an irregular heartbeat; bipolar pacemakers are generally not affected by the small electromagnetic fields created by dental equipment.

Bleeding on gentle probing—represents bleeding from the soft tissue wall of a periodontal pocket where the wall of the pocket is ulcerated (i.e., where portions of the epithelium itself have been destroyed).

Blinding—the assignment of a subject to a study group without the subject and/or the investigator knowing the assignment.

Blunted papilla—a papilla that is flat and does not fill the interproximal space.

Bone grafting—the surgical procedure that involves elevating periodontal flaps, identifying and cleaning periodontal bone defects, preparation of the tooth root, and placement of some material that is selected to encourage the body to rebuild alveolar bone.

Bone resorption—bone loss due to osteoclastic activity.

Bruxism—forceful grinding of the teeth.

Bulbous papilla—a papilla that is enlarged and appears to bulge out of the interproximal space.

C

Calcium channel blockers—medications used to control high blood pressure; these medications are associated with gingival overgrowth in some patients.

Calculus—see dental calculus.

Cancellous bone—the latticelike bone that fills the interior portion of the alveolar process (between the cortical bone and the alveolar bone proper). It is also known as spongy bone.

Candidiasis—an infection with a fungus, usually *Candida albicans*. *C. albicans* usually is a harmless inhabitant of the mouth, but may cause infections under certain circumstances such as the use of antibiotics, xerostomia, diabetes mellitus, and suppression of the immune system. Also known as oral thrush.

Cell junctions—specialized connecting bodies that attach one cell to another.

Cell plasma membrane—a continuous sheet that forms the outer boundary of the cell.

Cell wall—a tough protective layer that surrounds a bacterium and helps it to maintain its overall shape. The composition of the cell wall is an important characteristic used in identifying and classifying bacteria. See also gram-negative bacteria, gram-positive bacteria.

Cementoenamel junction (CEJ)—the area where the cementum and enamel meet on the cervical region of the tooth.

Cementum—a thin layer of hard, mineralized tissue that covers the surface of the tooth root. **Acellular cementum** is the portion of the cementum that does not contain living cells. **Cellular cementum** is the portion of the cementum that contains cementocytes; found primarily in the apical third of the root.

Change agent—a role in which the dental healthcare provider uses communication skills, education, and other resources to help a patient make desired changes in behavior.

Chemical plaque control—the use of chemical agents for the control of microorganisms at specific sites.

Chemical signals—a primitive communication system of chemicals used by the microcolonies within a biofilm to communicate with each other.

Chlorhexidine—an antimicrobial agent used to inhibit colonization of microorganisms on the surfaces of the mucous membranes and teeth.

Chronic—a condition that develops slowly and persists for a long period.

Chronic inflammation—a long-lived inflammatory response that continues for more than a few weeks.

Chronic periodontitis—a bacterial infection resulting in inflammation within the supporting tissues of the teeth, progressive destruction of the periodontal ligament, and loss of supporting alveolar bone. It is characterized by pocket formation and/or gingival recession. It is the most frequently occurring form of periodontitis. This type of periodontitis was previously known as adult periodontitis.

Circumscribed—a condition that is confined to a small area.

Clenching—the continuous or intermittent closure of the maxillary teeth against the mandibular teeth.

Clinical—the signs and symptoms of a condition or disease that can be observed by a clinician.

Clinical attachment level (CAL)—the distance from the cementoenamel junction (CEJ) to the junctional epithelium as measured with a periodontal probe.

Clinical attachment loss—an estimate of the actual amount of histologic attachment loss.

Clinical decision-making—see decision making.

Clinical practice guidelines—a detailed description of a process of patient care management designed to assist health care providers in identifying the preferred treatment for a condition.

Clinically relevant—a finding from a research study that is important enough to affect patient treatment decisions (to cause a clinician to incorporate it in future patient treatment).

Coaggregation—the ability of new bacterial colonizers to adhere to the bacteria that are already attached to the dental pellicle.

Col—a valleylike depression in the portion of the interdental gingiva that lies directly apical to (beneath) the contact area. The col is not present if the adjacent teeth are not in contact or if the gingiva has receded.

Collagen fibers—nonelastic fibers that are highly resistant to tension; most abundant fibers in connective tissue.

Communicable disease—any disease that is transmitted from one person to another. Destructive periodontal microorganisms can be passed between parent and child and between spouses through saliva.

Communication—the imparting or conveying of knowledge or information from one person (the source) to another (the receiver).

Complement system—a complex series of proteins circulating in the blood. Complement facilitates phagocytosis and kills bacteria directly by puncturing the bacterial cell membrane.

Compliance—the extent to which a patient's behavior is in accordance with the health advice that he or she has received from a healthcare provider. A patient who does not follow recommendations for daily self-care would be described as **noncompliant**. A patient who meets regularly scheduled periodontal maintenance appointments would be described as **compliant**.

Comprehensive periodontal assessment—an intensive clinical periodontal assessment used to gather the information needed to make a periodontal diagnosis.

Congenital—a condition that is present at birth.

Connective tissue—fills the spaces between the tissues and organs in the body. It is made up of a large amount of extracellular matrix and relatively few cells.

Connective tissue grafts—a periodontal surgical procedure that requires harvesting a donor section of connective tissue, usually from the palate. The connective tissue graft can be placed partially under a flap created at the site to be grafted.

Connective tissue papillae—fingerlike extensions of connective tissue that extend up into the epithelium.

Consultation—a process in which the help of a specialist is sought in the planning and implementation of a care program.

Contagious—disease that may be spread by direct or indirect contact.

Continuous progression theory—a theory of disease progression that suggests that periodontal disease progresses throughout the mouth in a slow and constant rate over the adult life of the patient.

Control groups—subjects in a clinical trial who did not receive the active treatment.

Controlled-release delivery device—a device placed directly into the periodontal pocket that is designed to produce a steady release of an antimicrobial agent over several days within the periodontal pocket.

Coronal—toward the crown end of the tooth.

Cortical bone—the bone that forms the hard, outside wall of the mandible and maxillae on the facial and lingual aspects.

Corticosteroids—cortisol-like medications used in the treatment of many conditions, such as arthritis, colitis, asthma, certain cancers, Addison's disease, and in organ transplants to suppress the body's immune response to the transplanted organ. These are strong medications that have serious side effects.

Cotherapist—a term used to underscore the patient's vital role in the control of periodontitis.

Cratered papilla—a papilla that appears to have been "scooped out" leaving a concave depression in the midproximal area.

Crevicular fluid—see gingival crevicular fluid.

Critical thinking—decision making that involves careful assessment of all factors before accepting or reaching a conclusion.

Crohn's disease—a chronic inflammatory bowel disease of unknown origin.

Crown—a metal, ceramic, or ceramic-bonded-to-metal covering for a badly damaged tooth.

Crown lengthening surgery—surgery designed to create a longer clinical crown for a tooth by removing both some of the gingiva and some alveolar bone from the necks of the teeth.

Cyclosporine (SYE-kloe-spor-een)—an immunosuppressive agent used to reduce the body's immune response; used in patients who receive organ transplants.

Cytokine—powerful protein mediators produced by immune cells that influence the behavior of other cells. The cytokine (literally cell protein) is a molecule that transmits information or signals from one cell to another.

Cytoskeleton—the internal skeleton of the cell that allows the cell to maintain its own shape and gives the cell the capacity to move. The cytoskeleton is composed of a network of protein filaments.

Cytotoxic—having the ability to kill cells.

Cytotoxin—an agent that inhibits the function of cells.

D

Decalcification—the removal of calcium salts from a tooth.

Decision making—the use of information gathered during the clinical assessment to identify treatment strategies to meet the individual needs of the patient.

Dehiscence—a cleftlike defect in the cortical bone including the bone margin.

Dental calculus—mineralized bacterial plaque, covered on its external surface by nonmineralized, living bacterial plaque.

Dental implant—a nonbiologic (artificial) device surgically inserted into or onto the jaw bone to replace a missing tooth or act as an abutment to provide support for a prosthetic denture. Also see endosseous implant and subperiosteal implant.

Dental implant abutment—see transgingival abutment post.

Dental implant fixture—the titanium fixture is the portion of a dental implant that is surgically placed into the bone. The fixture will act as the root of the implant and needs 3 to 6 months to be fully surrounded and supported by bone.

Dental pellicle—a thin coating of salivary proteins that attach to the tooth surface within minutes after a professional cleaning.

Dental plaque—see bacterial plaque and biofilm.

Dental plaque-induced gingivitis—gingival inflammation of a periodontium resulting from dental plaque.

Dental prophylaxis—scaling and polishing procedures to remove coronal plaque, calculus, and stains for healthy patients and patients with gingivitis.

Dentinal hypersensitivity—a short, sharp painful reaction that occurs when some areas of exposed dentin are subjected to mechanical (touch of toothbrush bristles), thermal (ice cream), or chemical (acidic grapefruit) stimuli.

Dentogingival unit—a structural unit composed of the junctional epithelium and the gingival fibers that acts to brace the gingiva against the tooth.

Deplaquing—the disruption or removal of subgingival microbial plaque and its byproducts from cemental surfaces and the pocket space.

Desmosome—a buttonlike adhesion disk that connects two neighboring epithelial cells and their cytoskeletons together.

Diabetes mellitus—a disease in which the body does not produce or properly use insulin, a hormone that is needed to convert sugar, starches, and other food into fuel for use by the body.

Diffuse—inflammation of the gingival margin, papilla, and attached gingiva.

Disease sites—individual teeth or specific surfaces of a tooth that are experiencing periodontal destruction.

Down syndrome—a genetic condition characterized by varying degrees of mental retardation and multiple defects.

E

Edema—abnormal swelling resulting from fluid accumulating in the tissues.

Efficacy—the degree to which a treatment is beneficial when implemented under the usual conditions of a research investigation, usually a randomized clinical trial.

Elevate—in periodontal surgery, temporarily lifting the gingiva and underlying soft tissues away from the tooth roots and alveolar bone.

Embrasure space—the open space apical to the contact area between the proximal surfaces of two teeth. In health the embrasure space is filled by the interdental papilla (type I embrasure); in a type II embrasure the height of interdental papilla is reduced; in a type III embrasure the interdental papilla is missing.

Endocarditis—a bacterial infection caused by bacteria that adhere to the lining of the heart chambers and the heart valves.

Endodontic abscess—an abscess that results from an infection of the tooth pulp. (Compare with abscess of the periodontium.)

Endosseous implant—a type of dental implant that is placed into the alveolar and/or basal bone and protrudes through the mucoperiosteum. It is the most widely used type of dental implant.

Endotoxin—a major component of the cell walls of gram-negative bacteria that will initiate the host immune response. Also known as lipopolysaccharide.

Epidemiology—the study of the prevalence, incidence, and etiology of disease within the total population (rather than an individual).

Epithelial-attached plaque—a type of dental plaque found within a periodontal pocket that is loosely attached to the epithelium of the pocket wall. Also known as epithelium-associated plaque and loosely adherent plaque.

Epithelial attachment (EA)—the biologic mechanism that joins the junctional epithelium to the tooth. The components of the epithelial attachment are the hemidesmosomes and the internal basement lamina.

Epithelial pegs—see epithelial ridges.

Epithelial ridges—deep extensions of epithelium that reach down into the connective tissue. (The epithelial ridges also are known as rete pegs and epithelial pegs.)

Epithelium-connective tissue interface—the boundary where the epithelium and connective tissues meet. In most places the two tissues meet in a wavy, uneven junction.

Etiology—the study of all factors that may be involved in the development of a disease, including the nature of the disease agent, susceptibility of the patient, and the way in which the disease agent invades the patient's body.

Evidence-based care—the conscientious and judicious application of the current, best evidence from clinical care research in the management of individual patients.

Exacerbation—an active period of disease when all the signs and symptoms of the disease are present in all of their severity.

Exotoxins—harmful proteins released from the bacterial cell that act on host cells at a distance.

Extent—the degree or amount of periodontal destruction that can be characterized based on the number of sites that have experienced tissue destruction.

External basal lamina—the basal lamina that attaches the junctional epithelium to the connective tissue. Also see internal basal lamina.

Extracellular matrix—a material that surrounds the cells. The amount of extracellular matrix is abundant in the connective tissues and sparse in the epithelial tissues.

Extracellular slime layer—a protective barrier that surrounds the mushroom-shaped bacterial microcolonies of a biofilm. The slime layer protects the bacterial microcolonies from antibiotics, antimicrobials, and host defense mechanisms.

Exudate—pus. Pus represents dead white blood cells and can occur in any infection, including periodontal disease.

F

Facultative anaerobic bacteria—bacteria that can exist either with or without oxygen.

Familial—a trait, condition, or disease that occurs in members of the same family.

Fenestration—a windowlike defect in the cortical bone resulting in an isolated area of the root that is not covered by bone.

Fibroblast—a flattened connective tissue cell with a large nucleus that is responsible for the production and remodeling of the extracellular matrix.

Fibrosis—in dentistry, an increase of fibrous connective tissue in the gingiva as the result of chronic inflammation. Fibrotic tissue is often pink and initially may be mistaken for healthy tissue.

Finger-like radiolucent projections—radiolucent lines seen on a radiograph that extend from the crestal bone into the interdental alveolar bone caused by a reduction of mineralized tissue (bone) adjacent to blood vessel channels within the alveolar bone.

Flaps for access—periodontal flap surgery performed to provide access for improved treatment of tooth roots. Also known as modified Widman flap surgery.

Fluid channels—a series of channels that penetrate the extracellular slime layer of a biofilm, provide nutrients and oxygen for the bacterial microcolonies, and facilitate movement of bacterial metabolites, waste products, and enzymes within the biofilm structure.

Fluid lavage—the constant stream of fluid that runs through the ultrasonic handpiece and exits near the point of the ultrasonic instrument tip. This fluid lavage produces a flushing action that washes debris, bacteria, and unattached plaque from the periodontal pocket.

Food Guide Pyramid—a diagram that presents the recommended daily servings from the five major food groups.

Food impaction—the forcing of food (such as pieces of tough meat) between teeth, trapping the food in the interdental area.

Free gingiva—the unattached portion of the gingiva that surrounds the tooth in the region of the cementoenamel junction.

Free gingival graft—a periodontal surgical procedure that requires harvesting a donor section of tissue, usually from the palate. This donor tissue includes both the surface epithelium and some of the underlying connective tissue.

Free gingival groove—a shallow linear depression that separates the free and attached gingiva. (This line may be visible clinically but is not obvious in many instances.)

Fremitus—in dentistry, a palpable or visible movement of a tooth when in function. It can be assessed by gently placing your index finger against the facial aspect of the tooth as the patient either taps the teeth together or simulates chewing movements.

Full-mouth debridement—periodontal debridement completed in a single appointment or in two appointments within a 24-hour period.

Full-mouth disinfection—full-mouth debridement combined with the use of topical antimicrobial therapy.

Functional occlusal forces—the normal forces produced during the act of chewing food.

Furcation involvement—occurs on a multirooted tooth when periodontal infection invades the area between and around the roots resulting in a loss of attachment and alveolar bone between the roots of the tooth.

G

Generalized—a descriptive modifier used to describe the extent of periodontal disease. Generalized periodontitis involves more than 30% of the sites in the mouth. See also localized.

Generalized aggressive periodontitis—a form of aggressive periodontitis that usually occurs in persons younger than 30 years of age, but patients may be older; it is characterized by rapid tissue destruction around most teeth.

Generalized chronic periodontitis—a form of chronic periodontitis in which more than 30% of the sites in the mouth have experienced attachment loss and bone loss. Generalized chronic periodontitis was previously known as generalized adult periodontitis.

Gingiva—the tissue that covers the cervical portions of the teeth and the alveolar processes of the jaws. It is composed of a thin outer layer of epithelium and an underlying core of connective tissue.

Gingival crevicular fluid—a fluid that flows into the sulcus from the gingival connective tissue; the flow is slight in health and increases in disease.

Gingival curettage—a periodontal surgical procedure that involves an attempt to scrape away the lining of the periodontal pocket using a periodontal curet, often a Gracey curet. Gingival curettage normally is *not* a part of modern periodontal therapy.

Gingival diseases with modifying factors—the less common types of plaque-induced gingivitis. There are three main subcategories of gingival diseases with modifying factors: (i) gingival diseases modified by systemic factors, (ii) gingival diseases modified by medications, and (iii) gingival diseases modified by malnutrition.

Gingival epithelium—a stratified squamous epithelium designed to function in the wet environment of the oral cavity.

Gingival fibers—the network of ropelike collagen fiber bundles located coronal to (above) the crest of the alveolar bone. More correctly termed the supragingival fiber bundles.

Gingival hyperplasia—an enlargement of the gingiva due to an increase in the number of cells.

Gingival margin—the thin, rounded edge of free gingiva that forms the coronal boundary, or upper edge, of the gingiva. In health, the gingival margin contacts the tooth slightly coronal to the cemento-enamel junction.

Gingival necrosis—tissue death resulting in partial loss of interdental papillae, giving the appearance that the papillae have been punched-out or cratered.

Gingival papilla—see interdental papilla.

Gingival pocket—a deepening of the gingival sulcus as a result of gingival enlargement. There is no apical migration of the junctional epithelium or attachment loss.

Gingival recession—migration of the free gingival margin to a position apical to the cemento-enamel junction. Gingival recession is an indication of the apical migration of the junctional epithelium in the presence of disease or trauma.

Gingival sulcus—the space between the free gingiva and the tooth surface.

Gingivectomy—a surgical procedure in which some of the gingiva is excised (cut away) and removed.

Gingivitis—a bacterial infection that is confined to the gingiva. It results in reversible damage to the gingival tissues.

Gingivitis on a periodontium with no attachment loss—plaque-induced gingivitis that occurs on a periodontium that has no attachment loss (no destruction of periodontal fibers or alveolar bone).

Gingivitis on a reduced but stable periodontium—plaque-induced gingivitis that occurs in patients who have been successfully treated for periodontitis but who afterward develop gingivitis. In this instance, there is loss of attachment and alveolar bone (due to previous destruction of fibers and bone), but the periodontium currently is stable and not undergoing any additional attachment loss.

Graft—see bone graft, connective tissue graft, and free gingival grafts.

Gram-negative bacteria—bacteria with double cell walls that do not stain a purple color when stained with a dye known as crystal violet. Believed to play an important role in the tissue destruction seen in periodontitis.

Gram-positive bacteria—bacteria with a thick, single cell wall that retains a purple color when stained with a dye known as crystal violet.

Gram stain—a process for staining microorganisms used to identify and classify bacteria into two groups based on their cell wall composition. Gram-positive bacteria stain purple, and gram-negative bacteria stain pale red.

Granules—sacs, found in the cytoplasm of certain white blood cells, filled with potent chemicals that allow the cells to digest microorganisms.

Granulocytes—leukocytes filled with granules.

Ground substance—a gel-like substance that holds the cells and fibers together.

Guided tissue regeneration—the periodontal surgical procedure in which periodontal flaps are elevated, bone defects are identified and cleaned, tooth roots are treated, and barrier materials are placed to control the usually rapid growth of epithelium into the wound.

H

Hemidesmosome—a half-desmosome that connects the epithelial basal cells to the basal lamina.

Hepatitis—inflammation of the liver.

Histology—study of the microscopic structure and composition of tissues.

Horizontal bone loss—an even pattern of alveolar bone destruction seen in periodontitis.

Horizontal tooth mobility—see mobility.

Host—an infected individual. In the case of periodontitis, the host is an individual with periodontitis.

Host defense mechanisms—a group of body-protective systems that guard the body against infective microorganisms.

Host immune response—the reactions of the immune system to infective microorganisms.

Human immunodeficiency virus (HIV)—the virus that causes acquired immune deficiency syndrome (AIDS).

Hyperplasia—see gingival hyperplasia.

I

IL-1 genotype—a specific genetic marker that puts a person at a higher risk for periodontal disease.

Immune system—the body's most important line of defense against attacks by bacteria, viruses, fungi, and parasites.

Immunosuppression—reduction of the immune responses.

Immunosuppressive drugs—agents that interfere with the ability of the immune system to respond; these drugs are used to avoid organ rejection after organ transplantation.

Implant—see dental implant.

Inactive disease site—a disease site that is stable, with the attachment level of the junctional epithelium remaining the same over time.

Incidence—the number of new disease cases in a population that occur during a given interval of time (e.g., new cases per 100,000 persons per year).

Infection—the invasion of the body tissues by pathogenic organisms that multiply and cause disease.

Inflammation—the body's reaction to injury or invasion by disease-producing organisms. The inflammatory response is a protective body response that focuses host defense components at the site of the infection to eliminate microorganisms and heal damaged tissue. Also see acute inflammation and chronic inflammation.

Inflammatory mediators—biologically active compounds secreted by immune cells that stimulate the inflammatory response. Inflammatory mediators of importance in periodontitis are the cytokines, prostaglandins, and matrix metalloproteinases.

Inflammatory response—redness, warmth, swelling, pain, and loss of function produced in response to infection.

Informed consent—an agreement by the patient to proposed treatment after he or she has a full understanding of the nature, purpose, and potential harmful effects of the treatment.

Infrabony pocket—a type of periodontal pocket in which the junctional epithelium, which forms the base of the pocket, is located apical to (below) the crest of the alveolar bone. The pattern of bone destruction is vertical (uneven loss of bone).

Insurance coding—a standardized system that assigns a unique code to each dental service. Coding was conceived to provide consistency and specificity for reporting dental treatments for insurance billing purposes.

Interdental col—see col.

Interdental gingiva—the portion of the gingiva that fills the area between two adjacent teeth apical to (beneath) the contact area. The interdental gingiva consists of two interdental **papillae**, one facial papilla and one lingual papilla.

Interleukins—cytokines that play an important role in periodontitis, such as interleukin-(IL)-1, IL-6, and IL-8.

Intermittent disease progression—a theory of disease progression that suggests that periodontal disease is characterized by periods of disease activity and inactivity (remission).

Internal basal lamina—the basal lamina that attaches the junctional epithelium to the tooth surface. Also see external basal lamina.

Interproximal bone—the area of bone that lies between the proximal surfaces of two adjacent teeth. The interproximal bone is also known as the interdental septum.

Interradicular bone—the bone between the roots of a multirooted tooth.

J

Junctional epithelium (JE)—nonkeratinized stratified squamous epithelium at the base of the sulcus that attaches the gingiva to the tooth.

K

Keratin—fibrous protein found in skin and nails.

Keratinized layer—the outermost (surface) layer of epithelial cells; these cells have no nuclei and form a tough resistant layer on the surface of the skin; the most heavily keratinized epithelium of the body is found on the palms of the hands and soles of the feet.

L

Lamina dura—the continuous white (radiopaque) line around the tooth root as seen on a radiograph. Also known as the alveolar bone proper.

Learning style—an individual's characteristic ways of processing information, feeling, and behaving in learning situations.

Lesion—an injury or wound.

Leukocytes—white blood cells.

Level of the mucogingival junction (MGJ)—determined by measuring the distance from the free gingival margin to the mucogingival junction, on the external surface of the gingiva. The level of the mucogingival junction is used in determining the width of the attached gingiva. Also see mucogingival junction.

Lipopolysaccharide (LPS)—a major component of the cell walls of gram-negative bacteria that will initiate the host immune response; also known as cellular endotoxin.

Local environmental risk factors—oral conditions or habits that increase an individual's susceptibility to periodontal infection.

Localized—a descriptive modifier used to describe the extent of periodontal disease. Localized periodontitis involves 30% or less of the sites in the mouth. See also generalized.

Localized aggressive periodontitis—a form of aggressive periodontitis that has its onset around the time of puberty and is characterized by rapid tissue destruction around the permanent first molars and incisors.

Localized chronic periodontitis—a form of chronic periodontitis in which 30% or less of the sites in the mouth have experienced attachment loss and bone loss. Localized chronic periodontitis previously was known as localized adult periodontitis.

Long junctional epithelium—the primary pattern of healing through repair that occurs after periodontal debridement; there is no new formation of periodontal ligament or bone.

Loss of attachment—the destruction of connective tissue fibers and alveolar bone in periodontitis.

Lymphocytes—small white blood cells that play an important role in recognizing and controlling foreign invaders. The two main classes of lymphocytes are B-lymphocytes and T-lymphocytes.

Lysosomes—granules filled with strong bactericidal and digestive enzymes that can kill and digest bacterial cells after phagocytosis.

M

Macrophages—are large leukocytes with one kidney-shaped nucleus and some granules. These highly phagocytic cells produce high concentrations of products (MMPs and PGE_2) that enhance both connective tissue and bone destruction.

Maintenance—see periodontal maintenance.

Malpractice—professional negligence that is the cause of injury or harm to a patient, resulting from care that is *below* the standard of care expected in the profession.

Marginal—inflammation of the gingival margin and papilla.

Marginal plaque—the supramarginal plaque that is in direct contact with the gingival margin. Marginal plaque is important in the development of gingivitis.

Matrix metalloproteinases (MMPs)—a family of at least 12 different enzymes produced by various cells of the body. These enzymes can act together to break down the connective tissue matrix.

Mediators—biologically active compounds that stimulate the inflammatory response such as cytokines, prostaglandins, and matrix metalloproteinases.

MEDLINE—a database of more than 11,000,000 biomedical references indexed by the National Library of Medicine and available through PubMed at no charge.

Melanin—brown to black pigment in the gingival epithelium.

Membrane attack complex—a protein unit that is part of the body's immune system and is capable of puncturing the cell membranes of certain bacteria.

Meta-analysis—a comprehensive, systematic review of the literature to find relevant studies, assess the quality of the data, and to present the data in an organized fashion.

Microbes—tiny living organisms such as bacteria, viruses, protozoa, and fungi.

Microbial plaque—see bacterial plaque.

Microcolony—a tiny independent community of thousands of compatible bacteria clustered together in a sessile, mushroom-shaped colony within a biofilm.

Microorganism—any tiny living organism such as bacteria, fungi, protozoa, and viruses.

Mobility—the loosening of a tooth that may result from loss of attachment and alveolar bone. **Horizontal tooth mobility** is assessed by trapping the tooth between two dental instrument handles and applying alternating moderate pressure in the facial-lingual direction against the tooth first with one, then the other instrument handle. **Vertical tooth mobility** refers to the ability to depress the tooth in its socket and is assessed by using the end of an instrument handle to exert pressure against the occlusal or incisal surface of the tooth.

Moderate—a descriptive modifier used to describe the severity of periodontal disease. Moderate periodontitis exhibits 3 or 4 mm of clinical attachment loss. See also slight and severe.

Modified Widman flap surgery—see flaps for access.

Monocyte—a large leukocyte that develops into a macrophage when it leaves the blood stream and enters the connective tissue.

Mouth breathing—the process of inhaling and exhaling air primarily through the mouth, rather than the nose; often occurs while the patient is sleeping.

Mucogingival junction—the clinically visible boundary where the pink attached gingiva meets the red, shiny alveolar mucosa.

Mucogingival surgery—periodontal surgical procedures designed to augment the gingiva. Also referred to as periodontal plastic surgery.

Multifactorial etiology—a disease, such as periodontal disease, that results from the interaction of many factors. Etiologic factors for periodontal disease include bacterial, local, and systemic factors.

N

Necrosis—death of tissue.

Necrotizing periodontal diseases—a destructive infection of periodontal tissues that involves tissue necrosis. Also see necrotizing ulcerative gingivitis and necrotizing ulcerative periodontitis.

Necrotizing ulcerative gingivitis (NUG)—a painful infection, primarily of the interdental and marginal gingiva, characterized by partial loss of the interdental papillae (punched-out papillae), gingival bleeding, and pain.

Necrotizing ulcerative periodontitis (NUP)—a painful infection characterized by necrosis of gingival tissues, periodontal ligament, and alveolar bone. NUP is an extremely rapid and destructive form of periodontitis that can produce loss of periodontal attachment within days.

Neutrophil abnormalities—hereditary deficiencies in neutrophil function or cell number that can lead to overwhelming systemic bacterial infection and are often associated with increased susceptibility to severe periodontal destruction.

Neutrophils—phagocytic leukocytes that have many granules, called lysosomes, present in their cytoplasm. Neutrophils play a vital role in combating the pathogenic bacteria responsible for periodontal disease. Also known as polymorphonuclear leukocytes (PMNs).

New attachment—a term used to describe the union of a pathologically exposed root with connective tissue or epithelium.

Nifedipine (nye-FED-I-peen)—a calcium channel blocker used as a coronary vasodilator in the treatment of hypertension, angina, and cardiac arrhythmias that can be associated with gingival overgrowth.

Nonkeratinized layers—inner layers of epithelial cells; these cells have nuclei and act as a cushion against mechanical stress and wear

Nonplaque-induced gingivitis—gingivitis that is not caused by bacterial plaque and does not disappear after plaque removal; it can result from such varied causes as viral infections, fungal infections, dermatologic (skin) diseases, allergic reactions, or mechanical trauma.

Nonresponsive sites—sites that show continued loss of attachment and may exhibit clinical signs of inflammation and/or bleeding upon probing following appropriate treatment.

Nonsurgical periodontal therapy (NSPT)—all the nonsurgical measures used to help control gingivitis and periodontitis, including mechanical and chemical bacterial plaque removal, plaque control, and periodontal debridement of the subgingival and supragingival tooth surfaces and pocket space.

Nucleus—contains all the chromosomal DNA of the cell.

Nutrition—the study of food and drink as related to the growth and maintenance of the body.

O

Occlusal adjustment—when the dentist makes minor adjustments in a patient's bite to minimize the damaging forces of trauma from occlusion.

Occlusal trauma—excessive occlusal forces that cause damage to the periodontium.

Occlusion—contact of opposing teeth.

Operculum—a flap of gingival tissue covering a portion of the crown of a partially erupted tooth.

Opportunistic infection—an infection, in a person whose immune response is reduced, caused by an organism that ordinarily does not infect persons with healthy immune systems.

Opsonization—the process of coating a microorganism with antibodies or a complement protein to make it easier for phagocytes to recognize, engulf, and destroy it.

Oral implant—see dental implant.

Oral irrigation—the in-home use of a pulsating water stream created by a mechanized device and a standard tip designed to be placed at a 90-degree angle on the tooth near the gingival margin or a specialized tip designed to be placed beneath the gingival margin.

Oral prophylaxis—see dental prophylaxis.

Osseointegration—the histologic term for the direct contact between alveolar bone and the surface of a dental implant. An implant will fail without stable osseointegration.

Osseous defect—a deformity in the alveolar bone.

Osseous surgery—periodontal surgery to modify the bone level or shape of the bone.

Osteoblast—a cell that is associated with the formation of bone.

Osteoclast—a cell that is associated with the resorption of bone.

Osteoporosis—a condition of decreased bone mass. Osteoporosis leads to fragile bones that are at an increased risk for fractures.

Osteoradionecrosis (ORN)—a complication resulting from radiation of the jaw that renders the oral bone less capable of resolving trauma or infection and can result in severe destruction of bone.

Outcome measures—investigation end points in a clinical trial that have a measurable component (such as the presence or absence of bleeding upon probing).

Overhanging restoration—an area of a restoration where an excess of restorative material projects beyond the tooth surface.

P

Pacemaker—a device surgically placed in the chest of a patient to regulate an irregular heartbeat. Newer pacemakers are bipolar and are generally not affected by the small electromagnetic fields created by dental equipment.

Papilla—see interdental papilla.

Papillary—inflammation of the interdental papilla only.

Parafunctional—occlusal forces that result from tooth-to-tooth contact made when not in the act of eating.

Pathogenesis—the sequence of events that occurs during the development of a disease or abnormal condition.

Pathogenic—capable of causing disease in human beings.

Pathogenicity—the ability of a disease-causing agent to produce a disease.

Pathologically deepened sulcus—another term for a periodontal pocket.

Patient compliance—see compliance.

Peer-reviewed—professional journals that use a panel of experts to review research articles for study design, statistics, and conclusions.

Pericoronitis—an infection in the soft tissue surrounding the crown of a partially erupted tooth. Also known as operculitis.

Peri-implant disease—pathologic changes in the periodontal tissues that surround a dental implant.

Peri-implant gingivitis—plaque-induced gingivitis (with no loss of supporting bone) that occurs in the gingival tissues surrounding a dental implant.

Peri-implant tissues—the periodontal tissues that surround a dental implant.

Peri-implantitis—chronic periodontitis in the tissues surrounding an osseointegrated dental implant, resulting in loss of alveolar bone.

Perimucosal seal—adaptation of the epithelium to the titanium abutment post of a dental implant. Also known as the biological seal.

Periodontal—a term used to describe the structures situated around a tooth.

Periodontal debridement—the removal or disruption of bacterial plaque, its byproducts, and plaque-retentive calculus deposits from coronal surfaces, root surfaces, and within the pocket space and tissue wall, as indicated, for periodontal healing and repair. Calculus is removed only because it is a breeding ground for bacterial plaque and conservation of cementum is a goal of periodontal debridement.

Periodontal diagnosis—the identification of the type of gingival disease or periodontitis based on the clinical features of the disease (e.g., plaque-induced gingivitis or chronic periodontitis).

Periodontal disease—a bacterial infection of the periodontium. Periodontal disease that is limited to an inflammation of the gingival tissues is called gingivitis. Periodontal disease that involves the gingiva, periodontal ligament, bone, and cementum is called periodontitis.

Periodontal dressing—a protective material used to cover periodontal surgical wounds.

Periodontal fiber bundles—the principal fibers of the periodontal ligament.

Periodontal flap—a surgical procedure in which the dentist makes incisions around the necks of the teeth and lifts the gingiva and underlying soft tissues away from the tooth roots and away from the alveolar bone. Most periodontal surgical procedures require performing periodontal flaps.

Periodontal ligament (PDL)—a layer of soft connective tissue that covers the root of the tooth and attaches it to the bone of the tooth socket.

Periodontal maintenance—an ongoing program designed to assist the patient in maintaining periodontal health. Also referred to as supportive periodontal therapy.

Periodontal osseous surgery—a surgical procedure in which bone contours are corrected to mimic healthy alveolar bone contours.

Periodontal pathogens—bacteria that are capable of infecting the tissues of the periodontium.

Periodontal plastic surgery—see mucogingival surgery.

Periodontal pocket—a pathologic deepening of the gingival sulcus as the result of the apical migration of the junctional epithelium and the destruction of alveolar bone and periodontal ligament fiber bundles.

Periodontal regeneration—restoration of the architecture and function in healing periodontal tissues.

Periodontal screening and recording (PSR)—an efficient easy-to-use screening system for the detection of periodontal disease.

Periodontal screening examination—a periodontal assessment used to determine the periodontal health status of the patient and identify patients needing a comprehensive periodontal assessment. (Also see comprehensive periodontal assessment.)

Periodontics—the dental specialty concerned with the prevention and treatment of periodontal disease.

Periodontist—a dentist who has completed advanced training in periodontics and who specializes in the diagnosis and treatment of periodontal disease.

Periodontitis—an inflammatory disease process that results in some extent of permanent destruction to the tissues of the periodontium, including the loss of gingival connective tissue, destruction of the periodontal ligament, and resorption of alveolar bone.

Periodontium—the functional system of tissues that surrounds the teeth and attaches them to the jawbone. These tissues include the gingiva, periodontal ligament, cementum, and alveolar bone.

Periodontology—the study of the periodontium in health and disease.

Periosteum—a layer of connective tissue covering the outer surface of bone; it consists of an outer layer of collagenous tissue and an inner layer of fine elastic fibers.

Phagocyte—a leukocyte that is able to surround, engulf, and digest microorganisms.

Phagocytize—the act of engulfing and digesting microorganisms.

Phagocytosis—the process by which leukocytes engulf and destroy microorganisms.

Phenytoin (FEN-i-toyn)—an anticonvulsant medication used to control convulsions or seizures in the treatment of epilepsy.

Placebo—an inactive or harmless substance, such as distilled water or sugar, used in experimental clinical trials to compare the effects of the inactive substance with those of the experimental drug or treatment.

Plaque—see bacterial plaque.

Plaque-induced gingivitis—gingival inflammation of a periodontium resulting from dental plaque.

Pocket—see periodontal pocket.

Pocket epithelium—the epithelial lining of a pocket characterized by the presence of epithelial ridges and ulcerations.

Polymorphonuclear leukocytes (PMNs)—phagocytic leukocytes that have many granules, called lysosomes, present in their cytoplasm. PMNs play a vital role in combating the pathogenic bacteria responsible for periodontal disease. Also known as neutrophils.

Porphyromonas gingivalis—a gram-negative bacterium that has been identified as an etiologic agent of periodontitis.

Pregnancy tumor—a noncancerous lump that may form on the interdental gingiva during pregnancy. Also known as a pregnancy-associated pyogenic granuloma.

Premedication—any medication given before anesthesia or an invasive procedure.

Prevalence—refers to the number of cases of a disease, such as periodontal disease, that can be identified within a specified population at a given point in time.

Primary herpetic gingivostomatitis—a painful oral condition that results from the initial infection with the herpes simplex virus (HSV).

Primary trauma from occlusion—excessive occlusal forces on a healthy periodontium.

Probing depth—the distance in millimeters measured from the *free gingival margin (FGM)* to the base of the sulcus or pocket as measured with a calibrated periodontal probe.

Prognosis—a prediction of the probable outcome of a disease.

Prostaglandins—a series of powerful lipid mediators of inflammation. Prostaglandins of the E series (PGE) play an important role in the bone destruction seen in periodontitis.

Prosthesis—an appliance used to replace missing teeth.

Pseudomembrane—a gray layer of tissue that covers necrotic areas of the gingiva; associated with necrotizing periodontal diseases.

PSR code—the code assigned to each sextant for the periodontal screening and recording (PSR) examination. See periodontal screening and recording.

Pus—a collection of dead white blood cells that result from the body defense mechanisms involved in fighting the infection. Also see exudate.

Q

Quadrant—one of four sections into which the dental arches can be divided.

Quantitative synthesis—a combining of data from several research studies to determine the overall relevance of the information.

R

Radiolucent—materials and structures that are easily penetrated by x-rays.

Radiopaque—materials and structures that absorb or resist the passage of x-rays. These structures absorb most of the x-rays so that very little of the x-rays reach the radiograph.

Random burst theory—a theory of periodontal disease progression that suggests that patients experience short periods of destruction of about 4 to 7 months alternating with short periods of disease inactivity lasting for 4 to 7 months.

Randomization—the unbiased assignment of subjects or objects in a research study to a control or experimental group on a random basis.

Randomized clinical trial—a study in which a group of subjects that is receiving an experimental treatment is compared with a control group that is receiving a placebo or an alternative treatment.

Reattachment—the reunion of the connective tissue and root that have been separated by incision or injury, but *not by disease*; the attaching again of the connective tissues of the gingiva and/or periodontal ligament under such conditions as surgical flap procedures or tooth replantation or transplantation.

Recall—see periodontal maintenance.

Recession—see gingival recession.

Recurrent disease—new signs and symptoms of destructive periodontitis that reappear after periodontal therapy because the disease was not adequately treated and/or the patient did not practice adequate self-care.

Reevaluation—a formal step in nonsurgical therapy that is designed to gather information to be used in several critical clinical decisions regarding future care of a patient with chronic periodontitis.

Refractory disease—destructive periodontitis in a patient who, when monitored over time, exhibits additional attachment loss at one or more sites despite appropriate, repeated professional periodontal therapy and exercising satisfactory self-care as well as following the recommended program of periodontal maintenance visits.

Regeneration—the biologic process by which the architecture and function of lost tissue is *completely* restored.

Reliability—the extent to which a test measurement or device produces the same results with different investigators, observers, or administration of the test over time. If several tests produce the same result, the measurement is considered reliable.

Remission—an inactive period of disease when the signs and symptoms of a chronic infection may partially or completely disappear.

Repair—healing of a wound by formation of tissue that does not truly restore the original architecture or original function of the body part.

Resective—a periodontal surgical procedure designed to remove damaged periodontal tissues.

Resorption—see bone resorption.

Rete pegs—see epithelial ridges.

Risk assessment—the identification of risk factors associated with dental disease to determine which patients are more or less likely to prevent or control their dental disease.

Risk factors—conditions, habits, or diseases that increase an individual's susceptibility to periodontal infection. Proven periodontal risk factors include smoking, stress, diabetes, and genetic influences.

Root caries—decay on the root surfaces.

Root planing—a treatment procedure designed to remove cementum or surface dentin that is rough, impregnated with calculus, or contaminated with toxins or microorganisms.

S

Safety—a term for treatment that produces therapeutic benefits that outweigh any potential harm that is caused by the treatment.

Scaling—instrumentation of the crown and root surfaces of the teeth to remove plaque, calculus, and stains.

Secondary trauma from occlusion—normal occlusal forces on an unhealthy periodontium that was previously weakened by periodontitis.

Severe—a descriptive modifier used to describe the severity of periodontal disease. Severe periodontitis exhibits 5 mm or more of clinical attachment loss. See also moderate and slight.

Severity—the seriousness of a disease, determined by the rate of disease progression over time and the response of the tissues to treatment.

Sextant—one of six sections into which the dental arches can be divided.

Sharpey's fibers—the ends of the periodontal ligament fibers that are embedded in the cementum and alveolar bone.

Signs—those features of a disease that can be observed or are measurable by the clinician. Examples include gingival erythema (redness), edema, bleeding, loss of attachment, mobility, and loss of alveolar bone support.

Silent disease—a disease, such as periodontitis, that usually does not cause symptoms in the patient. A silent disease can exist in patients who are totally unaware of its presence.

Slight—a descriptive modifier used to describe the severity of periodontal disease. Slight (mild) periodontitis exhibits 1 to 2 mm of clinical attachment loss. See also moderate and severe.

Slough—necrotic tissue that can be shed from portions of the body, such as the sloughing of gingival tissue seen in necrotizing ulcerative periodontitis.

Stability—the ability of a chemical plaque control agent to remain stable at room temperature and have a reasonable shelf life.

Standard of care—a written statement describing the actions or conditions that direct patient care and can be used to evaluate performance.

Statistical significance—tells whether the observed outcome from one therapy is better than a comparative therapy in a research study.

Stippling—the dimpled appearance, similar to an orange peel, that may be visible on the surface of the attached gingiva.

Stratified squamous epithelium—epithelial sheets that form the surface of the skin and the mucous membranes of the body, including the oral mucosa.

Stress reduction protocol—methods used to reduce the stress experienced by a patient during dental treatment, including shorter appointments, early morning appointments when the patient is well rested, maintaining excellent pain control during treatment, and providing for postappointment pain control.

Subclinical—a histologic stage of a disease that only can be detected microscopically; there are no clinically visible signs at this stage of disease progression.

Subgingival irrigation—the in-office flushing of pockets performed by the dental hygienist or periodontist.

Subgingival plaque biofilms—the dental plaque biofilm that forms below the gingival margin and is associated with periodontitis.

Subperiosteal implant—a type of dental implant that is placed on the surface of the bone beneath the periosteum. See also endosseous implant.

Substantivity—the ability of a chemical plaque control agent to be retained in the oral cavity and be released slowly over time with a continued antimicrobial effect.

Sulcular fluid—see gingival crevicular fluid.

Sulcus—see gingival sulcus.

Sulcus with increased depth—a periodontal pocket with clinical attachment levels that remain the same or decrease over time.

Supportive periodontal treatment—another term for periodontal maintenance.

Suppuration—the formation of pus.

Suprabony pocket— a type of periodontal pocket in which the junctional epithelium, which forms the base of the pocket, is located coronal to (above) the crest of the alveolar bone. The pattern of bone destruction is horizontal (even loss of bone).

Supragingival fiber bundles—the network of ropelike collagen fiber bundles located coronal to (above) the crest of the alveolar bone. Also known as the gingival fibers.

Supragingival plaque biofilms—the dental plaque biofilm that forms above the gingival margin.

Suture—a stitch taken to repair an incision, tear, or wound. **Nonresorbable suture material** does not dissolve in body fluids and must be removed by the dental team. **Resorbable suture material** is designed to dissolve slowly in body fluids, but the material sometimes does not dissolve well in saliva.

Symptoms—those features of a disease that are noted by the patient. Examples of symptoms include pain, "itching" gums, blood on the bed pillow, and a bad taste in the mouth.

T

Therapeutic—a product that is beneficial in the treatment of a disease or condition and/or in maintaining a state of health.

Therapy—the treatment of a disease or condition.

Tissue—a collection of similar cells acting together to perform a particular function. The tissues in the human body can be classified into four types: epithelial, connective, nerve, and muscle.

Titanium—a biocompatible metal commonly used for dental implants.

Tongue thrusting—the application of forceful pressure against the anterior teeth with the tongue.

Tooth-attached plaque—a type of plaque found within a periodontal pocket that is attached to the tooth surface.

Toxin—a poison.

Transgingival abutment post—a titanium abutment post of a dental implant that protrudes through the tissue into the mouth and supports the restorative prosthesis (crown or denture) to the implant fixture. The titanium abutment is extremely biocompatible (not rejected by the body) and allows tissue healing around the implant.

Trauma from occlusion—excessive occlusal forces that cause damage to the periodontium.

Treatment plan—a sequential outline of the services and procedures to be carried out by the dentist, dental hygienist, and the patient that are designed to restore the periodontal health of the patient.

Trench mouth—a lay term for necrotizing ulcerative periodontitis.

Triangulation—a widening of the periodontal ligament space (PDLS), as seen on a radiograph. Triangulation is caused by the resorption of bone along either the mesial or distal aspect of the interdental (interseptal) crestal bone.

Trifurcation—the area of a root where the tooth divides into three roots.

Trigeminal nerve—the nerve supply to the periodontium.

Tumor necrosis factor—a cytokine that plays an important role in periodontitis.

U

Unattached plaque—a type of plaque found within a periodontal pocket that is not attached to either the tooth surface or the epithelium of the pocket wall.

V

Validity—the degree to which a measurement is appropriate for the question being addressed by a research study or that it measures what it is intended to measure.

Vertical bone loss—an uneven pattern of alveolar bone destruction seen in periodontitis.

Vertical tooth mobility—see mobility.

Virulence factors—mechanisms that enable biofilm bacteria to colonize, invade, and damage the tissues of the periodontium. Virulence factors may be structural characteristics of the bacterium itself or substances produced and released into the environment by bacteria.

W

World Health Organization (WHO) probe—the probe recommended for use in performing the periodontal screening and recording screening examination. It has a colored band (called the reference marking) located 3.5 to 5.5 mm from the probe tip.

X

Xerostomia—dryness of the mouth due to inadequate production of saliva.

J

Junctional epithelium, 8, 18, 24
  apical migration of, 40, 45
  basal lamina of, *25*
  gingivitis relating to, 43
  microscopic anatomy of, 25, *26*
  periodontal disease relating to, 39
  periodontitis relating to, 45
  periodontium relating to, 42
Junctional epithelium-connective tissue
      interface, 26

K

Keratin, 17
Keratinization, 18, 20, 23, 24
Keratinized epithelial cell, 20
Keratinized layer, 18
Kidney disease and hemodialysis, 209, 220

L

Lamina, basal. *See* Basal lamina.
Lamina bone, 197
Lamina dura, 200, *200*
Laser, use of, 425–426
Legal issues, documentation and insurance
      reporting relating to, 407, 408–409
Legal responsibility, 180, 181
Lesions
  nonplaque-induced gingival, 156–158
  periodontal-endodontic, combined, 143
  traumatic, 158
Leukemia, 209, 221
Leukemia-associated gingivitis, 154
LGE (linear gingival erythema), 116, 124,
      158, *158*, 158*b*
Liability, definition of, 407, 408, 409
Linear gingival erythema. *See* LGE.
Lipopolysaccharide. *See* LPS.
Liver disease, 209, 219
Local contributing factors, for periodontal
      disease, 100–112, *127*, 128–129
  direct damage caused by
    faulty restorations and appliances, 110,
      110, 111, 206, *206*
    food impaction, 108, *109*
    occlusal forces, *107*, 107–108, *108*
    patient habits, 109, *109*
  mechanisms of, 102, 102*t*
  plaque pathogenicity increased by
    undisturbed plaque growth, 106,
      106
  plaque retention increased by

dental calculus, 101, *103*, 103–104
tooth morphology, 104–105, *105*
Local delivery, 340, 341
Local delivery mechanisms, 427
Localized, 390, 391
Localized aggressive periodontitis, 162, 170,
      170, 170*b*
Localized chronic periodontitis, 162, 167
Localized inflammation, 146, 150
Localized periodontal disease, 239, 243
LONESOME DOC, 431, 432
Long junctional epithelium, 252, 259, 314,
      319
Long-cone paralleling technique, for
      radiographs, 201
Long-gray scale-low contrast images, of
      radiographs, 201
Loss of attachment, prevalence of, 59, *59. See
      also* Attachment loss.
LPS (lipopolysaccharide), 68, 80
Lymph nodes, 14
Lymphatic system, periodontium and, 1, 14,
      14
Lymphocytes, 86, 90, *90*
Lysosomes, 86, 89

M

Macrophages, 86, 90, *91*
Maintenance
  of dental implant patient, 375–387
  of dental implants, 381–385, 425
  periodontal, 239, 244*t*, 245, 252, 257,
      357–374, 359*b*, *360*, 361*t*
  of Stages of Change Model, 289, 293, 295
Maintenance phase, periodontal, 239, 244*t*,
      245, 360, *360*
Maintenance stage, 289, 293, 295
Malnutrition, 146, 155
Malpractice, 407, 408–409
Mandible, *10, 11*
Mandibular arch, *28*
Marginal inflammation, 146, 150
Master treatment plan, 239, 244, 244*t*
Matrix metalloproteinases. *See* MMP.
Medications
  gingival diseases modified by, 146, 155,
      155*b*
  systemic, 115, 117, 124–126
MEDLINE, 225, 230, 431, 432
Membrane attack complex, 86, 92
Menstrual cycle-associated gingivitis, 154
Microbiology, of periodontal disease, 67–83
Microscopic anatomy
  of alveolar bone, 33–34, *34*